Social Policy, the Media and Misrepresentation

The often misleading ways in which radio, newspapers and television report poverty, homelessness, education, health and disability are of crucial and growing concern to those studying social policy and the media. Such concerns are heightened in the political context of a government that is clearly committed to promoting its policies via media-based advertising and news management.

Social Policy, the Media and Misrepresentation is a radical collection of chapters by distinguished academics, journalists and broadcasters, which examines various aspects of news media reporting of social policy and the influences of such coverage on the processes of policy making and implementation. It offers an appraisal of the complex inter-relationships between news media, news sources, the content of media coverage of social policy and its impact on audiences, public opinion and policy makers. With detailed case studies, the various chapters explore:

- social work and child protection
- housing and homelessness
- the charity and voluntary sectors
- poverty and welfare policy
- health (including HIV/AIDS) and mental health
- education and crime and juvenile justice.

Social Policy, the Media and Misrepresentation establishes that media reporting of social policy illustrates a growing problem for policy making in democratic states when citizens are so poorly served by media with information about policy issues.

Bob Franklin is Reader in the Sociology of Media Communications at the University of Sheffield.

Social Policy, the Media and Misrepresentation

Edited by Bob Franklin

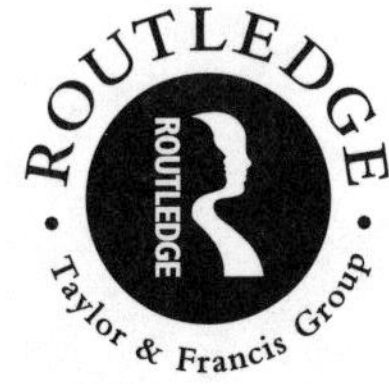

First published 1999 by Routledge
11 New Fetter Lane, London EC4P 4EE

Simultaneously published in the USA and Canada
by Routledge
29 West 35th Street, New York, NY 10001

Routledge is an imprint of the Taylor & Francis Group

Typeset in Garamond by M Rules
Printed and bound in Great Britain by Biddles Ltd, Guildford and Kings Lynn

British Library Cataloguing in Publication Data
A catalogue record for this book is available
from the British Library

Library of Congress Cataloging in Publication Data
Social policy, the media and misrepresentation / edited by Bob Franklin.
p. cm.
Includes bibliographical references and index.
1. Government and the press—Great Britain. 2. Social problems—Press coverage—Great Britain. 3. Mass media—Political aspects—Great Britain. 4. Mass media—Social aspects—Great Britain. 5. Journalistic ethics—Great Britain. 6. Press and politics—Great Britain. I. Franklin, Bob, 1949– .
PN4748.G7S69 1999
302.23'2'0941—dc21 99–24844
CIP

ISBN 0–415–20106–3 (hbk)
ISBN 0–415–20107–1 (pbk)

Contents

Figures and tables

Figures

Tables

Contributors

Meryl Aldridge is Senior Lecturer in the School of Sociology and Social Policy at the University of Nottingham. Her main research and teaching interest is in the sociology of news media. Publications include *Making Social Work News* (1994) and several articles on media representations of social work issues.

David Brindle is Social Services Correspondent of the *Guardian*. He is a former labour correspondent of the *Financial Times*, which he joined from the *Coventry Evening Telegraph*. He was social services correspondent of the year in 1997.

David Deacon is a lecturer in Communication and Media Studies in the Communications Research Centre, Department of Social Sciences, Loughborough University. He is co-author of a number of books including: *Taxation and Representation: The Media, Political Communication and the Poll Tax* (with Peter Golding 1995) and *Mediating Social Sciences* (with Natalie Fenton and Alan Bryman 1997).

Simon Duncan is Reader in Applied Social Studies at the University of Bradford and held the Holdsworth Fellowship at Manchester University for 1998–9. Publications include *The Local State and Uneven Development* (1987), *Lone Mothers and Paid Work: Gendered Moral Rationalities* (co-author 1999), and co-editor/contributor to *Single Mothers in an International Context* (1997). He chairs the European Science Foundation Network 'Gender Inequality and the European Regions'.

Rosalind Edwards is Reader in Social Policy at the Social Sciences Research Centre, South Bank University. Publications include *Mothers and Education: Inside Out?* (co-author 1993), *Lone Mothers and Paid Work: Gendered Moral Rationalities* (co-author 1999), and co-editor/contributor to *Single Mothers in an International Context* (1997). She is also co-editor of the *International Journal of Social Research Methodology: Theory and Practice*.

Vikki Entwistle is a Senior Research Fellow in the Health Services Research Unit at the University of Aberdeen, where she is currently working on issues relating to patient involvement in health care decision making. At the NHS Centre for Reviews and Dissemination at York University she helped to develop research-based consumer health information materials about treatment options and undertook several projects to investigate media coverage of health issues.

Bob Franklin is Reader in Media Communications in the Department of Sociological Studies at the University of Sheffield. He is co-editor of *Journalism Studies*. Publications include: *Social Work, The Media and Public Relations* (co-editor 1991), *Newszak and News Media* (1997), *Making the Local News: Local Journalism in Context* (co-editor 1998) and *Hard Pressed: National Newspaper Reporting of Social Work and Social Services* (1998).

Peter Golding is Professor of Sociology and Head of the Department of Social Sciences at Loughborough University. He is co-editor of the *European Journal of Communication*. Publications include: *Images of Welfare: Press and Public attitudes to Poverty* (co-author 1982), *The Political Economy of the Media* (co-author 1997); *Cultural Studies in Question* (co-editor 1997).

Tony Jeffs works in the Community and Youth Work Studies Unit in the Department of Sociology and Social Policy at the University of Durham. He has published extensively about education, youth work and youth policy. He has recently published a book about the life and work of Henry Morris and is preparing a study of the settlement movement.

Bill Jordan is Professor of Social Work at Huddersfield University and Reader in Social Studies at Exeter University. He is the author of some twenty books of political thought, social theory and social work. His latest book, *The New Politics of Welfare: Social Justice in A Global Context*, was published in 1998.

Jenny Kitzinger is Senior Research Fellow at Glasgow University. She is co-author of *The Mass Media and Power in Modern Britain* (1996) and the *Circuit of Mass Communication* (1997) and co-editor of *Developing Focus Group Research: Politics, Theory and Practice* (1998).

John Muncie is Senior Lecturer in Criminology and Social Policy at the Open University. His most recent books include *Criminological Perspectives* (1996), *The Problem of Crime* (1996) and *Youth and Crime: A Critical Introduction* (1999).

Greg Philo is the Research Director of the Media Unit at Glasgow University. He has written widely in the area of media and communications. His recent books include *Media and Mental Distress* (edited) (1995), *Message Received* (edited 1999) and *Cultural Compliance* (co-edited 1999).

Steve Platt is a freelance writer, who has covered housing and social affairs issues for more than twenty years. He is a former editor of *Roof* and the *New Statesman*.

Ann Pointon is a disability consultant and trainer with a background in broadcasting, having been employed at the BBC for twenty years. She chairs BECTU's Disabled Members' Network, is a member of the Executive Committee of the Trade Union Disability Alliance (TUDA), a member of the National Council of the Campaign for Press and Broadcasting Freedom and a member of the Arts Council of England's Lottery Advisory Panel on Film. Her publications include, *Framed: Interrogating Disability in the Media* (co-edited 1997), *Disability and Television: Guidelines on Representations for Producers* (1992).

Jenny Secker is Senior Research Fellow with the Centre for Mental Health Services Development at Kings College London. Before joining CMHSD in 1977, she was specialist Research and Evaluation Officer at the Health Education Board for Scotland, where she collaborated with Greg Philo on research into the media and health.

Trevor Sheldon is a professor at the University of York, and Co-Director of the York Health Policy Group. He is the former director of the NHS Centre for Reviews and Dissemination, a national body responsible for putting together and disseminating research intelligence for the public and decision makers in the National Health Service. In 1993, Trevor was part of the team that developed the national formula for allocating resources to health authorities for hospital and community health services.

Miri Song is a Korean-American woman who now lives and works in Britain. She is a lecturer in Sociology at the University of Kent. Her research interests include theorising on ethnicity and cultural identity, migration and immigrant family adaptation, young people and dynamics around racism(s). She is author of *Helping Out: Children's Labour in Ethnic Businesses* (1999).

Andy West has been a youth worker, a youth counsellor and a rights worker, a university lecturer and latterly a research and development officer for Save the Children. He has worked with young people around issues of housing, unemployment, homelessness and abuse. His recent work includes participatory research with young people leaving care in England, and with street children, rural children and children from slums in Bangladesh.

Kevin Williams is Senior Lecturer in the Centre for Journalism Studies at Cardiff University. His most recent published work includes *Get Me a Murder a Day! A History of Mass Communication in Britain* (1997). He has co-authored *The Mass Media and Power in Modern Britain* (1996) and the *Circuit of Mass Communication* (1997).

Introduction

Misleading messages: the media and social policy

Bob Franklin

'Social policy', Polly Toynbee argues, 'makes neither news nor history unless', she suggests appending an important qualification, 'there is some crisis' (*Guardian*, 13 January 1999). Her observation concerning the paucity of social policy news combined with the suggestion that the media tend to report social policy issues in highly critical, if not apocalyptic, terms are both affirmed by this collection of essays. Peter Golding, for example, reporting the findings of an analysis of media coverage of policy between 1996–97, confirms that social policy reports constitute only 11 per cent of all domestic news coverage in national newspapers, radio and television (see Chapter 9). This relative neglect of social policy is curious on at least four grounds. First, public expenditure on social policy is substantial, amounting to £214 billion in 1996, with £107 billion being spent on social security, £43 billion on health, £39 billion on education, £15 billion on public order and safety and £10 billion on housing and community amenities (Social Trends 1998: 120). Second, social policy has significant implications for almost every citizen. Education alone involves almost a quarter of the population directly: 13 million as pupils and students with a further one million as teachers and ancillary workers (see Chapter 10). Citizens' needs for housing, employment, pensions and health services are similarly universal. Third, social policy is a key concern for media audiences; especially during elections. A study of the 1997 general election ranked Europe (25 per cent), health (20 per cent), education (18 per cent) and pensions (9 per cent) as voters' four highest policy preoccupations, measured by the frequency with which these issues were raised with party candidates (Butler and Kavanagh 1997: 120). Finally, social policy is a central ingredient in all governments' policy agendas. If defence, foreign affairs, transport and agriculture are excluded, social policy effectively becomes coterminous with government policy: social policy, moreover, undoubtedly ranks among the most contentious of government policy arenas. Given these indicators of the high news salience or 'news value' of social policy issues, the reluctance of the media to report such policy concerns seems curious.

Toynbee's second observation, that social policy 'makes news' when there is a crisis, tells only part of the story. What Toynbee neglects to mention is how frequently media reporting is central to the *construction* as well as the *reporting* of crises. Headlines such as 'Fraud busters make a dawn swoop on welfare scroungers' (*Sunday Mirror*, 29 March, 1998) and '£2 billion blitz on dole cheats' (*Daily Mail*, 10 July 1995) transform the social problem of unemployment into a public crisis, if not moral panic, about welfare scroungers (see Chapter 9). *Sun* headlines denouncing '£200-a-day beggars' (28 October 1998) similarly shift the problem of homelessness into a crisis about beggars or, in Jack Straw's widely reported phrase, 'aggressive beggars, winos and squeegee merchants' (see Chapter 6). Policy discussions about the growing number of lone mothers are likewise reconstructed in media discourses into an alleged crisis posing both moral and financial threats to society. The programme title 'Babies on Benefit' betrayed much about the assumptions informing *Panorama*'s approach to this policy issue (20 September 1993). The media judge black lone mothers to pose a particular threat: a *Sunday Express* feature, headlined 'The ethnic timebomb', claimed that 'almost six in ten black mothers are bringing up children on their own, urged on by the benefit system' (13 August 1995) (see Chapter 15).

While a crisis is not always necessary to generate social policy coverage, reporting tends to focus overwhelmingly on the shortcomings of policy decisions and their implementation and certainly provides credence for the widely held journalistic maxim that 'bad news is to journalism what dung is to rhubarb' (Jacks 1986 quoted in *UK Press Gazette*, 10 February).

Social services, for example, traditionally suffer a bad press, while social workers are routinely 'press ganged' by journalists alleging a by now well known litany of 'sins' (see Chapter 5, Aldridge (1994); Franklin and Parton (1991)). A review of national press reporting during 1997–98 identified social workers as 'incompetent bunglers' (*Sun*, 15 October 1997) who 'fail to intervene' (*Observer*, 10 August 1997) or 'intervene ineffectually and help to create a costly dependency culture' (*Mail*, 28 March 1998). They are the 'faceless cohort of unjudgemental social workers' (*Daily Telegraph*, 13 August 1997) who lack 'common sense values' (*Guardian*, 23 December 1997). Social workers are also 'negligent' and 'take your kids away' (*Sun*, 19 January 1998). They 'sexually abuse youngsters in their care' (*Mail*, 5 December 1997), 'physically abuse clients' (*Independent*, 30 October 1997) and refuse to foster children with couples who are 'too old, too overweight or because they smoke' (*Mail*, 13 April 1998). They 'suffer from the pernicious doctrine of political correctness' (*Daily Telegraph*, 27 March 1998); they are trendy Blairite, *Guardian*-reading, bleeding heart multiculturalists' (*Daily Mail*, 28 September 1997). Social workers are the 'great blunderbuss (and blunder is usually the right word) of the social services' (*Mail on Sunday*, 28 September 1997). Their work with children is 'haphazard and inconsistent' (*Independent*, 25 June 1998) and, on occasion, parents have only been able to 'watch in horror and disbelief as their weeping children were dragged from their beds and taken away by "care" workers in frightening dawn raids' (*Mail on Sunday*,

1 February 1998); in short, social services 'have taken over' (*Sun*, 25 February 1998).

This unrelenting press criticism and misrepresentation of social work has important consequences. It demoralises social workers, influences their professional practice and, by helping to shape public opinion, impacts ultimately on social policy concerning social workers and their clients. The timing and policy ambitions of the Children Act 1989, for example, identify the legislation as the progeny of Cleveland and an attempt to placate media-generated public anxieties about the relationship between children, their parents and the state (Lyon and Parton 1995).

Similarly disparaging headlines and media coverage, with all the attendant implications for public opinion and policy prescriptions, are evident in other areas of social policy. Media reporting of mental health, for example, is too frequently conducted via stigmatising and stereotyped descriptions of people as 'loonies, nutters, psychos, divs, morons and mongs': words which Focus on Health, an umbrella group seeking changes to broadcasting and newspaper regulation to improve coverage, believes constitute 'an agenda of prejudice' (*Press Gazette*, 10 April 1998: 11). Philo and Secker argue, moreover, that the close association between violent behaviour and mental illness, which is stressed so prominently in media reports, has been instrumental in reshaping the policy of care in the community in ways which, standing the previous policy on its head, are designed to ensure 'compliance from those who resist voluntary engagement with the mental health services'. In policy terms, this media agenda of prejudice is judged to have triggered a 'knee jerk response' to 'ill considered fears' (Chapter 8).

Press reporting of the Bulger case offers another example of the potential for the media to stimulate policy developments (see Chapter 11, Franklin (1996a) and Franklin and Petley (1996)). The immediate policy response to media coverage of the trial of Bobby Thompson and Jon Venables was the opportunistic and punitive 'back to basics' captured in John Major's regrettable injunction that 'we must learn to understand a little less and to condemn a little more' (*The Times*, 22 February 1993): ironically, the policy promptly collapsed under the burden of sexual scandal surrounding the government. Bill Jordan argues, however, that media coverage had substantial, if somewhat delayed, policy consequences and 'shaped the specific form of communitarianism – backward looking, nostalgic, authoritarian and focused on social control – that now drives New Labour's programme' (see Chapter 12).

Press coverage of the Bulger case also prompted shifts in criminal justice policy. The media demonising of children and young people as inherently 'evil', combined with contemporary media images of children as beyond the control of the police, the courts and the criminal justice system, triggered populist policy responses from politicians in both major parties. During the 1990s, a mood of 'authoritarian populism' encouraged the revisiting of earlier policy preferences for the management and containment of young people notwithstanding a plethora of research studies illustrating the futility of such measures (Cavadino and Dignan 1997; Newburn 1996). In the run-up to the 1997 general election, Labour's intention to be 'tough on crime and tough on the causes of crime' became its most widely known soundbite. In government, the Crime and Disorder Act of 1998, with its emphasis on boot camps, tagging, curfews, parenting orders and the abolition of *doli incapax*, has been a central plank in Labour's legislative programme (see Chapter 11 and Franklin 1999).

Media reporting of education has provided further images of children 'out of control' and childhood 'in crisis'. The murder of headteacher Philip Lawrence, coupled with the closure of the Ridings school in Halifax, fed the growing public frenzy about policies to contain and control children (Lumley 1998). The moral panic about young people and education was in many senses a literal media artifice. A *Panorama* film crew, for example, photographed a journalist making a notice announcing 'school closed' and hanging it on the Ridings' school gates: antics worthy of *Globelinks*' rogue reporter Damien Day (see Chapter 10). Newspapers' lack of veracity was matched by a lack of measure. A story in the *Sun* headlined, 'Sex attack on sobbing miss shuts hell school', reported how 'a woman teacher was sexually assaulted by a boy of 14' and revealed that the 'shameful attack happened as thugs already banned from the school rampaged through the classrooms reducing teachers to tears' (*Sun*, 1 November 1996). Tony Jeffs explains that many such stories were fabricated by journalists whose news gathering activities included following staff, harassing governors, using a hoist to film in classrooms and 'paying students to misbehave, let off fireworks and recount fictitious behaviour' (see Chapter 10).

The 'dumbed down' media agenda

These misleading messages about social policy have been exacerbated by two significant developments within news media during the 1990s: first, the change in traditional news values which has become known as the 'dumbing down' of news (see Chapter 2) and second, the radical shift in national newspapers' political allegiances since the mid-1990s.

The increasingly competitive market in which print and broadcast journalism are obliged to operate has prompted a revision of editorial priorities in which the need to entertain audiences and readers has superseded the need to inform them: news has increasingly become part of the entertainment industry. This 'dumbing down' of news media has involved the trivialising and sensationalising of news coverage accompanied by a greater emphasis in news stories on human interest rather than the public interest, the prominence of 'softer' consumer stories above 'hard' policy-centered news and a preference for short, pithy news items above sustained, lengthy and detailed analysis. 'Infotainment' has increasingly become the staple diet of news bulletins (Franklin 1997).

One consequence of this development, according to some observers, has been that the distinction between the editorial styles of the tabloid and broadsheet newspapers has 'virtually disappeared' (Sampson 1996: 44). Editor Alan Rusbridger believes that the *Guardian* has moved sufficiently in a tabloid direction to warrant its redesignation as a hybrid 'broadloid'. But differences between broadsheet and tabloid newspapers are still apparent, although they are certainly blurring. So far as coverage of social policy is concerned, such differences are evident in the extent of coverage, its critical character and its editorial style and presentation. But even these three broad indicators reveal considerable overlap in tabloid and broadsheet coverage, illustrating increasingly complex patterns of editorial style.

Analysis of reporting of social services and social work in national newspapers during 1997–98, for example, revealed that the three broadsheet dailies in the study *(Daily Telegraph* (158), *Guardian* (342) and *Independent* (161)) published more than four times (661) as many reports about social services as the three tabloid newspapers (*Daily Mail* (60), *Mirror* (84) and the *Sun* (19)): a total of 163 reports (Franklin 1998: 15). The study also revealed tabloids' tendency to be more critical than broadsheet newspapers in their reporting of social services. Stories were designated 'adverse', 'beneficial' or 'neutral' depending on their expressed attitude to social services. In broadsheets, 49 per cent of coverage was identified as adverse, 11.1 per cent beneficial and 39.8 per cent neutral: in the tabloids 64 per cent was adverse, 4.4 per cent beneficial and 31.6 per cent as neutral. Tabloids such as the *Sun* (73.8 per cent adverse, 7.9 per cent beneficial and 18.3 per cent neutral) and the *Daily Mail* (66 per cent adverse, 2.3 per cent beneficial and 31.7 per cent neutral) were particularly critical in their appraisals of social services while the broadsheet *Guardian* was most benign (43.2 per cent adverse, 12.7 per cent beneficial and 44.7 per cent neutral). But despite its reputation as the 'social workers' friend', the *Guardian* remains critical of social services and publishes three times as much adverse as beneficial coverage (Franklin 1998: 13).

This leads directly to a final difference between tabloid and broadsheet coverage. Tabloids prefer a more robust, dramatic and Manichaean style of editorial which attempts to present issues in a 'them and us' format which identifies and distinguishes innocent victims from guilty perpetrators. Press coverage of the government report into the Rikki Neave case illustrates these differences of editorial style. The *Guardian* headlined its story: 'Managers face criticism for Rikki tragedy', the *Daily Telegraph* preferred the more dramatic: 'Rikki Neave report – three years on and children still at risk', while the *Sun* couched its headline in more characteristically tabloid style: 'Bunglers – kids still in danger' (all dated 15 October 1997).

A second consequence of this 'dumbing down' process has been the ascendancy of the columnist above the journalist. According to the distinguished editor C.P. Scott's well-known maxim, journalists report 'facts' and the separation of 'facts' from mere 'opinion' is judged to be 'sacred'. But the success of columnists is measured by the size of their mailbag. At best, hyperbole is at a premium: at worst, bigotry and bile seem too frequently to have become the tools of the columnists' trade. For columnists, measured analysis and discussion of social policy is rare, while social problems understood as the wrongdoing of individual demons is rife. Vilification is often the columnist's response. Consider the following unhappy extract from Tony Parsons' discussion of homelessness: *Street trash; beggars of Britain.*

> Punk beggars, drunk beggars, beggars with babies. Beggars in shell suits and beggars in rags. Beggars stinking of cheap lager with snot on their chin and a mangy mutt on the end of a piece of string. Lots of them. And gypsy beggars who try to stuff a ratty flower in your buttonhole with the sentimental line – 'For the children', coos some obese old hag. Old beggars too shagged out to beg, young beggars who look like they could run a four minute mile if they ever made it up off their fannies . . . All kinds of beggars everywhere and they will be with us forever now. They have no shame. Because begging is no longer taboo . . . My father's generation was incapable of begging . . . of all the taboos, *don't beg* was the greatest of all. You could sleep with your sister before you went begging . . . Now begging is a vocation. Soon beggars will have agents and accountants who will write off the food for their dogs-on-a-rope against tax. How low can you go? The British have become a nation of nappy wearers . . . We owe it to ourselves to walk past them, metaphorically gobbing in the grubby palms of their outstretched hands, chanting our protest against a world that is ever changing for the worse. No change, we say, no change. Just say no change.
>
> (Parsons 1995: 239–243)

The consequences of dumbing down are equally evident in television journalism. Serious investigative news journalists have been replaced by a nightly parade of carefully coiffured newsreaders who, Peter Sissons alleges, were focus-group tested for their 'viewer friendliness' as part of the BBC's extensive 'news review' (*Guardian*, 31 August 1998: 3). Newsreaders' reports, delivered in enthusiastic 'tabloid' tones and interspersed with ever greater numbers of previews of 'stories still to come' or restatements of 'tonight's major headlines', offer news 'in a more accessible style' which provides insights into the most recent miraculous developments in cloning technology, the latest celebrity or government minister to 'come out', or the spin-doctored scraps from the Westminster table. More stories, shorter stories, consumer stories and human interest stories are all seemingly preferred to more sustained policy analysis. In Britain, like America, news bulletins are moving down-market with such pace that 'television journalism' risks becoming an oxymoron.

The removal of the *News at Ten* from the prime-time slot it occupied for 34 years, in order to show uninterrupted films, confirmed for many observers the low priority attributed to television news in the highly competitive television schedules (*Guardian*, 20 November 1998). Documentary programming has not been exempt. Many broadcasters regret the demise of investigative documentaries and their replacement by the more populist 'docusoaps' exploring the intimacies of life below decks on a cruise liner, the daily conflicts of a traffic warden, as well as insider views of life working in a well-known Liverpool hotel (Fitzwalter 1998).

The second significant development in news media with implications for social policy has been the recent but quite remarkable shift in newspapers' partisan allegiances. At the time of the 1992 general election, there were 8.7 million readers of pro-Conservative newspapers with only 3.3 million readers of newspapers supporting the Labour Party. By 1997, however, six of the ten national dailies and five of the nine Sunday national papers were recommending readers to support Blair: a readjusted partisanship which left only 3.4 million readers of pro-Conservative papers, but 8.6 millions reading pro-Labour papers (Norris 1998: 122). This shift in newspapers' partisan allegiances reflects voters' disillusionment with the Conservative Party, newspapers' need to reflect their readers' views in their editorial and Labour's long-term campaign objective to 'win over' the Murdoch press (Franklin 1996b: 19). An additional factor is undoubtedly (Labour supporter) Lord Hollick's purchase of (Conservative supporter) Lord Stevens' United Newspaper group which prompted Pauline conversions in the political sympathies of the *Daily Express*, the *Sunday Express* and the *Daily Star* and illustrated neatly proprietors' rather than editors' influence over significant aspects of newspapers' editorial content. This growing ideological congruence between New Labour, certain newspapers and the reading public, has undoubtedly been reinforced by Labour's strong commitments to media presentation of policy and its well-resourced strategies for news management of policy discussions (see Chapters 1 and 2).

In these changed circumstances, Labour might anticipate that coverage of its policies, including social policies, would be more supportive and less critical than a decade ago. But support for a political party is only a single element in a newspaper's broader ideological position and its approach to policy questions. Many tabloids such as the *Daily Mail*, as well as the greater part of the Murdoch press, remain hostile to collectivist solutions to social problems, any further commitment of public expenditure to resolve social problems, any expansion in the role of the state in the provision of social and welfare services, or any closer involvement with European systems of welfare or legislative programmes. Consequently, governments which advocate policies involving any confrontation with these ideological commitments can expect vigorous and vocal opposition from certain sectors of the press.

Press partisanship is certainly highly influential in shaping media reports of social policy. An example of coverage of the same story by newspapers from opposing sides of the ideological/party divide is illustrative. In December

1997, the *Daily Mail* and the *Guardian* both reported the government's proposal to replace the Central Council for Education and Training in Social Work (CCETSW) with a more general Social Care Council. The distinctive language and style of the two reports illustrates the divergent ideological postures of the newspapers to social services: interestingly, some of the similarities in the two reports signal the reliance of both accounts on a press release from Paul Boateng's press office.

> 'Social workers face shake up' – The training body for social workers is to be wound up as part of the government's plans to regulate the million people employed in social care. Ministers announced yesterday that the body, which has been criticised for perpetuating 'politically correct' values in social work, would be replaced under the plans.
>
> (*Guardian*, 23 December 1997)

> 'Dogma is ditched for social workers' – The council which supervises the training of social workers is to be abolished by government, it has been announced. The move follows a series of disastrous incidents involving social services departments, and damning reports which attacked social workers and their managers.
>
> (*Daily Mail*, 23 December 1997)

The media misrepresentation of social problems and policy solutions outlined above, in tandem with developments in news media which signal that coverage might offer ever more misleading messages, suggests that the closer involvement of the media in the policy process has become a crucial concern for students of social policy. It has, moreover, become an essential strategy for any organisation with policy ambitions (whether government, interest groups or media themselves) to try to influence the news agenda in support of those ambitions, since news media are increasingly becoming the most significant public forum for debates about social policy (see Chapters 1, 3 and 4).

The book in outline

Social Policy, the Media and Misrepresentation examines and analyses various aspects of news-media reporting of social policy and the influences of such coverage on the processes of policy making and implementation. It offers an appraisal of the complex interrelationships between news media, news sources, the content of media coverage of social policy and its impact on audiences and policy makers. The various chapters explore media reporting of specific social policy areas such as social work and child protection, housing and homelessness, poverty and welfare policy, health and mental health, education and criminal justice. Other chapters provide detailed case studies of media reporting focusing on the impact of coverage of the James Bulger case on New

Labour's policy agenda, media images of disability, the media framing of paedophiles, media representations of lone mothers and the reporting of young people in care.

The broad concern of this book is to consider and evaluate, via these social policy case studies, a number of distinctive perceptions of the role of the media in the policy processes of democratic states. One view suggests that the press constitute a fourth estate, a watchdog which is highly critical of government and its activities; consequently relationships between journalists and politicians are essentially adversarial. On this account, the media are judged to perform a central role in securing accountable and responsible government. They provide the public with a flow of communications about policy making and implementation which guarantees not simply a well-informed public (the idea of the informed citizen) but, eventually, a rational policy-making process.

An alternative perception is highly sceptical about many of the assumptions underlying this view of media. Relationships between politicians and journalists, it is alleged, are increasingly collusive rather than adversarial. The media, rather than providing a vehicle for critical and radical appraisals of government and the policy process, are merely conduits for the burgeoning flood of handouts emanating from the expansive numbers of public relations experts, press officers and spin doctors employed by government, political parties and a range of specialist interest groups with policy agendas to promote.

These trends are enhanced by recent changes in the approach of news media to policy-centred 'hard news' coverage mentioned above. Competitive markets and a regulatory regime which constrains media with a 'lighter touch', have steered media increasingly in the direction of the provision of entertainment rather than information. Journalists' coverage of policy concerns seems increasingly to be distorted by the prism of human interest which, in tandem with news values emphasising sensational and sometimes ill-measured commentary, articulates a clear moral and political agenda. In these circumstances, media may obfuscate rather than clarify policy choices; press partisanship, the influence of news sources and journalists' news values may combine to systematically exclude certain policy options rather than setting the widest possible policy agenda before media audiences.

For their part, journalists and broadcasters have tended to be sceptical of both accounts and place much greater credence in 'cock up' rather than 'conspiracy' when seeking to identify the factors central to the construction of news agendas. It is the pressures of deadlines, the shortages of news space or programme time, the availability of information, the constraints of the laws of libel and competition with other news sources that shape the eventual character of news media content; in brief it is the way in which journalism is organised which is crucial in explaining the content of media messages (Randall 1996: 5).

Social Policy, the Media and Misrepresentation provides readers with evidence derived from a series of case studies to allow them to adjudicate between these competing perceptions of the role of media and their influence on the twin processes of policy making and policy implementation. The book has three further ambitions: first, to explore the complex relationship between news media and their sources of news located in a wide range of public and private sector institutions and agencies; second, to examine and analyse media coverage of specific social policy issues; third, to illustrate the impact of media reporting of social policy issues on specific audiences, the general public, policy elites and, via all three, the policy process. In brief the concern is to explore the production, intention and reception of media messages about social policy.

Part I focuses on the production of social policy news. Bob Franklin argues that the Labour government is devoting extensive and unprecedented resources to the tasks of news management and media-based advertising campaigns to establish a hegemonic position as the primary definer of policy discussions in news media. The suggestion that the government marketing and promotion of policy has crossed the line, which separates policy promotion from propaganda, is also considered (Chapter 1).

From the perspective of a specialist correspondent, David Brindle suggests that the production of news about social policy is 'much more chaotic' than 'readers ever imagine' while stressing that 'the process of putting together a newspaper or, for that matter, a TV or radio programme – is not without structure'. Brindle outlines the journalist's working day, discusses the journalist's relationships with news sources, identifies the major constituents of a 'good' story, bemoans the difficulties of working as a specialist correspondent and the 'worrying trend' of growing influence for 'government spin doctors' which he argues 'cannot be healthy for proper scrutiny of decision making' (Chapter 2).

David Deacon analyses media reporting of the voluntary sector, but is concerned primarily with the publicity strategies of voluntary and charitable organisations. He identifies the factors which are crucial in shaping the extent and character of their relationships with news media and concludes that media reporting of voluntary organisations 'confirms a strong linkage between media access' and an organisation's 'economic power' with journalists likely to 'prioritise *big charity* over *little charity* and *established* over *emerging* voices' (Chapter 3).

Kevin Williams explores the production of news about HIV/AIDS, arguing that media coverage was crucially shaped by the evident conflicts 'between specialist correspondents and general reporters', as well as the competition between 'powerful and official sources' (the Health Education Authority) and 'alternative or non-official sources' (the Terrence Higgins Trust) for media access: such access was central to efforts to 'shape media accounts and influence the policy process' (Chapter 4). Subsequent chapters also explore aspects of the production of social policy news. Vikki Entwistle and Trevor Sheldon, for example, discuss the significance of health correspondents' perceptions about what makes a good 'health' story and examine the role of the Department of Health's 'good news unit' and 'rebuttal unit' in the construction of health policy news (Chapter 7), while John Muncie stresses the significance of official news sources such as the police, the courts and the Home Office in the construction of crime news (see Chapter 11).

Many of the chapters explore media representations of social problems and policy solutions. Meryl Aldridge, for example, examines the contradictory media representations of social workers who are encouraged to intervene more often and decisively to prevent incidents of child deaths but, in the context of cases of alleged child sexual abuse such as Cleveland and the Orkneys, are excoriated by the media for intervening too often and too effectively (see Chapter 5). Steve Platt explores the media tendency to distinguish 'deserving' from 'undeserving' homeless people with the former exemplified by Cathy in Ken Loach's powerful drama, *Cathy Come Home* and the latter by young homeless people in the 1990s who appear in media accounts as 'beggars' and 'scroungers' and who, in the words of one ex-MP, should be 'hosed from the streets' (Chapter 6).

Vikki Entwistle and Trevor Sheldon identify a number of sometimes competing interpretive frameworks shaping health news which have prompted a recent focus on stories which challenge the traditional authority of senior practitioners, stories about technological developments which promise cures for ailments (from cancer to Viagra) and stories concerning the rationing of health services to people who are very ill: illustrated by the case of Child B who was refused treatment for leukaemia (Chapter 7). Greg Philo and Jenny Secker analyse and regret the media reporting of mental illness through the use of terms like 'mad', 'maniac' and 'psycho' and the unjustifiable association in media accounts of mental illness with violent behaviour (Chapter 8).

Peter Golding explores the 'intense scroungerphobia' which characterised press reporting of poverty and social security in the 1970s and the persistence of such reporting in the 1990s. Headlines such as 'Irish fiddler takes British tax-payer for £1 million' (*Mail on Sunday*, 20 July 1997) and '£1.4 bn benefit fraud is tip of iceberg' (*Daily Telegraph*, 10 July 1995) continue to provide the political context for the Blair government's commitment to 'think the unthinkable' and reform social security provision and expenditure (Chapter 9). Ann Pointon analyses press responses to the radical new images of disability, promoted by disabled activists in their struggle to win civil rights (Chapter 14), while Tony Jeffs explores 'the negative reporting of events at specific schools' such as Risinghill and Summerhill, media preoccupations with particular types of schools such as comprehensives and 'failing schools' as well as the evident media preference for representing school students as 'thugs' who are 'out of control' (Chapter 10). Jenny Kitzinger 'highlights the positive as well as the negative impact of coverage' of the crisis centring on the release of paedophiles into the community and argues that the media framing of paedophiles as 'stranger danger' ignores both the scale and nature of sexual violence especially within the family (Chapter 13). Ros Edwards, Simon Duncan and Miri Song explore media representations of lone mothers as either a social threat or a social problem (Chapter 15) while Andy West identifies media images of young people, especially young people in care, which associate them with 'courts and crime' and stigmatise them as 'burglars and prostitutes': one young person commented, 'they make us out to be monsters' (Chapter 16).

Finally, some chapters explore the implications of press coverage for the policy process; some argue for a clear, although not direct or simple, connection between media reporting and policy developments. Bill Jordan, for example argues for a significant influence for media coverage of the Bulger case on the failed Conservative policy of 'back to basics' as well as more recent statements of New Labour welfare policy (Chapter 12). John Muncie suggests the 'demonising' of children, endemic in the reporting of the Bulger case, 'helped to mobilise a moral panic about youth crime in general, . . . legitimised a series of tough law and order responses to young offenders' and has significantly shaped developments in criminal justice policy embodied in the Crime and Disorder Act 1998 (Chapter 11). Ann Pointon argues that much of the impetus behind the Disability Discrimination Act 1995, was provided by the radically revised images of disability which were highly attractive to the media and replaced the previous media stereotypes of disabled people as 'pitiable and pathetic' (Chapter 14), while Greg Philo and Jenny Secker argue for 'clear links' between media representations of people with mental health problems and 'public attitudes to community care' and suggest that media reporting has 'played some part in fuelling opposition to the policy' (Chapter 8). Simon Duncan, Ros Edwards and Miri Song suggest that media images of lone mothers which represent them both as a social threat or social problem, 'are significant components in the policy process' because of their role in defining issues and setting agendas around lone motherhood (Chapter 15).

These diverse accounts of the production, intention and reception of media messages about social policy illustrate the growing significance of media in the policy process and generate a number of consensual conclusions. First, the production of media messages about social policy is crucially affected by journalists' and broadcasters' relationships with their news sources. These relationships are changing as organisations with policy objectives increasingly try to influence media news agendas in order to achieve those policy ambitions. Second, many media messages about social policy are misleading: news media frequently misrepresent social problems and fail to present policy solutions accurately, fairly and impartially. Third, these misleading messages are influential in shaping public perceptions of social problems as well as the effectiveness of particular policy remedies. Finally, since politicians are responsive to public anxieties about policy issues and pressures for policy change – and because politicians no less than ordinary viewers and readers take note of media accounts – misleading media representations of social policy may ultimately influence the policy process. In the light of these conclusions, Toynbee's observation that 'social policy makes neither news nor history unless there is some crisis', is only partially correct. The identified crisis, moreover, is a crisis of journalism which, in turn, prompts a growing crisis for policy making in democratic states when citizens are poorly served by the media with information about social issues.

References

Aldridge, M. (1994) *Making Social Work News*, London: Routledge.

Butler, D. and Kavanagh, D. (1997) *The General Election 1997*, Basingstoke: Macmillan.

Cavadino, P. and Dignan, J. (1997) *The Penal System*, London: Sage.

Cohen, N. (1998) 'The death of news', *New Statesman* 22 May, 18–19.

Fitzwalter, R. (1998) *The Decline of the Documentary*, London: Campaign for Quality Television.

Franklin, B. (1996a) 'From little angels to little devils: changing media representations of children and childhood', *Community Care*, 24 October.

—— (1996b) 'Why the sun does not shine on Mr. Major', *Parliamentary Brief*, March, 18–21.

—— (1997) *Newszak and News Media*, London: Arnold.

—— (1998) *Hard Pressed: National Newspaper Reporting of Social Work and Social Services*, London: Reed Publications.

—— (1999) 'Children's rights: media misrepresentation and social policy', in C. Cuninghame (ed.) *Doing Rights*, London: Save the Children.

Franklin, B. and Parton, N. (1991) *Social Work, the Media and Public Relations*, London: Routledge.

Franklin, B. and Petley, J. (1996) 'Killing the age of innocence: newspaper reporting of the death of James Bulger', in J. Pilchar and S. Wagg (eds) *Thatcher's Children? Politics, Childhood and Society in the 1980s and 1990s*, London: Falmer Press, 134–154.

Lumley, K. (1998) 'Teeny thugs in Blair's sights: media portrayals of children in education and their policy implications', *Youth and Policy* 61, 1–11.

Lyon, C. and Parton, N. (1995) 'Children's rights and the Children Act 1989', in B. Franklin (ed.) *The Handbook of Children's Rights: Comparative Policy and Practice*, London: Routledge, 40–55.

Newburn, T. (1996) 'Back to the future? Youth crime, youth justice and the rediscovery of "authoritarian populism"', in J. Pilchar and S. Wagg (eds) *Thatcher's Children? Politics, Childhood and Society in the 1980s and 1990s*, London: Falmer Press, 61–77.

Norris, P. (1998) 'The battle for the campaign agenda', in A. King (ed.) *New Labour Triumphs at the Polls*, London: Chatham House.

Parsons, A. (1995) 'Street trash: beggars of Britain', in A. Parsons *Dispatches from the Front Line of Popular Culture*, London: Virgin Books.

Randall, D. (1996) *The Universal Journalist*, London: Pluto.

Sampson, A. (1996) 'A crisis at the heart of our media', *British Journalism Review* 7(3): 42–56.

Social Trends 1998 (1998) London: HMSO.

Toynbee, P. (1999) 'The quiet achievers', *Guardian* 13 January, 16.

Part I

Producing Social Policy News

Chapter 1

Soft-soaping the public?

The government and media promotion of social policy

Bob Franklin

On 17 September 1998, the *Guardian* published a rather curious and enigmatic photograph of David Blunkett enjoying a pint of beer, ensconced behind the bar of the Queen Vic on the set of BBC's popular soap opera *EastEnders*. Soap stars Patsy Palmer (Bianca) and Sid Owen (Ricky) were pictured on either side of the politician, although their pose signalled a preference for reading above drinking. Bianca's favoured 'literary tipple', held carefully to display the cover title, was Bill Bryson's *Notes from a Small Island*; Ricky's more controversial but popular choice was John Gray's *Men are from Mars, Women are from Venus*. The logos emblazoned on the actors' T-shirts, which announced the beginning of the National Year of Reading (NYR), identified the policy context for this particular photo opportunity.

Such occasions have become routine events for government ministers and central to the process of policy presentation. The current emphasis on the media packaging of policy means that ministers are more likely to be seen on television opening a new hospital building or feeding their children beefburgers during a food scare than engaged in more traditional activities such as debating at the despatch box in the House of Commons. But the photo opportunity at the Queen Vic was only a modest part of an extensive campaign to promote the National Year of Reading: the first in a series of television advertisements had been broadcast the previous evening. The Queen Vic was a particularly apposite setting for the campaign launch because the soap opera was introducing a new story line which involved the character Grant Mitchell reading to his baby daughter Courtney. Government press officers working on the campaign had also persuaded drama producers to feature story lines about literacy in other popular soap operas including *Brookside*, *Coronation Street*, *Hollyoaks* and *Grange Hill* over the coming year.

These advertising campaigns are undoubtedly problematic because of the extent to which their pre-packaged policy messages are injected into light entertainment programmes and soap operas, rather than being confined to more conventional advertising formats such as posters and leaflets. The campaign launch certainly proved controversial. Under the headline 'Big brother Blunkett is accused', the *Daily Mail* quoted a Conservative spokesperson who denounced 'this government intervention into the world of television soap operas' as an 'Orwellian nightmare' which the 'licence payer would reject as propaganda on the telly' (*Daily Mail*, 17 September 1998). The government promptly dismissed the allegation claiming the purpose of the campaign was to 'raise public awareness' about literacy problems. Conservative protestations of 'big brother', moreover, smacked of hypocrisy on at least two counts. First, it was a succession of Conservative governments which prompted the spiralling of government advertising budgets throughout the 1980s to peak at £200 million in 1988–89 (Cobb 1989: 12). Second, governments' determination to use soap operas to sell policy as well as soap was neither confined to, nor initiated by, the Labour party. Conservative Home Secretary Kenneth Baker used *Brookside* to promote anti-drug policies in the early 1990s and even the BBC radio soap *The Archers* was initially broadcast as a public information service for farmers and featured story lines initiated by the Ministry of Agriculture (Carroll 1998: 4).

There is certainly a long history in the UK of parties and governments using the media to promote their policies to the voting public. The Labour Party, for example, established its first Press and Publicity Department as early as October 1917 (Hollins 1981: 146) while debates within the party, about whether election campaigns should be 'image' rather than 'issue' driven, began in the 1920s (Wring 1997: 13–14). Some elder statesmen have always considered it to be axiomatic that successful policy implementation entails media promotion. Tony Benn, for example, in his *Years of Hope* diary, reproached Aneurin Bevan for his 'absurd idea that all publicity is unimportant and that all you need is the right policy' (Benn 1994: 190). William Beveridge, aided by his friend Frank Pakenham (Lord Longford) – a journalist and Beveridge's public relations adviser – achieved an early understanding of the significance of publicity, media management and even the use of soundbites, in helping to shape a climate of public opinion favourable to certain policy options. An important factor in the public reception of the Beveridge Report was that Beveridge, through broadcasts, articles and half-leaks – he was an occasional member of the massively popular radio *Brains Trust* – had made very certain that the world knew it was coming. He had repeatedly referred publicly to 'equality of sacrifice' and the possibility of 'abolishing poverty'. In March 1942, more than six months before the report, *Picture Post* could write 'everybody has heard of Sir William Beveridge'. As early as April 1942 a Home Intelligence report noted 'Sir William Beveridge's proposals for an "all-in" social security scheme are said to be popular' and by the autumn Home Intelligence was recording that 'three years ago the term social security was almost unknown to the public as a whole. It now appears to be generally accepted as an urgent post war need. It is commonly defined as a decent minimum standard of living for all' (Timmins 1996: 41).

Given this historical context, the conclusion of a study of the government's media campaign to promote the poll tax, which argued that 'the marketing of government activity has become a central activity of modern statecraft' seems unexceptional (Deacon and Golding 1994: 7). Politicians' longstanding but ever increasing use of the media to inform and persuade about policy, has been variously described as the 'packaging of policy' (Franklin 1994), the 'modern publicity process' (Blumler 1990), the activity of the 'public relations state' (Deacon and Golding 1994), a central feature of 'designer politics' (Scammell 1995), the 'Americanization' (a clumsy word but a more dubious concept) of British political communications (Negrine 1996) which entails the 'selling of politics' (Rees 1992), or what Bayley calls the 'politics of Labour camp' where, following Susan Sontag, camp is defined as 'the consistently aesthetic experience of the world . . . which incarnates a victory of "style" over "content", "aesthetics" over "morality", of irony over tragedy' (Bayley 1998: 7). This presentational emphasis in government communications has both detractors and advocates (McNair 1998).

Critics argue that when policy is packaged in this way relationships between government and the media become collusive, rather than adversarial. Worse, news media risk becoming little more than delivery services for government policy messages, carefully crafted by press officers working in the various departments of state and conveyed to readers and viewers who mistake them for the products of an independent and assiduous journalism (see Chapter 2). In these circumstances the media may confuse rather than clarify policy choices as governments try to structure news agendas in ways that exclude the discussion of certain policy options rather than placing the widest possible policy agenda before audiences and readers. But supporters object that designer democracy 'heightens the awareness and interest of voters' (Scammell 1995: 18) and suggest that 'an advertisement which electors look at and understand contributes more to political education than a dreary statement of policy which no one reads' (Harrop 1990).

What is undoubtedly new amid this longer-term trend is the Labour government's commitment to expanding the involvement of media in the processes of policy making as well as policy implementation. To date, governments' use of the media has been confined to the presentation of policy. The purpose of media campaigns has been to win public acceptability for policy initiatives and facilitate their implementation. But the new government seems to believe that the presentation of policy is at least as significant as the substantive policy content and that consequently the facility with which policy options lend themselves to media presentation is now a crucial ingredient in policy making. 'What they can't seem to grasp', a senior Labour spin doctor confided shortly after the 1997 general election, 'is that communications is [sic.] not an after thought to our policy. It's central to the whole mission of new Labour' (Gaber 1998: 13). It was Peter Mandelson who articulated this new role for the media most cogently, when he argued that the government's assessment of whether or not a policy was capable of clear presentation had become a touchstone of its acceptability to government and its merit as policy. 'There are some who still denigrate the presentation of policy as a diversion from its substance, as a superficial and unnecessary coating to the main product', he argued,

> I take the opposite view . . . if a government policy cannot be presented in a simple and attractive way it is more likely than not to contain fundamental flaws and prove to be the wrong policy. Once those flaws surface, the unattractive alternatives are sticking with it or overturning policy in which significant political capital might have been invested. We do not intend to fall into that trap.
>
> (Mandelson 16 September 1997)

This chapter examines the unprecedented prominence which the current government has given to the media in the policy process. Labour uses the media to promote policy initiatives via advertising, as well as to manage and orchestrate public discussions of policy developments. The obvious concern is that, by promoting policies in this way, the government is blurring, if not crossing, the very significant divide which separates the legitimate activity of providing information about government policy from the wholly unacceptable activity of using publicly funded public relations and promotional agencies to persuade the public to particular policy choices: in brief the divide which separates policy marketing from propaganda. The Labour government undoubtedly glosses too quickly and too glibly over the many complexities involved in distinguishing propaganda from the welcome and democratic ambition of 'raising public awareness'.

Flogging policy like soapflakes: government policy advertising

Government advertising budgets expanded threefold during the 1980s reaching the staggering annual expenditure of £200 million by the close of the decade (Cobb 1989: 12). Since 1983, the government had trailed marginally behind Unilever and Proctor and Gamble as the third largest UK advertiser, but the expenditure of £76 million on promoting the privatising of the electricity industry, with the additional £40 million for the campaign to sell off the water industries, helped to secure the government pole position by 1989 (Blair 1989: 4). Government policies seemed to be no easier to sell than soapflakes: indeed advertising budgets have been considerably greater. The growth in government advertising was certainly spectacular and prompted criticism both for the scale of the public expenditure involved as well as the alleged bias and partisanship of much of its content (Anderson 1988; Franklin 1994). Advertising on this scale, however, enjoyed a precedent in the postwar Attlee government's expenditure on advertising to win public support for the original policy of nationalising what were then the privately owned industries of coal, gas and electricity (Scammell 1995: 231 and Wildy 1985): a notable and costly irony.

The advertising boom revisited: Conservative and Labour campaigns

The campaigns to privatise industries were not the only triggers for a burgeoning of advertising expenditure under successive Conservative governments during the 1980s. The timing was propitious. Growing unemployment prompted the Department for Trade and Industry's (DTI) 'Action for jobs' campaign, the Department of the Environment launched a vigorous campaign to promote its 'community charge' initiative, while the emergence of AIDS and a worsening drug abuse problem prompted a series of high profile, and lavishly resourced, health education campaigns (Deacon and Golding 1994; Franklin 1994, see also Chapter 4). Some government departments revealed a particular enthusiasm for promoting policy via advertising. During 1987–88, for example, expenditure at Social Services reached £24 million, exceeded £32 million at the Manpower Services Commission, while the then Department of Employment allocated £11.3 million to advertising. Certain departmental budgets spiralled upwards, and at a pace! At the Department of the Environment advertising costs expanded from £1,163,093 in 1986 to £24.6 million a year later: the repackaging of the Department of Trade and Industry as the 'Department of Enterprise' along with other promotional initiatives increased the departmental advertising budget from £1,785,000 in 1986–87 to £31,276,000 in 1988–89 (Franklin 1994: 107–108). Government advertising reached a peak in 1988–89 but declined slowly throughout the 1990s.

The greater part of this government advertising expenditure was channelled through the Central Office of Information (COI), a specialist agency created to advise governments about publicity and marketing campaigns, press work, publications and advertising and to supply the necessary staff (journalists, press officers, radio producers, film makers and editors) and services to implement them (Garner and Short 1998). Government departments purchase advertising through the agency because its substantial expenditure enables the COI to negotiate considerable discounts which in 1997–98 amounted to almost £23,709,000 (COI 1998: 7). Some sense of the extent and nature of government advertising at the time, is revealed by the COI expenditure of £150 million on government publicity, which purchased 32,965 advertising slots on television and placed 9246 advertisements in print media. The COI also conducted more than 100 publicity campaigns for different government departments, produced 1800 publications, produced more than 140 films, videos and television commercials and mounted more than 140 exhibitions during 1987–88 (Cobb 1989: 13).

Much of this publicity was uncontentious and focused on recruitment advertising, social persuasion campaigns ('Don't drink and drive at Christmas') and public information advertising perhaps announcing new benefit entitlements. But during the 1980s, opposition MPs and other critics alleged that government advertising was moving away from its traditional focus on public information in the direction of promoting the policy of the governing party. Four other significant shifts in government advertising originate in the 1980s but continue to shape the current patterns of expenditure: a notable increase in expenditure on television advertising (from 25 per cent in 1970 to 46 per cent in 1997): a considerably enhanced budget for promoting economic and social policy; a shift from expenditure on overseas to domestic publicity, as well as a striking tendency for advertising expenditure to increase in the year prior to general elections – evident in every election since 1964 (Scammell 1995: 207–14)

The election of Labour in 1997 has triggered a renewed government commitment to expenditure on policy promotion which has, in turn, marked a renaissance in the fortunes of the COI at both national and regional levels (Baird 1997: 13). Nationally, during 1997–98, for example, the COI devised and implemented a number of 'fully integrated' campaigns including the publicity for the 'New Deal' which involved all aspects of promoting the policy from 'securing media coverage on regional television and in the press' to 'delivery of the "New Deal" in Job Centres' and the development of relevant web site materials (COI 1998: 3). Regionally, the COI's eleven regional centres have been subject to a communications audit which concluded that the COI 'is well placed for providing a very extensive network to reinforce key Government messages' (Baird 1997: 13).

This typically systematic and comprehensive Labour approach to policy promotion has been costly. During 1997–98, Malcolm Bruce and Margaret Ewing posed a series of parliamentary questions inquiring about levels of 'total expenditure on all forms of publicity and advertising' in each of the major government departments. The replies revealed that costs of publicity and advertising costs were: £15.5 million at the Scottish Office (HC Debs (House of Commons Debates), vol. 313 cols. 266–7); £962,854 for the Lord Chancellor (HC Debs vol. 303, cols. 109–11); £1.3 million at the Department of International Development (vol. 302 cols. 613–4); £8,109,000 at the Northern Ireland Office (HC Debs (vol. 302 cols. 616–7); £40.97 million at the Ministry of Defence (HC Debs vol. 302, cols. 441–9); £19,429,000 at Environment, Transport and the Regions (HC Debs vol. 301 cols. 618–9); £436,774 at the Foreign and Commonwealth Office (HC Debs vol. 301 cols. 395–6); £9,216,000 at the Department of Trade and Industry (HC Debs vol. 301 cols. 413–5); £17,724,255 at Social Services (HC Debs vol. 301 Col. 443); £22,124,000 at the Treasury (HC Debs vol. 301 cols. 113–4); £16,210,000 at the Department of Health (HC Debs vol. 301 col. 14); £609,000 at Culture, Media and Sport (HC Debs vol. 300 cols. 641–2); £9,080,593 at the Home Office (HC Debs vol. 300 cols. 530–1); £2,015,000 at the Welsh

Office (HC Debs vol. 300 col. 520); £17.4 million at the Department for Education and Employment (HC Debs vol. 300 cols. 530–1); £218,700 for the Attorney General (HC Debs vol. 302 col. 578) and £1,518,790 for the Chancellor of the Duchy of Lancaster (HC Debs vol. 302 col. 377).

The aggregate expenditure of £165,323,966 is a substantial sum which almost rivals the peak advertising budgets of the Thatcher governments of the late 1980s. Four observations make this expenditure even more noteworthy. First, expenditure has held up remarkably well despite the shrinking state sector. The greater part of the advertising budgets of the 1980s funded the privatising campaigns which no longer feature centrally in government policy. The evident consequence of the 'privatising' of nationalised industries has been precisely to diminish the state sector but with no visible effect on the size of advertising budgets. Second, by bulk purchasing through the COI, government departments secured a discount of 32.6 per cent on advertising expenditure and consequently the above-cited figures underestimate by approximately one third the media value as well as the quantity of advertising actually purchased by government. Third, since April 1984 the COI has been obliged to bid for the publicity work of government departments in competition with private-sector agencies such as Saatchi and Saatchi. In 1997–98, only eleven departments purchased publicity and advertising services through the COI with a total spend of £110,680,000 (COI 1998: 5). The remaining £55 million spent by government departments was allocated to private-sector marketing and PR agencies, which represents a substantial growth in the fortunes of these companies. Finally, the advertising budgets for social policy departments (Social Services £17.7 million, Education and Employment £17.4 million and Health £16.2 million) are among the most substantial and surpassed only by those for Defence (£41 million), the Treasury (£22.1 million) and the Environment (£19.5 million).

Sea changes and soap operas: the National Year of Reading

These advertising budgets, although generous, signal little of the flavour of specific campaigns. The promotion of the National Year of Reading (NYR), mentioned at the beginning of this chapter, is worth exploring in more detail because it illustrates many of the typical features of what the marketing industry has come to describe as an 'integrated campaign'. The National Year of Reading was launched amidst considerable media razzmatazz on 16 September 1998: the planning of the campaign had begun a year previously. The overall aim of the campaign is 'nothing less than a sea change in the nation's attitude to reading' (DfEE 1998a: 2). More specifically, the objective is to 'ensure that by the year 2002, 80 per cent of all 11 year olds will reach the standards expected of their age in English' (DfEE 1998a: 3); such ambitions seem uncontentious if not laudable.

Labour commissioned the public relations consultancy Hill Knowlton to be responsible for the planning and day-to-day implementation of the campaign. Hill Knowlton's qualifications for handling such accounts are exemplary. The Conservative government had commissioned the company in 1988 to 'raise the public profile and public image' of the water companies in the run-up to privatisation: another 'integrated campaign'. Extracts from a strategy document from that campaign, entitled *Tactics*, were published in a Labour opposition report which revealed that Hill Knowlton's plans included: 'placing' an item in *Tomorrow's World* about using trout to monitor water quality (agreed one year in advance of the broadcast); training celebrities such as Chay Blyth, Duncan Goodhew and Sharron Davies in the industry's objectives and securing guest appearances on *Wogan* and breakfast television; organising a wet T-shirt competition in the *Sun*; the inclusion of promotional material in the scripts of soap operas like *EastEnders*, arranging contributions to LBC phone-ins, as well as contributing feature items to the *Jimmy Young Show* and *Women's Hour*' (Blair 1989: 3). The two campaigns share more than a passing similarity.

NYR, like its predecessor, has managed to persuade scriptwriters and directors of peak-time soap operas to include story lines in these popular dramas which promote the key ambitions of the campaign. *EastEnders* and *Coronation Street*, for example, agreed to feature stories about adult literacy problems while 'children's television favourites such as *Hollyoaks*, *Grange Hill* and *Brookside* will carry plotlines promoting reading as "fun" and "cool" pastimes to dispel the myth among youngsters that only boffins enjoy books' (Lepkowska 1998). Television producer Phil Redmond has given the scheme his enthusiastic backing (*Guardian*, 17 September 1998: 4). When literacy related stories are featured in *Brookside*, programmes will be 'followed up with a helpline, *Brookside* learning materials and a *Brookside* video. When viewers phone the helpline they will be referred on to their local Brookie Basics Centre where they can improve their literacy in a relaxed setting' (*The National Year of Reading Update* October 1998: 4).

Soap operas may be the most desirable programming to access for promotional purposes but NYR was also promised coverage 'in a wide range of popular programmes such as *Ready Steady Cook* and *Esther*', in Channel 4's *Big Breakfast* and in BBC television and radio programming for schools such as *Look and Read* and *Words and Pictures* (DfEE 1988b: 6–7). This 'free' access to prime time audiences has been supplemented by paid advertising with a budget of £1.8 million. The first in a series of television advertisements, part of a campaign entitled *A Little Reading Goes a Long Way* and designed to encourage fathers to read to their children, was broadcast the evening before Blunkett's photo opportunity at the Queen Vic and carefully timed to coincide with Manchester United's game with Barcelona in the European Champions League: a scheduling which guaranteed maximum target audience reach.

The NYR launch on the *EastEnders* set was promptly followed by a press conference attended by Ken Follett, Estelle Morris and Phil Redmond: other celebrity backers include the Spice Girls, Chris Evans, John Cleese, Olympic champion Linford Christie and jockey Richard Dunwoody. Such celebrity firepower guarantees press interest but, in the spirit of a 'belt and braces' approach, the DfEE distributed 5,000 'press packs' 'containing highlights of the events that will be taking place around the country'. Perhaps unsurprisingly, the *National Year of Reading Update* was able to confirm that 'media coverage has been incredible and we are delighted with the enthusiastic way in which the press has greeted the launch of the year' (September 1998: 1). Other elements in the marketing mix included the production and distribution of glossy leaflets and booklets (by the tens of thousands), 'Roadshow' events in city centres typically involving local media, the creation of a NYR web site and the organisation and promotion of a variety of national (National Poetry Day and National Children's Book Week) and local events including the 'Babies' Book Day' in Oxfordshire. Bolton MBC distributed 'reception class packs' to 4,000 children and their carers sponsored by McDonalds. Throughout the year, the campaign activities were closely monitored and new events planned, with feedback provided by a national network of focus groups, that most favoured of New Labour policy forums (*National Year of Reading Update*, October 1998).

This flurry of promotional activity was funded largely from the public purse with the DfEE meeting the £1.8 million bill for television advertising with a further expenditure of £750,000 to help fund local initiatives. But the campaign also relied on funding partnerships with the private sector. Sainsburys, for example, sponsored the national Bookstart campaign and made a commitment to distribute a million books by the year 2000 at a cost of £6 million. For some sponsors, the National Year of Reading undoubtedly offered irresistible merchandising opportunities. The involvement of Walkers Snack Foods and McDonalds, for example, alongside Golden Wonder's offer of four free joke books in return for tokens collected from the company's 'Wotsits' snack food wrappers, appears *prima facie* less than disinterested.

The purpose of outlining details of the NYR campaign is less to criticise than to illustrate the extent of the government's advertising and public relations activities to promote what are politically relatively minor and 'low key' policy issues such as literacy. But NYR raises significant concerns about whether a government is marketing policy in a way which risks moving in the direction of propaganda: even if it is doing so unconsciously. The National Year of Reading was certainly not a politically contentious policy arena: unlike the earlier campaign to privatise the water industry. Nor is it necessary to endorse the bizarre – not to mention publicity seeking – criticisms of the Conservative spokesperson who accused 'Big brother Blunkett' of holding views 'straight out of 1984', to feel some unease about the extent to which soap operas and other popular television light entertainment programmes are being used as vehicles for government policy messages (*Daily Mail*, 17 September 1998). The deployment of such a public relations strategy has become commonplace. A report by the think-tank Demos, for example, recommended the further use of television soap operas to promote socially desirable practices such as 'good parenting' (Straw 1998). Perhaps more worrying is the legitimacy which this use of television for propaganda has achieved; certainly it no longer seems to warrant comment. Reporting Blunkett's photo opportunity at the Queen Vic, the *Guardian* expressed few misgivings about the government's plans to 'mobilise all the propaganda weapons of popular culture to improve the nation's reading skills' (*Guardian*, 17 September 1998). The NYR and similar campaigns raise at least two other issues. The first concerns the extent of public knowledge about the scale and costs of these campaigns. It is uncertain, for example, whether the public is aware that during 1997–98 the government spent in excess of £165 million on advertising and promoting its policies. Second, there is surely some doubt about whether these substantial sums of public money are most effectively and properly spent in the publicising, rather than the provision, of particular services: £165 million could provide a good number of school buildings and new teaching jobs. The campaign to promote NYR, moreover, presents a particular irony: namely central government is spending money on advertising campaigns to encourage reading at a time when local government – in the teeth of local opposition – is closing libraries to meet centrally imposed spending targets!

Advertising and marketing campaigns represent only a single strand in the government's strategy for policy presentation. Undoubtedly more significant both for promoting policy, but also constraining criticism of policy, are the various ways in which the government seeks to manage media reporting of its activities.

Doing the dirty work: New Labour and news management

Alastair Campbell the Prime Minister's Press Secretary can deploy considerable resources to the task of news management. Like all previous Press Secretaries, since Francis Williams was first appointed by Attlee in 1945, Campbell briefs the lobby twice daily which provides an opportunity to give the government's spin on the policy concerns of the day to the 200 most senior political journalists at Westminster. He can also call upon the skills of the 1,000 press and public relations specialists in the Government Information and Communications Service (GICS), which includes the 300 press officers working in the COI's national and regional offices, the six staff in the newly established Strategic Communications Unit (SCU) at Number 10, as well as the growing band of 'specialist' media advisors who work closely with senior ministers in the various government departments (Franklin 1998a). The poor public reputation of these advisors is a notable irony given that their prime role is to secure favourable media coverage of policy. A *Sunday Times* profile of Charlie Whelan, an advisor at the Treasury until January 1999, quoted 'a senior Labour source' (usually a coded phrase for the PM's Press Secretary) who commented 'politics is a dirty business and all politicians have a sort of dark or sinister side. You need someone to do your dirty work and that is what Charlie Whelan does for Gordon Brown' (*Sunday Times*, 19 December 1997). Campbell would be well placed to know. Clare Short offered him similar acclaim. 'Campbell', she suggested, 'does the dirty work' but, she added reflectively, 'with the PM's approval' (*Observer*, 22 February 1998: 3).

Whether news management constitutes 'dirty work' is a moot point, but it is certainly a rather furtive and clandestine activity. Occasionally journalists break cover to provide an insider's account of government–press relations: Nicholas Jones' *Soundbites and Spin Doctors* is invaluable for the light it shines into particularly murky corners (Jones 1995). Journalists may also expose particularly blatant examples of news management or 'deliberate misinformation'. In February 1998, for example, when the government was being heavily criticised for announcing planned cuts to Disability Living Allowances (DLA), Whitehall began briefing the media about alleged benefit fraud by disabled people, prompting newspaper headlines that almost £1 billion a year was being paid to people who were not entitled to benefit. The briefing was little more than a diversionary strategy to diffuse the growing public criticism of cuts to DLA (*Guardian*, 9 February 1998: 6). A recent study of national newspaper coverage of social services provided rare evidence underlining the importance of government press offices in shaping social policy news. More than 500 news sources contributed to press coverage during the year-long study, but the twenty most influential sources provided the quotations used in more than a quarter of the press coverage. The five sources most frequently cited by journalists accounted for more than 13 per cent of sources quoted in press reports: a quite remarkable 'strike rate'. The effectiveness of the press offices at the Home Office and the Department of Health in sourcing news reports guaranteed that Paul Boateng and Frank Dobson were the two most regularly quoted sources of news about social issues during 1997–98 (Franklin 1998b: 19).

Since 1997, Labour has undoubtedly tried to develop in government the highly effective structures and processes for news management which served the party so well in opposition. It has tried to incorporate the 'Millbank media machine' into government: and with some evident success. In his evidence to the inquiry into the Government Information and Communication Services, Sir Richard Wilson, the Cabinet Secretary, claimed 'there is a more systematic determined effort to co-ordinate in a strategic way, presentation of government policies and messages in a positive light across the whole of government, than I can remember since the time I have been in the civil service' (Select Committee on Public Administration 1998: xii). This news management strategy has entailed three ambitions: the increasing centralisation and control of communications at Number 10, a more disciplined and assertive relationship with journalists, and, the growing politicisation of the GICS.

The 'cancer at the heart of government': the central control of communications

Centralising communications at Number 10 under the control of the Prime Minister's Press Secretary has been the key priority in Labour's communications strategy. The purpose of structuring communications in this way is to ensure the government's supremacy as the unequivocal 'primary definer' of policy issues in media discussions. Central control has become tight. Mountfield's report on government communications noted that 'all major interviews and media appearances, both print and broadcast, should be agreed with the No. 10 Press Office before any commitments are entered into. The policy content of all major speeches, press releases and new policy initiatives should be cleared in good time with the No. 10 private office' and finally, 'the timing and form of announcements should be cleared with the No. 10 Press Office'. The Number 10 press office also co-ordinates the work of departmental press offices, via a weekly meeting of information officers which is chaired by Campbell, to 'secure a timely and well ordered flow of departmental communications and to see how best departmental communications can play into the broader Government messages and themes' (Mountfield 1997: 7).

The establishment of the Strategic Communications Unit (SCU) in January 1998 has provided Campbell with further news management resources. The SCU, which includes two special advisors (David Bradshaw and Philip Bassett are both ex-*Mirror* journalists), is responsible for 'pulling together and sharing with departments the government's key policy themes and messages' (Select Committee on Public Administration 1998: para 19): i.e. keeping government spokespeople 'on message'. The unit liaises with media management organisations in individual departments, such as the Strategy and Communications Directorate in the DfEE, to co-ordinate government policy messages (see Chapter 10). The SCU appears to operate according to the old propaganda maxim that if you say something often enough, people will begin to believe it. Consequently its core task is 'inserting common phrases into ministerial speeches and coming up with soundbites for media interviews to demonstrate the supposedly collective will of government' (Preston 1998: 8). The SCU's activities are complemented by 'Agenda', a new computer system, operational since 25 February 1998, which 'helps to co-ordinate government's publicity activities' by listing 'forthcoming newsworthy events, lines to take, key departmental messages and themes and ministerial speeches' (Select Committee 1998a: xiii and Appendix 12).

The government's 'communications day' begins with a 9 am meeting attended by the most significant communications staff including Alastair Campbell, Jonathan Powell the Prime Minister's Chief of Staff, specialist advisers from the Treasury and the Deputy Prime Minister's Office as well as representatives from the Cabinet Office and the Chief Whip's Office (MacAskill 1997: 8). The aim of the meeting, once again, is to ensure that strategy and presentation are 'in step' and to allocate people to resolve any specific policy presentation problems arising that day (Mountfield 1997: 8). Labour's determination to stay 'on message' requires that nothing is left to chance. The policy 'message' must be carefully scripted, meticulously rehearsed, universally endorsed by party and government, centrally co-ordinated and favourably presented in the news media. These communications demands have prompted predictable tensions both within Labour's own ranks and between the government and news journalists.

In March 1998, for example, Harriet Harman and Frank Field were faxed by Alastair Campbell and instructed not to give any media interviews because of growing rumours of a split between them over welfare policies. Campbell also chastised Harman and asked her for an 'explanation why the interviews with the *Guardian*, *Women's Hour* and *World At One* were not cleared through this office' (*Guardian*, 30 March, 1998: 5). In July 1998, when Frank Field, the Minister for Welfare Reform, left the government, following the first reshuffle, there were further clashes. Shortly after his resignation, Field was subjected to an 'assault by the government's increasingly unattractive publicity machine' (Hattersley 1998: 14) which denounced him as an 'impractical, abstract theoretician . . . incapable of running a department or translating ideas into workable policy' (*Observer*, 2 August 1998: 1). Field had become the latest in a succession of Cabinet ministers including Clare Short, Frank Dobson, Chris Smith and the 'psychologically flawed' Gordon Brown, to be systematically and publicly rubbished by the Prime Minister's Press Secretary via the lobby. Field responded by describing the Number 10 press office as 'the cancer at the heart of government' (*Jimmy Young Programme*, BBC Radio 2, 3 July 1998). The occasion was 'one of the bitterest briefing wars of this government' (*Observer*, 2 August 1998: 1). Further 'difficulties' arose in November 1998 when Labour's new General Secretary drafted a code of conduct for members of the NEC which contained a number of restrictive clauses as well as a general ruling that NEC members should 'agree to inform the party press office and to seek their advice before discussing NEC business with the media'. After a brief protest, the 'code' was redesignated as 'guidance' but the requirement for NEC members to consult Millbank before giving interviews to journalists remains (*Guardian*, 18 November 1998: 15).

The 'resignation' of Charlie Whelan in January 1999, amid allegations that he leaked information about Peter Mandelson's loan from Geoffrey Robinson, consolidated this process of centralisation. A key dissenting outpost of spin within the broader new Labour project was silenced. This centralised control of communications at Number 10 has also met opposition from the news media and prompted, in government perceptions, the need for tougher, less congenial attitudes towards journalists and broadcasters.

Dealing with the 'awkward squad': Labour's relationships with journalists

Journalists and broadcasters can respond to the government's news management initiatives in one of two ways. If they accept the government line, they can anticipate being rewarded with minor 'exclusives' and enjoying access to senior politicians for interview and comment. But any journalists who 'sign up for the awkward squad' find their bids for interviews denied, along with their access to 'breaking stories and exclusives' (Gaber 1998: 14). Little wonder some journalists are 'desperate to stay in favour' (MccGwire, 17 October 1997: 11). In short, the government is playing an old-fashioned game of carrots and sticks (Ingham 1998: 9–14), although some commentators believe that 'with new Labour . . . the game is played with an unprecedented degree of nastiness' (Gaber 1998: 14).

Another reason informing some journalists' uncritical coverage of Labour's policies and performance in government is the belief that their proprietor Rupert Murdoch has agreed a pact (albeit perhaps an implicit pact) with Tony Blair. Murdoch is allegedly exacting a demanding price for his newspapers' support for Labour since the 1997 general election: a period characterised by an extraordinary degree of non-decision making in media policy. There has been no legislation to outlaw Murdoch's predatory pricing of *The Times*, for example, nor any legislation to restrict press invasion of privacy, nor any effective regulation of Sky's pole position in the race for supremacy in the digital television market. Some journalists argue that Blair is conceding too much policy ground in return for the editorial quiescence of the Murdoch press. 'We have a Prime Minister', Nick Cohen argues, 'who cannot control his tongue when Rupert Murdoch's posterior passes by' (*New Statesman*, 22 May 1998: 20).

But sticks are more commonplace than carrots in this news management game. In October 1997, Campbell circulated a memo to all Heads of Information in the GICS arguing that 'media handling' (his preferred term for media relations) must become more assertive. 'Decide your headlines', he insisted, 'sell your story and if you disagree with what is being written argue your case. If you need support from here [Downing Street] let me know' (Timmins 1997: 1). For the 'awkward squad' the 'handling' has certainly become rough! Journalists are bullied, publicly harangued and excluded from important but informal government news briefings. Andrew Marr, when editor of the *Independent*, was the subject of a negative briefing by Labour sources. His options were presented starkly: Marr was told 'you are either with us or against us' (MccGwire 1997: 11). Complaints from the Number 10 press office can allegedly halt even the most distinguished journalistic careers. Rosie Boycott's withdrawal of an offer of the political editor's job at the *Daily Express* to Paul Routledge was believed by journalists to be the result of Routledge straying off message by publishing a biography of Gordon Brown which was critical of Tony Blair.

Broadcast journalists, especially those working at the BBC, are subject to similar pressures to secure their editorial compliance: pressures exemplified by the 'Humphreys problem'. A letter from David Hill, then the Labour Party's Head of Communications, threatened to sever all relations with the *Today* programme after John Humphreys' particularly searching interview with Harriet Harman about proposed cuts to benefits for lone parents. The letter, which was promptly leaked, is remarkable for its overtly threatening style, the use of military metaphors, as well as the belief that it is appropriate for politicians to dictate the style and content of broadcast interviews: interesting too is the assumption that media interviews should 'benefit us'. 'The John Humphreys problem', Hill began, 'has assumed new proportions after this morning's interview with Harriet Harman. In response we have had a council of war and are seriously considering whether, as a party, we will suspend co-operation when you make bids through us for government ministers . . . Frankly none of us feels this can go on . . . We can see no benefit to us. We need to talk as this is now serious' (quoted in the *Guardian*, 13 December 1997: 12). But even spin doctors with Campbell's energy, undoubted competence and bullying mentality cannot police every broadcaster's potentially critical indiscretion: consequently some journalists suggest the 'object of the [news management] exercise is to implant a self censor in every BBC brain' (*Guardian*, 9 February 1998: 8).

Labour and the GICS: 'hell bent on radical change'

In government, Labour has access to the resources and services of the GICS which is staffed by approximately 1000 career civil servants whose press and public relations activities are governed by a code of conduct (The Whitehall Red Book) designed to guarantee their political impartiality and independence from any government trying to use them as propagandists for government policy. For the GICS, the traditional civil service value of neutrality is at a premium. 'Press officers', according to the Red Book, must 'establish a position with the media whereby it is understood that they stand apart from the party political battle, but are there to assist the media to understand the policies of the government of the day' (Cabinet Office 1997: para 11).

One consequence of 'assisting the media' in this way, by presenting 'the government's policies in their best light', is that 'some advantage naturally accrues to the party in power': this is 'entirely proper' (Select Committee 1998: xv). For the civil service press officer, however, it is never appropriate to 'justify or defend those policies in Party political terms, to use political slogans, expressly to advocate policies as those of a particular political Party or directly attack (although it may be necessary to respond to in specific terms) policies and opinions of opposition Parties and groups' (Select Committee 1998a: xv). By contrast, 'special advisors' such as the Prime Minister's Press Secretary Alastair Campbell, 'are not bound by the usual requirements that civil servants should be able to assist governments of "whatever complexion" and that they should be "impartial"' (Select Committee 1998a: xv). The Select Committee on Public Administration, investigating concerns that the Labour government might be using the GICS in ways which offend these demarcations between 'civil servants' who provide 'information' and 'special advisors' who are employed as 'propagandists', concluded that there 'is a very fine line between the promotion and defence of government policy and the promotion and defence of the ruling party's policies'; the Committee further agreed that the policing of that line was a matter for the Prime Minister's Press Secretary's 'own judgement' (Select Committee 1998a: xv). Since 1997, however, civil servants have expressed growing concerns that this 'line' is too frequently crossed: the 'judgement' of the Prime Minister's Press Secretary too frequently exercised injudiciously. Senior information officers have warned about the 'creeping politicisation of the GICS' (Select Committee 1998a: 80). The former Head of Information at the Northern Ireland Office (NIO) has described the process as one in which the Labour Government seems 'hell bent on radical change' (Select Committee 1998a: 85). The government's response has been to argue that it wishes merely to 'modernise' the GICS to ensure 'it is equipped to meet the demands of a fast changing media world' (Mountfield: para 2). A number of developments have given rise to civil service concerns.

First, the new government has appointed an unprecedented number of special advisors to promote government policy. Political correspondent Andrew Rawnsley wrote about 'an influx of Labour Apparatchiks into posts traditionally occupied by career civil servants' (*Observer*, 1 June 1997). The dramatic use of language is appropriate rather than hyperbole. The thirty-two advisors employed by John Major's administration promptly swelled to sixty posts within the first six months of the Labour government at an additional cost of £600,000 (a 44 per cent increase over Conservative expenditure) (Franklin 1998: 11). A pay award to special advisors in December 1998, moreover, raised Campbell's salary to £91,014 per annum: more than a senior cabinet minister's; the total wages bill for the seventy current advisors is £3.5 million (*Guardian*, 17 November 1998: 5). This is a substantial sum, paid from the public purse, to underwrite partisan propaganda emanating from government departments.

Second, there has been a remarkable turnover in senior staff at the GICS. In the year since May 1997, twenty-five heads of information and their deputies, from a total of forty-four such senior posts, have resigned or been replaced: the Select Committee on the GICS confirmed this was 'an unusual turnover' (Select Committee 1998: xviii). The reasons for these staff changes ranged from 'a lack of personal chemistry' between information officer and minister to a relationship which was 'unsustainably poor', but also included 'the desire of ministers for information officers to be less neutral than they thought was compatible with their regular civil service terms of employment' (Select Committee 1998a: xviii). Andy Woods, retired head of information at the

Northern Ireland Office argues that there has been a 'culling' of heads of information and their replacement 'in key positions of professional civil servants by "politically acceptable" temporary bureaucrats', a process he labels the 'Washingtonisation' of the civil service (Select Committee 1998a: 86).

Third, the proliferation of special advisors is creating a 'two tier structure of information' in which the advisors have become the dominant partners over civil servants (Select Committee 1998a: ix). Advisors are chosen by ministers and typically have worked closely with them over a number of years: they are trusted and close allies. By comparison the heads of information are part of the inheritance of government and judged to be rule governed, uncommitted and insufficiently motivated. Predictably, the significant communications priorities are allocated to the advisor leaving the civil service press officer with less consequent day-to-day matters. Jill Rutter, who resigned as head of information at the Treasury, complained that Charlie Whelan had 'taken over three quarters of her job' (*Daily Telegraph*, 6 December 1997: 3).

Finally but undoubtedly the most significant change at the GICS has been the need to 'get on message', i.e. to propagandise for the government. The pressure for change has been quite overt. Campbell's memo to heads of information confirmed that the central ambition for GICS publicity is that the 'government's four key messages' must be 'built in to all areas of our activity'. Labour is 'a modernising government', a government 'for all the people', which is 'delivering on its promises' with 'mainstream policies' which are providing new directions for Britain (*Financial Times*, 9 October 1997: 1). The determination to incorporate these 'themes' into all communications activity requires press officers to be considerably more assertive in their relations with journalists and broadcasters. Some GICS officers have been unwilling to comply with what they considered to be nothing less than an ethical breach of their professional values; some preferred to 'retire'. Liz Drummond claimed that during her long career in the GIS she had been:

> schooled to a style of information and explanation; the ethos was 'facts are sacred, comment is free' and many press officers have privately expressed their uneasiness at being expected to switch to a more aggressive approach where seizing the agenda and occupying the front pages is apparently more important than the content, where events and announcements are relentlessly pushed rather than being left to find their own level according to their news value, and where those media outlets or individuals which did not adhere to the 'on-message' approach are penalised by intimidatory tactics and the threatened withdrawal of access and facilities. In such a climate presentation comes perilously close to propaganda and it is disappointing to lovers of free speech and a free press that so many parts of the media appear to have embraced the new style almost without criticism.
>
> (Select Committee 1998: 81–82)

These changes to the working protocols of the GICS prompted growing misgivings among parliamentarians, journalists and government press officers resulting in an inquiry into the Government Information and Communications Service in March 1998. The terms of reference for the inquiry were quite remarkable by conceding at the outset what the committee was set up to establish: namely whether or not the GICS is impartial. Consequently, the terms of reference suggested the Committee should try to establish not if the GICS *is* impartial, but 'the extent to which the GICS *should be* politically impartial' and the 'balance between delivering neutral information and giving a political spin' (Select Committee on Public Administration Press Release, 30 March 1998b, emphasis added). Given this starting point, the committee's conclusions were unlikely to be critical of government press operations, but the eventual outcome of the report's inquiries was unpredictably acrimonious.

An early critical report drafted by the clerk was modified radically by the committee's in-built majority of Labour members. The official report which was eventually published contained none of the original criticisms of Alastair Campbell and the Government Information and Communications Services nor the many proposals for reform. In the words of one committee member, the report 'could have been written by Alastair himself . . . on one side of A4 saying everything in the garden is rosy' (*Guardian*, 5 August 1998: 1). The combined opposition members of the committee (Conservative and Liberal Democrat members) denounced the redrafted report as 'whitewash' and its supporters as 'the glove puppets of Alastair Campbell' (*Guardian*, 7 August 1998: 4). The opposition members also decided on the very unusual strategy of publishing an alternative report which reinstated the original criticisms of, and recommendations for, the government information machine of which four are significant. First, tapes of lobby briefings should be 'routinely kept for 12 months' (xxxii) to check if Campbell has been misleading journalists. Second, those advisors who 'undertake significant amounts of party political activity should be paid from party funds and not the taxpayer'. Third, the government should 'consider whether the Strategic Communications Unit' gives an undue advantage to the governing party' and, finally, that the House 'examine the concerns expressed by Madam Speaker on the sharp growth in "pre-briefing"' [i.e. 'leaking' or 'trailing'] of government policy statements to the press which undermines the authority of Parliament (Select Committee Report 1998a: xxxii–xxxiii). The major recommendation in the official report was the suggestion for a new code of conduct to define more clearly the government's relationships with the media. The code, to be drawn up and policed by Alastair Campbell, 'would make clear the obligations on special advisors and ministers to work closely with press officers in general and the Prime Minister's official spokesperson in particular' (Select Committee 1998a: xx). It seems nothing less than extraordinary, that the principal recommendation of a Select Committee inquiry into the politicising of the government information services should propose the further centralising of government communications under the control of the Prime Minister's Press Secretary, especially when that recommendation enjoys the support of only the government members of the committee. In this context, the description of the official report as 'whitewash' seems unexceptionable.

Soft-soaping the public about policy?

The media have enjoyed a growing significance in the processes of policy making and implementation since the election of the Labour government in 1997. The period has witnessed a resurgence in government advertising with budgets matching and, in some departments, superseding the peaks of Conservative expenditure in 1988–89, even though the public sector has subsequently contracted. This government commitment to the promotion of policy has triggered a notable flurry of newspaper, radio and television advertising, accompanied by billboard campaigns, the publication of leaflets and glossy booklets explaining policy developments and the promotion of policy via the new medium of the Internet. Government promotion of policy has also involved persuading scriptwriters and producers to include key policy themes into the storylines of mainstream television programming, especially the popular, high audience, soap operas. The campaign to promote the National Year of Reading is typical of the government's extensive commitment to 'integrated' campaigning to promote its policy ambitions.

The government's use of advertising has been buttressed by a renewed commitment to news management. New Labour is attempting to control and manage information flows about government activities and intentions, in order to define and frame policy debates, to a quite remarkable degree. It has developed new institutions and processes for news management to guarantee this 'packaging of policy'. It has centralised communications at Number 10 and imposed a severe communications discipline on members of the government, the Parliamentary Labour Party and its National Executive Committee. It has threatened journalists, briefed against them and publicly admonished them for interrogating ministers. The government has also expanded the numbers of partisan advisors to assist in the communications task of policy promotion. Labour rejects any suggestion that it is 'politicising' the government information service: governments and press secretaries always have. Labour prefers to couch its ambitions in the language of 'modernising' the service and achieving a 'closer integration of policy and its communication' (Mountfield 1997: 2).

But there is an obvious contradiction between Labour's rhetoric about being a listening and consultative 'people's government' legislating for the 'people's priorities' (Campbell's new and populist name for the Queen's traditional 'gracious speech' which opens every parliamentary session) and the reality of a government committed to the rigorous management and centralised control of information about policy. This tension is partly resolved by Labour's evident enthusiasm for recasting the relationship between government, media and citizens in significant ways. Labour's obsession with controlling the media seems to reflect a concern to use newspapers, radio and television to address voters directly while bypassing parliament, the traditional, but increasingly defunct, forum for debates and the close scrutiny of government policy. In this newly reconstructed relationship and 'in a new media age, new forms of dialogue must be created. Focus groups and market research are an essential part of this dialogue. So too are interactive party broadcasts and "Town Hall" meetings at which politicians can be questioned and held to account' (Gould 1998: 297–298). Labour, according to Mandelson, wishes to consult citizens about their policy preferences via 'plebiscites, focus groups, lobbies, citizen movements and the Internet'. It no longer seems necessary to debate policy in Parliament. What is required is 'a different style of politics' which is more responsive and more closely tuned to public choices and preferences (*Guardian*, 16 March 1998: 8). It is these choices and preferences which should inform policy. But the government's judgement about the independence and autonomy of citizens' policy choices risks appearing naive if not disingenuous. The government's growing enthusiasm for news management and the publicly funded advertising of policy initiatives makes politicians influential in shaping the very choices of citizens which they claim are driving the policy process. Citizens' policy preferences are not constructed in a vacuum but rely on information and opinion provided by the news media which are increasingly subject to news management and spin by the GICS, the COI and the Number 10 press office. It is undoubtedly easier for the government to persuade scriptwriters to endorse the merits of new policy initiatives than it is to win the support of critical, well-informed and organised groups of backbenchers during a Commons debate. While governments prefer to present, debate and promote their policies via the media rather than in Parliament, *EastEnders* will continue to offer soft soap as well as soap opera to its 20 plus million viewers three times a week.

References

Anderson, D. (1988) *The Megaphone Solution: Government Attempts to Cure Social Problems With Mass Media Campaigns*, London: Social Affairs Unit.

Baird, R. (1997) 'Keeping an eye on the COI', *Press Gazette*, 19 September, 13.

Bayley, S. (1998) *Labour Camp: The Failure of Style over Substance*, London: B.T. Batsford Ltd.

Benn, T. (1994) *Years of Hope: Diaries, Papers and Letters 1940–1962*, London: Hutchinson.

Blair, T. (1989) 'Privatisation advertising: a report', unpublished report by the then Shadow Spokesperson for Trade and Industry.

Blumler, J.G. (1990) 'The modern publicity process', in M. Ferguson (ed.) *Political Communication: The New Imperatives*, London: Sage.

Cabinet Office (1997) *Guidance on the Working of the Government Information Service*, London: HMSO.

Carroll, R. (1998) 'Producers "bombarded" with political storylines', *Guardian*, 17 September 1998, 4.

Cobb, R. (1989) 'Behind big brother', *PR Week*, 13 February, 14–15.

COI (1998) *COI Annual Report and Accounts*, London: HMSO.

Deacon, D. and Golding, P. (1994) *Taxation and Representation: the Media, Political Communication and the Poll Tax*, London: John Libbey.

DfEE (1998a) *National Year of Reading: How to Get Involved*, London: DfEE.

—— (1998b) *National Year of Reading: Getting Ready*, London: DfEE.

—— (1998) *National Year of Reading Update, Issues 1–8*, January to October 1998 London: DfEE.

Franklin, B. (1994) *Packaging Politics: Political Communications in Britain's Media Democracy*, London: Arnold.

—— (1998a) *Tough on Soundbites, Tough on the Causes of Soundbites: New Labour and News Management*, London: Catalyst.

—— (1998b) *Hard Pressed: National Newspaper Reporting of Social Work and Social Services*, London: Reed Publications.

Gaber, I. (1998) 'A world of dogs and lamp-posts', *New Statesman*, 19 June, 13–14.

Garner, B. and Short, J. (1998) 'Hungry media need fast food: the role of the Central Office of Information', in B. Franklin and D. Murphy (eds) *Making the Local News: Local Journalism In Context*, London: Routledge, 170–182.

Gould, P. (1998) *The Unfinished Revolution: How the Modernisers Saved the Labour Party*, London: Little Brown and Company.

Harrop, M. (1990) 'Political marketing' *Parliamentary Affairs* 43: 277–291.

Hattersley, R. (1998) 'Frank Response', *Guardian*, 3 August 1998, 14.

Hollins, T. (1981) 'The presentation of politics: the place of party publicity, broadcasting and film in British politics 1918–39', unpublished PhD thesis, University of Leeds.

Ingham, B. (1998) *Evidence to the Select Committee on Public Administration, The Government Information and Communications Service*, London: HMSO, HC770, 1–15.

Jones, N. (1995) *Soundbites and Spindoctors*, London: Cassell.

Lepkowska, D. (1998) 'Celebrities booked to improve literacy', *Times Educational Supplement*, 13 March.

MacAskill, E. (1997) 'Cabinet watch', *Red Pepper*, September, 34.

Mandelson, P. (1997) 'Coordinating Government Policy', a speech delivered to the conference 'Modernising the policy process', at Regents Park Hotel, 16 September.

MccGwire, S. (1997) 'A dance to the music of spin', *New Statesman*, 17 October, 11.

McNair, B. (1998) 'Journalism, politics and public relations: an ethical appraisal', in M. Kieran (ed.) *Media Ethics*, London: Routledge, 49–65.

Mountfield, Lord (1997) *Report of the Working Group on the Government Information Service*, London: Cabinet Office, HMSO.

Negrine, R. (1996) *The Communication of Politics*, London: Sage.

Preston, R. (1998) 'Corporate confusion becomes a sin of the past', *Financial Times*, 8 January, 8.

Rees, L. (1992) *Selling Politics*, London: BBC Books.

Scammell, M. (1995) *Designer Politics: How Elections are Won*, London: Macmillan.

Select Committee on Public Administration (1998a) *The Government Information and Communications Service: Report and Proceedings of the Select Committee together with Minutes of Evidence and Appendices*, London: The Stationery Office, HC770.

Select Committee on Public Administration (1998b) Press Notice 'The Government Information Service' 1997/98–20, 30 March 1998.

Straw, E. (1998) *Relative Values*, London: Demos.

Timmins, N. (1996) *The Five Giants: A Biography of the Welfare State*, London: Fontana.

Wildy, T. (1985) 'Propaganda and Social Policy in Britain 1945–51: Publicity for the Social Legislation of the Labour Government', unpublished PhD thesis, University of Leeds.

Wring, D. (1997) 'Political marketing and the Labour Party', unpublished PhD thesis, University of Cambridge.

Chapter 2

Media coverage of social policy

A journalist's perspective

David Brindle

When the playwright Arnold Wesker spent several months at the offices of the *Sunday Times*, gathering background material for his drama *The Journalists*, he decided to produce an account of his observations. The resulting slim volume caused such offence to some of those he observed that its publication was held up for five years. This was his conclusion:

> The journalist knows his world is among the least perfect of all imperfect worlds. Most are raring to get out and write books – the best of them do, frustrated by small canvases and the butterfly life of their hard earned thoughts and words.
>
> (Wesker 1977: 103)

Wesker was not, suffice to say, overly impressed by what he found. Indeed, his book conveys a sense of bemusement that grown men (as national newspaper journalists in the main then were) could want to subject themselves to such demeaning work. More than a quarter of a century later, many people outside the media seem still to share that view.

The industry has changed out of all recognition: relatively large numbers of journalists at all levels are women and not a few are black; and technological advance, long delayed while the trade unions remained strong, has transformed the job. Yet the popular image of journalism appears often to remain that of the unscrupulous, dog-eat-dog press of 1920s Chicago, immortalised on stage and screen in *The Front Page*. There is undoubtedly a fear of the media, but above all there is a lack of understanding. And nowhere is that lack more evident than in the world of social policy.

No tablets of stone

Probably the single most common misconception about what I do is that I do it to edict, or that it is at least pre-determined according to policy positions and protocols. One assumption is that my editor decrees which stories are to be covered, how they should be treated and what editorial line is to be taken.

Alternatively, because of the *Guardian*'s liberal image, other people assume such matters are thrashed out in policy discussions involving me and other colleagues. Either way, there is a widespread belief that I approach the working week with a shopping list of news and feature issues to be written about, and with detailed briefing on the angle to take on each. The reality is that papers are much more chaotic operations than their readers ever imagine. While it would be wrong to say there is no top-down editorial diktat, the great bulk of day-to-day decisions about coverage are taken by individual writers or desk editors without reference to colleagues, let alone the editor.

There are two circumstances in which the editor will insist on something being reported. One is when the paper is running a campaign on a particular issue, as with the *Independent*'s focus in the mid-1990s on the emerging pattern of abuse of children and young people in residential care over the previous thirty years. To sustain the momentum of such a campaign, developments which ordinarily might not meet the criteria for publication will be carried in what is, in effect, reserved editorial space. The other circumstance is what is known as an 'editor's must', a term laden with significance and with implied adverse consequences should expectations not be fulfilled. As the words suggest, they refer to a story that must be carried, no matter what. This can range from a pet hobbyhorse to something the editor half heard on the radio that morning. For many years, one national paper would regularly carry reports of the most obscure issues to do with sailing on the River Crouch in Essex. More common is an elliptical reference by the editor, of a deputy, to an 'interesting' issue. This will be taken by their lieutenants as a clear instruction to ensure the said issue is covered fully in the next edition.

By and large, though, journalists take on-the-run decisions about what to cover, and what not, on the basis not of any written or even verbal orders or guidelines but according to an almost intuitive sense of what is important and what fits the bill for the paper in question. For the *Guardian*, with its particular constituency, this means a greater-than-average interest (though not as great as people often think) in social policy issues. For the *Daily Mail*, with its well-known stance on 'traditional' family values, this means a bigger appetite for stories about marriage, divorce and abortion.

How it works

This is not to say that the process of putting together a paper – or, for that matter, a TV or radio programme – is without structure. On a national paper, the day begins with an editorial conference at which desk editors representing the various departments of news and features review that morning's product, assess the efforts of the competition and, usually, pat themselves on the back for a job well done. The conference then turns to the next day's issue, with each department – essentially home news, foreign, features, city and sport – outlining the events and issues they plan to cover. At this stage, the listing may simply be, 'Home Office press conference on crime figures', or it may be a more detailed, 'Crime up: Home Secretary to announce new measures'. (With the modern trend of pre-briefing, rare indeed is the announcement not already trailed in the press by government spin doctors.) And listing at this point does not necessarily mean that the proposed article will end up in print.

News and features lists change as the day goes on and plans can be torn up and rewritten well into the evening. Indeed, when the first editions of the dailies become available after 10 p.m. – there is a swap system among the main titles – good stories in the rivals are picked out, checked for veracity and written up for later editions. What is read in the first version of the paper in Cornwall and Scotland can, therefore, differ considerably from what is read in later versions in London.

Setting the leader line

While the morning meeting is the main planning forum, there are further, though smaller, editorial conferences as the day wears on and the pace of the operation picks up. These include a leader conference at which the senior journalists who write the editorial comments – usually not, contrary to popular belief, the editor – decide which issues to tackle. They may discuss what line to take, although much again is left to the individual's assumptions about the paper's values. Exceptionally, there may be a general debate among the staff about a leader line – on the merits of the Gulf War, for example – but the usual pattern is for the leader writer to discuss the issues with the relevant specialist correspondent.

As with so much else to do with the media, those on the outside, looking in, tend to overestimate the sophistication of what is a fairly crude process. In an analysis of the *Guardian*'s coverage of alleged ritual child abuse in Rochdale in 1990, Meryl Aldridge has remarked upon the fluctuating leader line: here supportive of social services, there critical in a 'very un-*Guardian*-like' way (see Chapter 5). She concludes that the position the paper eventually arrived at, supporting the families involved against social services, may have had a historical basis:

> Yet over Rochdale, after an initial struggle, the paper leapt to the parents' defence, ditching the concerns of its stereotype readership. One possible explanation of this apparent paradox is the newspaper's roots, as the *Manchester Guardian*, in the northwest. As a result, over Rochdale, it reacted more like a local paper than a liberal national broadsheet.
>
> (Aldridge 1994: 99)

The prosaic truth is that the varying leader line through the saga reflected the differing views of two leader writers. The apparent supremacy of one position in such situations results less from informal, intellectual debate, more from practical considerations such as one party going on leave.

Where news comes from

Whereas general reporters are assigned to stories chosen by a news editor, specialists typically propose stories to the news desk. Whether proposals are taken up depends on the individual news editor's view and the number of story ideas already on the newslist. Most days, I will put forward two or three ideas in the expectation of being asked to write one or two, of which one may get into the paper.

I rely heavily, indeed too heavily, for story ideas on institutional sources. That means Whitehall, leading professional associations and, increasingly under the contract culture, voluntary groups. Pressure not to miss a government announcement is an enormous incentive to do the job from your desk, and a corresponding disincentive to take time out to see social policy in practice. People are often surprised, and by implication disappointed, at how little I see on the ground of what I write about in the abstract. It is a failing I readily admit to, though I like to think I witness more practice than do most of my peers.

Other sources of material are the 'trade' press, the specialist weeklies or monthlies, and tip-offs from readers. The Thatcher/Major years, when there was a clampdown on the passing of information by public servants to the media, undoubtedly slowed the flow of tips and certainly that of confidential documents. It was on charges of breach of confidentiality that one of my best sources, nurse Graham Pink, was eventually disciplined by NHS managers in Stockport – though not, thankfully, before his powerful testimony of hospital elderly care had already had a profound impact on public and political opinion.

The Labour government elected in 1997 promised protection for whistleblowers, as in fairness had the Major administration. But experience of the first years of Labour rule suggested that public sector workers were, if anything, even less likely to pass information than they had been under the Conservatives. This obviously had some political basis, in that sources have very often been trade union activists who would at least have been giving Labour the benefit of the doubt, but it also suggested that there was to be no return to the days of brown paper envelopes arriving at newspaper offices by the sackful.

Working as a specialist

As a specialist, my job is to patrol the areas for which I am responsible. I am there to make sure that the paper does not miss stories that appear elsewhere, to produce exclusive stories of our own and to provide interpretation of, and sometimes informed comment on, emerging issues. I also see my role in part as acting as a bridge between the paper and the interest groups, professional and user, on my patch. In this respect, the trick is to be and remain a perfectly balanced bridge, leaning in particular not too far towards the 'client group', for want of a better term. The most heinous crime a specialist can commit is to go native, to become too closely identified with their professional sources. This is not generally a question of corruption, certainly not in social policy, but it can over time become easy to adopt professional perspectives on issues such as resource constraints – i.e. there is never enough – than to question the use of resources already available.

One information source that never dries up, sadly, is the constant stream of people dissatisfied, and very often angry, with the treatment they have received from public services. Indeed, the growth of a more consumerist attitude towards such services, in contrast to the gratitude of the '1945 generation' at having any services at all, seems to be fuelling dissatisfaction. I receive calls and letters every day, almost without fail, from people who feel at their wits' end with social security, the Child Support Agency, the NHS and, most often, social services. The most distressing approaches are those from parents who believe their children have unjustifiably been taken into care. Rarely can such complaints be explored, not least because of social services' reluctance to discuss them on grounds of client confidentiality. But it is difficult to find the time to look into any grievance. Contrary to widespread supposition, specialists in the press are very much one-person shows: there is no research backup and rarely any designated understudy on the general reporting staff. It would be quite possible to spend all the time pursuing readers' problems. In order to do the job, you end up pursuing almost none.

The good story

What makes a good story? It seems to be to the eternal bafflement of social policy professionals that good practice does not win headlines; that journalists are not falling over themselves to report, 'Child saved from abuse' or 'Patient treated successfully'. Social services journalist Anne Fry has it about right, 'A good story – contrary to popular social work belief – is not about some worthy policy development, practice initiative or social services personality. It is about raw emotion, disagreement between professionals and, best of all, culpability' (Franklin and Parton 1991: 66–67).

This came to a head, not for the first time and surely not for the last, in coverage of the early joint reviews of social services departments by the Audit Commission and the Social Services Inspectorate. While many of the first thirty review reports were positive, media attention focused on a handful that were critical, notably those on Sefton, Barking and Dagenham, Sheffield and Coventry. Social services leaders were angered by the imbalance and, at the 1998 social services conference, Rita Stringfellow, chair of the

Local Government Association's social affairs and health committee, publicly criticised the 'unhelpful' language being used by this writer and, indeed, by the newly-appointed chief inspector of social services, Denise Platt. Government ministers sought to blame the media for dwelling on the few negative reports, and ignoring the rest, but the fact was that the Whitehall publicity machine had deliberately played up the negative joint review reports in order to portray the Labour administration as tough on poor social work. If there was a media conspiracy, the politicians were very much party to it.

Culpability is very much top of the media agenda: witness the (usually frustrated) demands for at least one head to roll on publication of every inquiry report into a so-called 'care-in-the-community killing'. But other factors can serve to raise the level of interest in stories. Research for the Department of Health on communication and the risks to public health has identified ten 'media triggers' likely to make a story about a health risk a major one. They are:

1. Questions of blame
2. Alleged secrets and attempted cover-ups
3. Human interest through identifiable heroes, villains, dupes, etc. (as well as victims)
4. Links with existing high-profile issues or personalities
5. Conflict (between experts and/or between experts and the public)
6. Signal value: the story as a portent of further ills ('What next?')
7. Many people exposed to the risk, even if at low levels ('It could be you!')
8. Strong visual impact
9. Sex and/or crime
10. Snowballing of reportage: the fact that something is a major story is often itself a story, and this becomes self-fuelling as media compete for coverage.

Most of these factors can be said to have general application. But in the field of social policy, I would add an eleventh trigger: that the story has development potential, that it can be turned into something more than the sums of its present parts. One of the most hilarious, but at the same time cautionary, accounts of this has been written by sociologist Robert Burgess, now Vice-Chancellor at Leicester University. He had been awarded a research grant to lead a study of children's knowledge of nutrition, as part of the Economic and Social Research Council's Nation's Diet initiative. The first media treatment of this, in a regional daily paper, was fairly accurate. But as the story was picked up, sequentially, by news agencies and other papers, it became increasingly distorted into a shape more to the media's liking. In the end, the *Sun* reported:

> Din-dins prof hunts chip kids. A professor is to share bags of chips with kids for two years – to find out why they prefer junk food to school dinners.

> Sociologist Robert Burgess, dubbed Doctor Din-Dins, will visit schools around the country and follow children on lunchtime trips.
>
> (Haslam and Bryman 1994: 29)

In a similar vein, though mercifully less extreme, much of the media went into overdrive in December 1997 about the threat to the great British doorstep. This was supposedly posed by amendments to the building regulations to make homes wheelchair accessible. 'Hilda Ogden would be tearing out her curlers – they're planning to do away with the great British doorstep,' lamented the *Daily Mail*. The fact that the change would apply only to new properties was played down; that it was part of a bigger package to improve general accessibility and was supported by organisations including the Chartered Institute of Housing, the Royal Institute of British Architects and the Consumers' Association, was scarcely mentioned at all.

The converse of this compulsion to push stories beyond their natural limits is to be found in media coverage of the voluntary sector. Here is a burgeoning, £13 billion-slice of the economy, employing almost 500,000 paid staff and at least 3 million volunteers, delivering a fast-growing wedge of public services. Yet it is as if the media do not want the sector to have grown up.

Coverage remains very much stuck in a 1950s charity time warp of good-cause fundraising, lifeboats, guide dogs and helping sick children. Even on the broadsheet national papers, there is a clear antipathy to stories that treat the leading charities as the big businesses they now are. But stories exposing the 'fat-cat' salaries of charity bosses, earning in excess of £65,000 a year for running multi-million-pound operations, are lapped up.

As a specialist correspondent, the challenge is to survive within this environment, observing the unwritten rules about what is a good story and demonstrating obeisance to some of the (least objectionable) prejudices, while keeping faith with your constituency. The tension implicit in this can be very great. It has been with increasingly heavy heart over recent years that I have approached the task of covering inquiry reports on care-in-the-community homicides. On one hand, it has been clear that the reports have been revealing fewer and fewer insights into the underlying problems and have been contributing to a grossly distorted picture of mental health care. On the other hand, when the rest of the media are carrying the reports in full and gruesome detail, it is simply not an option to argue for no coverage. The compromise is to try to present the issues in as restrained and balanced a way as possible.

This is not to say that, by doing so, you are seeking to protect your professional contacts. Of course it is true that specialists rely on their contacts and cannot afford to risk being cut off by betraying confidence or reporting in an overly hostile manner. But it is impossible to avoid reporting critically, when justified, and experience suggests that most social policy professionals take a mature view of this. Over the past ten years, I could count on the fingers of one hand the number who have reacted so adversely to something I have written that further working relations have been damaged.

Playing the system

One of the lasting impressions of specialising in this field is how poor the social policy world appears to be at shaping the media agenda. If you remain purely reactive, as too many seem to, coverage tends to be framed by the trigger factors: blame, cover-up and so on. 'But you never print the good news!' comes the protest. And it is undeniably true, as discussed above, that you will never find a paper clearing page one for a graphic account of the successful rehabilitation of a young offender. But that is not to say that the promotion of positive images is a lost cause. For all the media bias against social workers, and there undoubtedly is such bias, the profession has in recent years been pleasantly surprised to find itself praised for its counselling and other work in the aftermath of civil disasters. Skilful, proactive handling of the media has even been known to turn near-catastrophe (in every sense) into a veritable public relations triumph, as in the case of the abduction and return of baby Abbie Humphries from the Queen's Medical Centre, Nottingham, in 1994.

So what kind of news and feature ideas am I looking for? The essential answer is anything which offers robust evidence, quantitative or qualitative, of the functioning of both society and the controls upon it. Social welfare agencies are sitting on a wealth of this kind of information, but very rarely do they seek to make use of it. Whitehall has recently woken up to this, beginning quite aggressively to market the social data series held by the Office for National Statistics. One result has been a much higher media profile for the various official surveys and one-off reports based upon them. While it would be absurd to suggest that a voluntary organisation could match the number-crunching of the Government's statistical arm, even the smallest charity is likely to have sound empirical evidence of the social issues it works with. Put into the public domain in the right way and at the right time, for timing is a great deal in successful use of the media, such evidence could be invaluable.

As regards promotion of good practice, the *Guardian* is unique among national papers in having a weekly supplement, *Society*, devoted to social policy in the broadest sense. Yet, with honourable exceptions such as the Joseph Rowntree Foundation, it is remarkable how few organisations seek to have their work highlighted in this way. This may reflect fear of being 'stitched-up' by the press, of being drawn on to territory you do not wish to discuss and of saying things you do not mean to say, but I believe the professional magazines encounter a similar reticence. In stark contrast to the private sector, where even the smallest advance of process is trumpeted abroad, those in the public service seem diffident to a fault.

Problems of client confidentiality

There is, however, understandable caution about publicity when it might involve identifying service clients. This is one of the principal causes of strain between the media and social policy practitioners. Papers, just as much as TV and radio, are these days looking to personalise policy stories. If you approach the news desk with a proposal to cover a research report, the first question will be, 'Are there any case studies?' Very often, availability of a case study will be the difference between the paper carrying a substantial article on a report or survey, and carrying nothing at all.

The problem of client confidentiality is clearly greater in some spheres than others. It is perfectly reasonable that people with mental health problems, for example, may be reluctant to be profiled in the press or interviewed by electronic media. But too many social welfare organisations assume automatically that none of their clients would want to be identified. Too often, no effort is made to find case studies or negotiate conditions by which their anonymity could be preserved. While news and features editors naturally prefer people to be named, and indeed pictured, when push comes to shove there is always room for pseudonyms and pictures in silhouette.

Some of the more media-wise charities have absorbed this lesson to good effect: it would be unthinkable of the NSPCC, for one, to issue a report without having lined up a selection of families and/or workers prepared to talk about their relevant experiences. Even MIND, the mental health charity, is now invariably able to find service-users willing to speak to reporters on one basis or another. Statutory service-providers remain way behind on this, however, and very often refuse even to ask clients about the possibility of co-operating with the media. If they did, they might very well be surprised by the response.

Missing the trick

Unfortunately, it is not just in terms of failure to help personalise issues that many social welfare organisations are missing a media trick. The bulk of my daily postbag goes straight into the wastebin, very often unread beyond the first couple of lines, because it is hopelessly irrelevant to the interests of a national paper. I receive astounding numbers of press releases about openings of day centres and health units, launches of training packs and Web sites, sponsored events and cheque presentations (complete with cheesy photographs), even though there is not a shred of evidence that my paper ever carries such things. Many, depressingly, come from public relations consultants doubtless charging fat fees for their special expertise in accessing the media.

I also receive considerable numbers of press statements written in jargon impenetrable even to me, let alone the general public, or put together in such an unappealing way that you might conclude there was some intent to discourage interest. This is the opening paragraph of a press release on a revolution in training for the 2 million people working in health and social care:

> The two National Training Organisations (NTOs) which are being established for the Personal Social Services and Health Care sectors will work together on key projects and initiatives. The two NTOs, whilst covering distinct areas, also have a range of shared issues and concerns which will benefit from joint working.

This, similarly, is the opening of a press statement on a prestigious international conference of experts on mental illness among older people. It shows all the signs of having been written by a committee.

> Today . . . experts in the care of the elderly discussed the enormous challenges which face both the developed and developing worlds in coping with the serious mental health problems of aging populations. They paid particular attention to the burden of dementia, the illness most devastating to the individual, distressing to the care-giver and demanding of society, which is estimated to affect some 22 million people worldwide.

It is vitally important to put in the first paragraph the main hook to lure journalists who will scan only a few lines. This is the opening of a press release from a leading insurance company:

> XXX have surveyed more than 1,000 customers on the issue of effective eyesight and discovered that nearly nine out of ten of those questioned feel that motorists should have their vision tested more regularly for road safety purposes.

Hardly very surprising, you might think. Nine paragraphs later, at the very end, the company spokesman is quoted, 'In our survey, nearly one in five of our over-50 customers felt they knew someone whose eyesight was poor enough to cause a danger to other road users, yet that person continued to drive.'

Many organisations fail to realise that the chances of getting something into the papers are much improved if the material relates to something of current debate. At the same time, there is a general lack of appreciation that, while papers can and do make last-minute changes to cover an emerging issue, most features are planned a week or two in advance. Almost weekly I am asked on a Monday if I can get something into *Guardian* (*Society*) forty-eight hours later. The short answer is no. The overriding problem I encounter, however, is a simple failure on people's part to read the paper: to look at what is carried, and what is not, and to tailor submissions accordingly. It may seem blindingly obvious, but it very often appears to be beyond even the most pricey public relations agency.

Worrying trends

Anybody reading the press closely for the past few years must have been struck by the changes that have taken place. Certainly any direct comparison of a broadsheet paper with an issue of the same title a decade ago is arresting. There are fewer stories, fewer words to the page and the overall content is a lighter, frothier mix. Pages are dominated by packages of words and pictures: a main article, though typically no longer than 600 words, together with a large photograph and usually a box or panel giving bullet points or a list of related facts (as in, 'Six other unhappy lottery winners' or 'Ten more celebrity alcoholics'). There is a new emphasis on the arts and a seemingly insatiable, if somewhat incestuous, appetite for stories about the media. Above all, there is a concentration on 'lifestyle' and consumer issues.

This trend, which some have called 'dumbing-down', has extended also to television and radio (Franklin 1997). It has made it increasingly difficult to win editorial space and airtime for policy matters, especially if they cannot be presented in terms that the media can easily assimilate. Some issues of considerable importance have gone almost wholly unreported in the media because of this. The Labour government's reforms of the NHS in 1999, for example, have simply been ignored by most papers and electronic media because of their complexity. As most people, and most news desks for that matter, never understood the Conservatives' NHS internal market system, it was argued, it mattered little if Labour's further change – introduction of primary care groups and trusts – therefore went unexplained and unexplored.

This carries all kinds of dangers, however. The lesson of the fiasco of the Child Support Agency in the early 1990s was that when the political process fails, producing unworkable legislation, and the media in turn fail to exercise proper scrutiny, the outcome is disastrous for society. Thus, too, the media excused themselves on grounds of the complexity of the issue. It is all very well devoting double-page feature spreads to searing questions of the day such as, 'Should men wear shorts?', but there are wider responsibilities to bear in mind.

The other important trend in recent coverage of social policy has been the rise of the spin doctor. The 1997 Labour government did not invent the black art, contrary to popular belief, but it certainly put it into practice with enthusiasm and ruthlessness (See Chapter 1). The significance is twofold. First, the rigorous briefing of favoured journalists ahead of a government policy announcement means that the 'line' is firmly established before any detail officially emerges. Should the details then fail to support that line, or suggest another, it is very difficult to swim against the tide. It is doubly difficult for TV journalists who, very often, have been tipped the wink to prepare background filming to support the line being briefed. With that film in the can, they are pretty much locked on to the line. And with TV following the line, it becomes even more unlikely that individual newspaper journalists will be able to argue for anything different. The influence of TV cannot be overestimated: it is not unknown for national papers to turn upside down their take on a story to fall in step with the BBC early evening bulletin.

The second significance of spin doctors is that they dislike specialist correspondents. We know too much. Much the preferred conduit for briefings is the parliamentary lobby, where what is said is not only unattributable, but supposedly never uttered, and where political journalists will generally take at face value what they are told. Ministers can in this way launch crackdown after crackdown, fly policy kite after kite, without ever being challenged too closely on detail, cost, or indeed whether they have already said as much, or something wholly contradictory, some time previously. Since the change of government, the number of opportunities for specialists to quiz ministers at press conferences or other events has fallen sharply. Access to departmental officials has also been curtailed. Again, the trend cannot be a healthy one for proper scrutiny of policy making, for the overall working of checks and balances.

Conclusion

When Arnold Wesker looked back on his stint at the coalface of journalism, he wrote that 'though someone must guard society from charlatans, exploiters and political fraudulence, yet, one wonders, how carefully are those guards chosen for their wise ability to distinguish between honesty and dishonesty. How "pure" can the soul be that trafficks in human blemishes?' (Wesker 1977: 104).

Journalism is a rough trade which attracts a rum mix of characters to practise it. Doing business with journalists, and placing trust in us, must come hard to those from more refined professional backgrounds. Yet the press, TV and radio are, and will remain, essential sounding boards for public services in an era of growing accountability. The world of social policy ignores the media at its peril. And the media, to be sure, will pay a heavy price if it ignores social policy.

References

Aldridge, M. (1994) *Making Social Work News*, London: Routledge.

Bennett, P. (1997) 'Communicating about risks to public health', unpublished research paper, Department of Health.

Franklin, B. (1997) *Newszak and News Media*, London: Arnold.

Franklin, B. and Parton, N. (eds) (1991) *Social Work, the Media and Public Relations*, London: Routledge.

Haslam, C. and Bryman, A. (eds) (1994) *Social Scientists Meet the Media*, London: Routledge.

Wesker, A. (1977) *Journey into Journalism*, London: Writers and Readers Publishing Cooperative.

Chapter 3

Charitable images

The construction of voluntary sector news

David Deacon

Introduction

It is an established social convention that personal acts of charity should be accompanied by a degree of modesty. But while individuals are expected to keep their altruism quiet, organisations thrive on publicity which is the life-blood of charitable and voluntary activity. It is essential for the economic viability of voluntary organisations and one of the key mechanisms by which they gain public credibility and exert political influence. Moreover, the significance of communication issues for the voluntary sector is increasing, for a range of social, political and economic reasons. This chapter explains why this is so and examines an important but neglected issue concerning public communication in this area: the role played by the mainstream news media in publicising different types of charitable and voluntary activity.[1]

The changing role of the voluntary sector

To understand why communication considerations have gained importance for voluntary organisations, it is necessary to appreciate the significant changes that have transformed their social, civic and political roles since the 1970s. This period has witnessed major retrenchments in the role of the state in welfare provision, prompted by spiralling costs of state provision during periods of economic uncertainty, and by a 'crisis in values' in the desirability of state intervention (Deakin 1987: 172). In this context, the voluntary sector has been 'rediscovered' by commentators across the political spectrum and in many different national contexts (Kuhnle and Selle 1992).

In Britain, voluntary provision has been actively encouraged by successive political administrations, albeit with slightly different inflections. In the statutory social welfare system of the 1970s, the rhetoric of community and participation heralded a new age for voluntary organisations. In particular, a new concept of statutory–voluntary partnership arose (Wolfenden 1978). In the 1980s and early 1990s, successive Conservative administrations sought to roll back the frontiers of the state, and the voluntary sector was expected to step into the breach, fortified by corporate and public altruism (Thatcher 1985; Major 1992). Since Labour's election victory in 1997, expectations of the sector remain high, although the rhetoric has shifted away from notions of the displacement of statutory provision, and back towards concepts of partnership (Noble 1997). Drawing on the recommendations of the Deakin Commission on the Future of the Voluntary Sector (Deakin 1996), the Blair government is now seeking to develop a 'compact' with the sector, in which policy makers in both central and local government are being urged to 'think voluntary' (*Guardian*, 18 February 1998).

As expectations of the sector have increased, so there has been a dramatic growth in the range of voluntary activity (although this proliferation should not be seen simply as a response to policy makers' growing demands). The Charity Commission (1998) lists 187,000 charities on its official register for England and Wales, commanding an income of £18.3 billion. In 1996 there were 10,000 new additions to the Commission's register, balanced by an equivalent number of closures and mergers (Charity Commission 1997). These figures underestimate the total range of voluntary activity, since there are many more agencies that conform to what could legitimately be described as voluntary agencies, but which are not registered as charities.[2]

This increased social presence and responsibility has brought considerable pressures and uncertainties for the sector. On a financial level, voluntary provision has altered significantly. First, statutory sector support has changed, most significantly in the emergence of a 'contract culture' where voluntary organisations are required to compete for government contracts to deliver public services (Taylor 1992). Second, government attempts to foster private support (through public, trust and corporate giving) have met with variable success. According to recent research, donations from the public fell by 20 per cent in real terms between 1993 and 1996 and the proportion of individuals donating fell from 81 per cent to 68 per cent for the same period (NCVO 1998). These losses, moreover, have not been offset uniformly by revenue from other sources, such as revenue from the National Lottery, corporate sponsorship, trading income and investment income. Between 1994 and 1997 there was a mere 2 per cent increase in the sector's income, with medium-sized charities recording a fall of 3.4 per cent.

Aside from the financial difficulties triggered by this decline in public giving, concerns have been expressed that it may be symptomatic of a deeper malaise in public attitudes towards the sector. Voluntary organisations and charities have traditionally attracted high levels of public support and approval, but some claim 'donor fatigue' is on the increase and that a generation gap may be opening up. According to NCVO research, younger people are becoming more 'consumerist' about charities than older age groups, and expect more feedback about what is achieved with their donations (Brindle 1998). Furthermore, despite a Home Office minister's recent insistence that 'Young people believe "it's cool to care"' (*Home Office News Release*, 28 January

1998), a study by the Institute of Volunteering Research found that 43 per cent of people aged 18 to 24 acted as volunteers in 1997, compared with 55 per cent in 1991. Additionally, the amount of time they spent volunteering dropped from 2.7 hours to 0.7 hours (Brindle 1998). These findings coincided with a report from Voluntary Service Overseas that revealed a rapid decline in recruits for the first time in 40 years (*Guardian*, 22 February 1998).

Consequently, growing numbers of voluntary organisations are having to compete ever more widely for a shifting and, in some senses, shrinking pool of resources. At the same time they are having to work harder to demonstrate their accountability and credibility to the public (Baird 1996). Added to these financial and social uncertainties are quandaries about the political functions appropriate to voluntary organisations. Although successive Conservative governments between 1979 and 1997 encouraged the growth of charities and voluntary organisations, they were less willing to accept an increase in their political influence (Golding 1992). Nevertheless, a broad consensus emerged within the sector that urged a more active, campaigning role for organisations (see NCVO 1990: Chapter 3).

A situation where voluntary organisations can be both agents of governmental policy as well as advocates of causes is a recipe for uncertainty. Advocacy may place groups in direct conflict with the institutions that support them. Furthermore, it can often take organisations uncomfortably close to the terrain of party politics, which – for groups with charitable status at least – raises a host of serious issues, as there are long-standing regulations prohibiting inappropriate political activities by charities. Despite a recent review and 'relaxation' of these rules (Charity Commission 1995), they remain stringent (Burt 1998).

It remains to be seen how political relations will develop between the voluntary sector and the new Labour administration, but it is highly unlikely that political tensions between statutory and voluntary sectors will evaporate. In June 1998, for example, there was a high profile spat between Clare Short, the Minister for International Development, and several of the major international aid charities over disaster relief in Southern Sudan. In the Minister's view, the high profile humanitarian appeals initiated in response to this crisis had 'muddled the message' about the problem, which she claimed was rooted in political and military instability in the region rather than a lack of resources. Furthermore, she felt overly emotive campaigning deflected attention away from development issues and fostered public pessimism and cynicism (*Independent*, 29 May 1998). In response, one senior representative from the Aid agencies argued that her attack was equivalent to 'blaming 999 crews because we have a lot of accidents' (*Daily Telegraph*, 29 May 1998).

Public communication and the voluntary sector: the growing imperative

Because of these general uncertainties in seeking funds, contributing to political debate and securing public trust, the need for voluntary agencies to communicate effectively with the general public and external agencies has become acute. Consequently, many voluntary and charitable organisations have sought to develop their publicity work, utilising marketing and PR techniques developed in the private sector. A recent survey by the Charities Aid Foundation (CAF) (Pharoah and Welchman 1997), however, found 'a very mixed picture of the extent to which charities are gearing up for the challenge of future public communications' (Pharoah and Welchman 1997: 27). The research identified a core group developing 'consistently more strategic approaches to communication' (ibid.: 28), which tended to be the larger, better resourced organisations. This supports earlier evidence of a concentration of PR and marketing activity at the affluent end of the sector (Fenton *et al.* 1993; Bell 1994; Deacon 1996).

What are the implications of this growing divide in voluntary sector initiated public communication? Some claim the growing slickness and persistence of some charitable marketing has inadvertently fuelled a growth in public apathy and 'donor fatigue' (Eastwood 1998), but there is little evidence to support this argument. For instance, the agencies which are most proactive in marketing terms have substantially increased their revenue from public donations over recent years, whereas it is the so-called 'Cinderella charities' (Rowe and Thorpe 1998) – the middle-income charities which are shown to be less able and inclined to grasp the promotional nettle – that have been hardest hit by the downswing in public giving. Research has also shown that the age group that is allegedly most remote and questioning in fund-raising terms (young people) tends to be least concerned about the growing professionalism of voluntary sector marketing (Gaskin *et al.* 1996: 10–11). This is perhaps not surprising, for if we are witnessing a shift from more static, habitualised patterns of charitable giving to a more 'consumerist' mentality (*NCVO News Release*, 22 January 1998), marketing will inevitably assume greater significance, as it is the structural means by which consumers are hailed by competing public and commercial interests.

One of the main conclusions of the CAF study was that small and medium-sized charities urgently needed 'to review their organisational skills and resources in relation to public communications' (ibid.: 28) to close the widening communication gulf. But given that 'cost' was consistently identified as the greatest inhibiting factor on the development and implementation of a concerted communication strategy, it is difficult to see how smaller organisations can hope to compete if required to subsidise their publicity work entirely on their own.

One possibility for reducing the public communication deficit would be for the smaller organisations to focus on a two-stage communication strategy: developing their public profile by increasing their presence in the mainstream media. Astute news management can often deliver a level of publicity that exceeds the purchasing power of even the most affluent agencies (McNair 1998: 154).

Aside from this obvious cost benefit, media coverage can deliver other significant advantages. Although it may lack the precision of the niche marketing adopted by some sophisticated agencies, its broad range offers opportunities to address 'unconverted' as well as 'converted' audiences. This can help to widen an organisation's communicative reach, and thereby assist in maintaining the diversity and vitality of its donor base. Significantly, the CAF survey noted a consistent failing of voluntary sector marketing was a tendency to target existing donors, rather than to explore new avenues. This exacerbates problems with falling response rates, market saturation and donor fatigue (ibid.: 7).

Media coverage can also confer status on an organisation and its work, and demonstrate its social value and political effectiveness. This is particularly valuable at a time when concerns about accountability in the sector are growing among the public. This 'halo effect' can also extend to governmental and other institutional elites: enhancing their receptivity to timely sponsorship requests, contract applications or grant bids, and increasing an organisation's political presence and leverage. The success of Greenpeace's campaign in 1995 in forcing Shell UK to rescind its decision to sink the Brent Spar oil-storage platform in the North Sea offers a dramatic illustration of the latter point. Initially, Shell thought it had won the political battle having convinced the British government and many senior scientific experts that the sinking would not lead to serious environmental degradation. In the event, it was forced to back down in the face of a growing storm of media and public outrage that can be attributed directly to the astute news-management activities of Greenpeace (Anderson 1997; Bennie 1998).

But media exposure can be a double-edged sword. Voluntary organisations are acutely dependent on public goodwill, and can therefore be damaged seriously by hostile coverage. But this threat actually increases the reasons why agencies should seek to develop their media relations, for effective news management is not just about publicising politically expedient information, but also limiting and deflecting media interest from damaging or threatening issues (Ericson *et al.* 1989). In David Hencke's judgement:

> Voluntary organisations who economise on press departments are courting trouble. At best they are letting their organisation and its work be ignored by the public. At worst they find themselves in grave difficulties if the media learn about serious problems and their work becomes a local or national scandal as a result of bad publicity.
>
> (quoted in Jones 1984)

There are other factors, however, that may dissuade voluntary agencies from courting the mainstream media too assiduously. The broad reach and relatively indiscriminate nature of media publicity can create pressures and difficulties for voluntary organisations, particularly those with more modest resources at their disposal. Smaller and medium-sized voluntary organisations often have to strike a difficult balance between not being ignored and not being overwhelmed, and there is always a risk that a sudden wave of publicity may increase demands for organisations' services that they are unable to meet (Deacon and Golding 1991: 84–86).

Additionally, media publicity loosens organisations' control over the terms of their public representation. On a basic level, this may lead to occasions where journalists misinterpret and misrepresent an organisation and its aims, perhaps by invoking political and social stereotypes that the organisation itself would want to avoid. Disability rights groups, for example, have long complained about the media's tendency to portray people with disabilities as either 'needy victims or total heroes' (Morrison 1997). On a more fundamental level, there is a danger that excessive concerns with publicity may start to distort an organisation's core values: a process described by Blumler (1989) as 'spurious amplification', where 'inflammatory rhetoric and extravagant demands to make stories more arresting, distort . . . what the group stands for' (Blumler 1989: 352).

These broad uncertainties surrounding the benefits and costs of mainstream media coverage are also being accentuated by changes in mainstream media systems. For example, the reappraisal of many of the founding precepts of 'public service' broadcasting in Britain has created worries as to how voluntary groups will fare in any future, diverse and market-led media system (NCVO 1989). More generally, there is the question of how the progressive infiltration of tabloid news values into other media sectors (Franklin 1997; Langer 1997; Bromley 1997) will affect media imaging of voluntary activity. Will journalists' growing predilection for prioritising 'human interest' over 'public interest' accentuate their receptivity to certain arenas of voluntary activity and diminish their interest in others?

These questions about the impact of long-term changes in media structures and values are beyond the remit of this discussion. First, because the processes are still unfolding, and second because there has been surprisingly little concerted investigation into the existing relationship between mainstream media and the voluntary sector. Without a clear idea of current trends in mainstream media representation of the sector, it is difficult to make any systematic appraisal of how things are changing.

The aim of the remainder of this chapter is to try to identify contemporary characteristics of media reporting of voluntary activity, by presenting the findings from research undertaken in the Department of Social Sciences, Loughborough University. The discussion looks in turn at media representations of the sector, the media relations of voluntary organisations and the perceptions of journalists about the value of voluntary agencies as news sources.

The voluntary sector in the news

The analysis of media coverage of voluntary organisations is based on content analysis of all voluntary sector-related news items found in a composite month of local and national broadcast and press coverage:[3] 3554 separate news and current affairs items were coded.

Four key trends emerged from the analysis of voluntary sector news. The first was that, in most news coverage, charity began at home and stayed at home. Ninety-four per cent of the voluntary organisations identified in the coverage were based in Britain, and 89 per cent were reported conducting their work in a domestic context. This parochialism varied, however, across the different media. National television news, for example, gave greatest coverage to agencies operating internationally (a third of all agencies reported), whereas local press coverage focused almost exclusively on domestic activity (94 per cent).

Second, certain key domains of voluntary activity dominated coverage. 'Health and medicine' was by far the most prominent arena of voluntary activity in news coverage, followed by 'children', 'animals' and the 'environment'. But there were also significant variations in the relative prominence of different arenas across media sectors. For example, whereas 'health and medicine' dominated voluntary sector coverage in the tabloids and the local press, it was less conspicuous in broadcast media and the national broadsheets. On the other hand, 'overseas relief and development' attracted significantly higher levels of coverage in broadcast media than in newspapers. What all sectors shared was a tendency to neglect many important areas of voluntary activity. Coverage of groups specifically representing ethnic minorities, for example, amounted to less than 1 per cent of the voluntary agencies that appeared, despite the growing social significance of the so-called 'black voluntary sector' in Britain (Qaiyoom 1992).

Third, voluntary organisations were far more likely to receive coverage for their deeds rather than their thoughts (see Table 1). There was twice as much coverage of the actions of voluntary agencies (tending to people's needs, fund raising, doing 'good works', etc.) than their comments (raising topics, adjudicating upon the views or actions of others, providing information, etc.). When voluntary voices were highlighted as commentators, their most common role was a 'signalling' one: highlighting issues and concern for wider public debate rather than directly engaging in the cut and thrust of political argument.[4] When organisations did enter the fray, they were most frequently reported in an adversarial manner – being more frequently featured criticising third parties than defending them or commenting dispassionately about them. Here again, there were clear variations across news media. The national tabloid

Table 3.1 Reasons for inclusion for voluntary agencies in news reporting

Reasons for inclusion	*All media* %	*National TV news* %	*National radio news* %	*National broad-sheets* %	*National tabloids* %	*Local TV news* %	*Local press* %
'ACTIONS'							
• Seeking resources	36	12	15	10	26	15	51
• Other voluntary actions	30	21	11	33	31	22	30
• Maladministration/ inefficiency	1	0	0.5	1	1	3	1
'COMMENTS'							
• Highlighting issues	12	20	21	21	15	20	6
• Criticising others	9	29	33	15	13	16	4
• Information providing	8	4	11	13	11	14	5
• Defending/ supporting others	2	7	3	2	2	3	1
• Commenting neutrally on others	2	7	4	4	1	5	1
• Responding to criticisms	0.5	1	1	0	0	3	0
(Number of reasons coded)	(6052)	(132)	(222)	(1151)	(851)	(239)	(3450)

Note: Numbers may not total 100 in all cases because of rounding up. Data refer to voluntary sector related coverage in news, features or editorial items only.

press and local press (particularly the latter), focused mainly on fund-raising initiatives and other 'good works'. In contrast, national TV and radio news gave greatest prominence to voluntary agencies as 'signallers' and 'critics'.

Finally, the research found remarkably little negative coverage of voluntary agencies and their work. Table 3.1 shows that issues related to voluntary sector 'maladministration or inefficiency' were hardly ever raised, and that organisations were only very occasionally featured in a defensive mode, responding to the criticism of others. As a related exercise, the study tried to establish some measure of the hostility or support articulated within news reporting. This involved noting the number of voluntary sector news items that included any form of commentary about voluntary organisations or issues. 'Commentary' was interpreted in very general terms: it could be an explicit editorial evaluation made by a journalist in the item, or the reported judgements of an 'accessed voice' (e.g. an acerbic comment from a politician). Furthermore, the comments could either be directed at specific voluntary actors or address issues related to the sector as a whole. Despite this very inclusive definition, instances of manifest commentary were found in only 4 per cent of the items coded. Most of these were addressed towards specific organisations, and the majority were positive in tone.

Collectively these findings suggest a surprisingly indulgent treatment of voluntary agencies in the news, but also a broad lack of interest in reflective debate about their actions, motives, opinions and functions.[5] This contrasts with media presentation of other non-official news sources. In reports of trade unions, for example, reporting critical questions about mandates and motives tend to be articulated prominently, as are broader discussions about the future of the movement in a changing industrial and political climate.

This combination of indulgence and neglect meant that many of the areas of voluntary activity and important policy debates about the sector remained largely hidden from public view. These absences were most apparent in particular media sectors, such as the local and populist media, which offered appreciably more constrained representations of voluntary activity, whether measured by location, arena or type of activity.

Content analysis, however, may be able to identify broad trends in coverage of the voluntary sector but it is not able to account for them. Such analysis, moreover, can only provide limited information about which organisations received coverage (because of the minimal details provided). To gain perspectives on these matters requires considerable assessment of the media strategies of organisations and the perceptions and practices of the journalists involved in the news production process. It is to these areas that this discussion now turns.

Voluntary organisations as news sources

To gain information on the media-related activities of voluntary organisations, a questionnaire was mailed to a random, stratified, cluster sample of 934 national and local voluntary organisations in Britain (see Deacon (1996)). The survey was conducted in 1993 and achieved a final response rate of 70.5 per cent (655 organisations).

The results established a high degree of media contact among respondents: only 13 per cent had not experienced any media contact in the previous two-year period and most were keen to attract more (only two organisations said they received too much media attention). Contact across different media sectors varied in two ways. First, organisations tended to enjoy most contact with the press, followed by radio and finally television. Second, local coverage far exceeded national reporting. Although these patterns are perhaps predictable – news-space is more limited in television than in other media, and in national media compared with local media – it is interesting to note how the publicity efforts of organisations mirrored this distribution of coverage. Whereas 62 per cent of organisations who had received press coverage said that they tended to initiate contact with the press, this proportion fell to 44 per cent among those who had received television exposure.

The survey also asked organisations to identify their motives for seeking media attention which were assigned to one of three broad headings. Use of the media to attract funds, grants and volunteers was categorised as 'resource motives'. Attempts to raise the public profile of an organisation, whether among supporters, the public or other political institutions were categorised as 'profile motives'. 'Issue motives' concerned those occasions when attempts were made to use the media to raise issues for broader public or political discussion. Although there is a degree of overlap between these categories, they are sufficiently distinctive to warrant their comparison. 'Resource motives' are the most inward looking and instrumental of all, being tightly orientated around the material needs of an organisation. 'Profile motives' are still self regarding, but have a certain external orientation, in that they are concerned with establishing the credentials of the organisation in the eyes of others. 'Issue motives' are the most outward looking and 'political' (in the broadest sense of the word), as they represent a conscious intention to use publicity to influence the actions and perceptions of others in ways that do not specifically focus around the organisation itself. Overall, the survey found that although issue, resource and profile motives were regularly cited by a wide range of organisations, profile motives were the most consistently emphasised.

When these general findings were disaggregated, clear structural divisions emerged in the media and publicity activities.[6] The better resourced organisations – as measured by annual budget, availability of paid staff, and range of activity (national rather than local) – reported the most media contact and appeared in more diverse media contexts. This greater presence can undoubtedly be explained in part by their significantly greater investment and professionalism in public communication activities. These organisations were by far the most likely to have designated media officers, to monitor media output, to distribute news releases and to produce other promotional material.

The findings also signalled, however, that this predictable relationship between economic power and media exposure is tempered by other factors. First, the survey assessed the regularity with which the organisation had formal contact with politicians and policy makers in government. It has been suggested that media exposure may be an indication of an organisation's political exclusion from the corridors of power (e.g. Rose 1989: 227), but this survey found that organisations that reported most regular parliamentary and central government contact also indicated the highest levels of media contact. When 'governmental proximity' was controlled, moreover, resourcing factors no longer remained consistent predictors of media contact. For example, organisations with paid staff who had the most regular central government contact were not significantly more likely to have gained media exposure than groups dependent on volunteers who had equivalent contact. In contrast, 'governmental proximity' retained a statistically significant link with media contact, even when the availability of paid employees remained constant.

Second, 'campaign-focused' organisations (as distinct from those principally concerned with 'caring/service/advice', 'self help' and 'other functions')[7] reported most contact across all media sectors and were more likely to have been featured as 'commentators' in hard news coverage. But they were no more professionalised than other organisations in their communication work, spent no more on publicity activities and only shared a broad enthusiasm for media attention. Where they did differ was in the motives they ascribed to their publicity seeking via the media. These proved to be significantly more externally orientated (i.e. 'issue' based). The same principle applied to the better-resourced, professionalised organisations, who also displayed consistently broader communicative agendas than smaller organisations. But multivariate analysis showed that 'organisational resources' and 'campaign-orientation' had independently significant links with media contact.

The fact that media contact cannot be exclusively explained by financial factors highlights the need to attend to another element in the generation of voluntary sector news: the mediating role of news professionals. As Bruck (1992: 142) rightly explains:

> In news analysis, we need to make the analytical separation between the discourses the media produce and the discourses they use as material to build on, to process and deliver. We need to be interested in the structures of transformation.

Let us now consider the role of the mediators.

Newsroom perspectives

To gain insights into journalists' perspectives thirty-eight semi-structured interviews were conducted with purposively selected national and local news professionals.[8] The interviews inquired about their exchange relationships with voluntary organisations, and their perceptions of the newsworthiness and credibility of this disparate range of sources.

Being good at giving news

> There are some charities that really have got no more idea than the man in the moon of how to communicate with the media.
>
> (National TV journalist)

Most journalists said they were having increasing contact with voluntary organisations in their work, but there were clear differences between local and national news professionals in their perception of the inherent newsworthiness of voluntary sector activity. Whilst national journalists paid lip service to the value and integrity of the sector, they saw it as having far less intrinsic news value than many other 'leadership arenas' (Seymour-Ure 1987), such as government, political parties and the trade union movement. In the local media, voluntary activity was more highly valued in its own right, as local 'good citizenry' was seen both as a reliable column filler for a quiet news day, and as a useful means for locating and 'localising' a programme or paper within its target region.

Despite this distinction and the positive comments all journalists made about the social contribution of voluntary organisations, most were highly antagonistic to the idea that voluntary organisations should receive special treatment in news reporting. In their view, it is legitimate to expect voluntary organisations to compete for their attention, by providing stories that recognised the demands and constraints of the news-selection process. Furthermore, many journalists criticised the inability of many voluntary agencies to provide information efficiently and to package it in 'interesting' ways. As one specialist social affairs correspondent complained:

> 'The sector as a whole is very naive in what it thinks the press can do for it, and what it can do for the press . . . Though I do get lots of approaches from smaller charities, they uniformly tend to be along the lines of "Can you give us a write-up for this or that?" Rather than by trying to stimulate our interest by saying "We are doing this and the reason you might be interested is because this reflects a general issue concerning a sector in society". And it's very heartening but very rare that I get an approach from a charity who are offering an idea that is going to work.'

Within this formulation, media prominence is seen as a measure of organisational competence, and if the media ignores organisations, it is because of their failure to respond to predictable market requirements. While not denying this is an important aspect, the suggestion made by several journalists that this is the sole mechanism that determines media presence is somewhat disingenuous, not least because it conveniently obscures the active and significant intervention made by journalists themselves in filtering, reworking and appraising media messages. Journalists do not just passively relay information, they need to translate it into news. Sometimes this simply involves the selective presentation of material that has already been 'pre-mediated' into an acceptable news account by news sources (Ericson *et al.* 1989: 6), at other times it involves actively reworking source material into new forms. Both tasks involve active judgements, and require the invocation of professional values to guide the editorial decision-making.

News values and the voluntary sector

Journalists repeatedly emphasised two important criteria that influenced whether a voluntary agency receives coverage. These were 'topicality' and 'generality'.

'Topicality' was the main criterion to test the value of voluntary sector information in 'hard news' terms (i.e. as 'information people should have to be informed citizens' (Tuchman 1972: 114)). Because the sector was not identified by the national media, in particular, as a significant leadership arena in its own right, it had to conform to news agendas determined by other powerful agencies and events. One consequence of this was that charities or voluntary organisations working in areas that became topical in the news agendas might suddenly find the media very receptive to their views and, indeed, be approached by journalists. Groups working in areas that are absent or marginalised from the mainstream news agenda, however, would find journalists far less receptive.

The second criterion was that of 'generality', reflecting journalists' interest in the broad relevance of a story. This was more of a 'soft news' test (i.e. dealing with 'human foibles and "the texture of human life"' (ibid.)). Although journalists, as mass communicators, can only ever imperfectly know their audience, their work is driven by a concern that they are talking to as wide a number of its constituents as possible, and in meaningful terms. This fixation with the general applicability of news had two implications for the reporting of voluntary activity.

First, it created a clear preference on the part of national journalists for those organisations with strong nationwide support. Second, it created a preference for those organisations that dealt with issues of a general rather than minority interest, and of an unproblematic and non-contentious nature.[9] This explains the predilection for 'cuddly charities' in news reporting (Hunt 1993): organisations that, as one broadsheet journalist put it, provide 'pictures of dogs . . . pictures of donkeys . . . stories about new units in hospitals . . . stories about new ways of helping sick children'. It also helps to account for the conspicuous absence of ethnic minority organisations from mainstream news reporting, particularly in the most popular media (who are most dependent upon achieving mass circulation). As one tabloid journalist candidly admitted,

> If it's something that affects a minority of the population then it is by definition a minority of our readership, and therefore it's, by definition, not going to get in the paper.

These news value-judgements demonstrate that media presence is not solely determined by the ability to deliver information regularly and coherently to news desks. The interviews also revealed, however, another range of judgements that guide news selection in this area. These concern journalists' perceptions of the credibility of different organisations.

Fair comments and half-truths: the hierarchy of voluntary sector credibility

In producing news, journalists seek to report the views and activities of 'authorised knowers' (Ericson *et al.* 1987), individuals or institutions who are seen to have some claim to speak authoritatively on public issues, because of their social, political or economic status. In the case of the voluntary sector, the issue of authoritativeness is less clear cut than it is with other sources. After all, anybody can set up a pressure group or a charity, and make inflated claims for their work.

Journalists made very clear distinctions when assessing the credibility of voluntary agencies, and these judgements had a significant influence on how and whether they were reported. Furthermore, they operated as a powerful filtering mechanism, which led to the automatic exclusion of voluntary agencies that were seen to lack credibility. This helps explain the remarkably uncritical coverage of voluntary groups in media coverage. In most cases a 'critique by exclusion' operated in which organisations deemed to have questionable motives or dubious competence were ignored rather than castigated: their lack of intrinsic news status militating against any sustained media scrutiny.

The issue of credibility also influenced those occasions when voluntary agencies were invited to comment on issues in the news. Journalists often welcomed the partiality of organisations who were prepared to enter the political fray, and make critical interventions on broader matters of public policy. Indeed, several journalists indicated that they increasingly relied upon certain voluntary agencies as a source of controversial comment, particularly in relation to government policy. This would partly explain the greater media prominence of campaign focused organisations, who were most orientated to external debate and therefore most likely to provide the controversial newsbites upon which mainstream media so centrally depend.

Journalists made clear distinctions concerning which organisations' views could be taken on their merits, which required further corroboration or balancing, and which should be completely ignored. On this point, many news professionals drew sharp distinctions between campaign orientated pressure groups and other types of voluntary and charitable agencies, particularly service providers. As one journalist explained, a pressure group 'is not sort of helping people in the way that a charity does . . . [Is not] a worthy cause which would make you think "yes!"' Pressure groups were seen to lack the involvement and support of an identifiable client group, which, in the journalists' eyes, lent authority to the views and opinions of those organisations that had such a base:

> Because of their breadth of experience and because they're in touch all the time with the sort of problem with which they're dealing, that sorts of transcends their particular thrust.
>
> (National TV journalist)

For this reason, campaign orientated groups were considered more useful as 'advocates' rather than 'arbiters' (Deacon and Golding 1994): a source of controversial reaction, rather than informed comment. By contrast, the views of caring and service providing organisations were often given greater credence, because they were seen to be based on practical experience rather than political opinions. By the same token, the greater the range and representativeness of an organisation, the more authority was attributed to its views, because this increased the breadth of interests it could claim to represent. Official links with, and recognition by, government also served to enhance estimations of an organisations' broader credibility.

Conclusion

This chapter has examined why issues related to public communication are gaining in importance for the voluntary sector in Britain. In particular, it has considered whether the mainstream media are accentuating or reducing divisions which may have a significant impact on the future financial viability and political influence of voluntary organisations.

The three-way analysis of media representations, organisations' media publicity strategies and the interventions of news professionals suggests that mainstream coverage tends to contribute to mainstreaming effects within the sector. News reporting offers a decidedly restricted view of voluntarism: marginalising contentious, minority or non-photogenic arenas, presenting organisations in an indulgent but largely anodyne and descriptive context, and engaging in little reflexive debate about the strategic role and needs of the sector. The survey of voluntary organisations' media strategies confirms a strong linkage between media access and economic power, while the interviews with journalists suggest that audience considerations and professional caution tend to encourage journalists to prioritise big charity over little charity, and established voices over emerging voices.

Additionally, the research illustrates how different factors combine to fashion patterns of inclusion and exclusion. The predominant portrayal of voluntary organisations as 'doing good works' in a 'soft news' context, for example, rather than as engaged political actors in a 'hard news' setting, is partly bound up with journalists' uncertainties about the authoritativeness of many voluntary agencies as commentators on public matters, but also reflects the reticence or inability of many voluntary agencies to engage consistently with the media in this potentially more controversial context. Furthermore, the research shows that newsworthiness is not just determined by the efficient distribution of publicity, but also the nature of the messages being produced. Smaller organisations, for example, appeared least able to invest in formal press and publicity work and prosecuted the most instrumental and limited communicative agendas. This combination inhibited their appeal to news professionals, who repeatedly criticised the failure of many voluntary agencies to extrapolate their messages effectively and to stress their broader significance.

This latter point highlights an essential problem for the suggestion that mainstream media coverage can somehow compensate for growing divisions in public communication paid for and initiated by organisations themselves.

Ironically, by seeking to use media publicity for instrumental purposes (fund-raising, volunteer recruitment, etc.), organisations inadvertently prepare the basis for their exclusion.

As a final point, it is important to acknowledge that these are tendencies rather than deterministic trends. The research also shows that strategic actions and effective political networking can compensate for limited financial resources and enable smaller organisations to win considerable media exposure. But there are limits on how far agencies are in control of their own media destiny. Astute media-centred campaigning may gain organisations prominence as 'advocates' of a particular viewpoint or interest group, but it cannot enable them to win status as 'arbiters' in news. This role is conferred by the news professionals and rests on their judgements about the political status and cultural capital of specific organisations. And in this respect, as in many others, the well resourced, the widely known and the well connected enjoy conspicuous and considerable advantages.

Notes

1 This media analysis is based on research funded by the ESRC (grant reference R000233193). In general the discussion draws on continuing collaborative research with Beth Walker, Peter Golding, Wendy Monk and Natalie Fenton in the Department of Social Sciences, Loughborough University.

2 Some estimates calculate a broader definition of voluntarism would increase the total to 350,000 organisations for England and Wales.

3 Sampling began on Monday 26 October 1992 and from that date every eighth day was sampled until 30 May 1993. All national daily and Sunday newspapers for each sample day were analysed, as were all daily and weekly newspapers published and distributed in four selected local regions: Norfolk, South Yorkshire, Hampshire and West Midlands. Thirty-three newspapers were coded in all. For the national broadcast sample, flagship news programmes from terrestrial channels were analysed (BBC1 9 p.m. news, ITN News at Ten, BBC2 Newsnight, C4 News, BBC Radio 4 World at One, BBC Radio 4 6 p.m. News, BBC Radio 1 News 92/3'). The local television sample comprised the main early evening regional BBC and ITV news programmes broadcast in each of the local sample areas, on each of the sample weekdays. An item was treated as 'voluntary sector-related' if it mentioned any organisation that was (1) non-profit making, (2) non-statutory, (3) non-party political, (4) not affiliated to a professional group and (5) had a formalised organisational structure.

4 The 'highlighting issues' category was used where a voluntary actor was featured requesting that 'something must be done' but did not direct criticisms towards, or make demands upon, specific institutions or individuals.

5 Of course, this is not to suggest that there is a complete absence of debate about the strategic role and needs of the sector in media reporting. It is noticeable, however, that what debate there is tends to be concentrated in specific public policy sections in 'up-market' broadsheets, such as the 'Society' section of the *Guardian*.

6 These divisions were even more stark than those exposed in the CAF survey of public communication. This is because the current survey sample included a more diverse range of voluntary organisations whereas the CAF study concentrated solely on charities with a total income of £300,000 or above [ibid.: 9].

7 For example intermediary organisations and grant making trusts.
8 Fifteen worked in the national media in Britain and twenty-three in local and regional media. A diverse range of media professionals was sampled across all media sectors: news editors, general reporters, specialist correspondents, producers and programme researchers.
9 This principle applied to the local media as much as the national media. The local media were concerned to address their local communities in their entirety, rather than particular sections.

References

Anderson, A. (1997) *Media, Culture and the Environment*, London: UCL Press.

Baird, R. (1996) 'Up front: how to decide who benefits', *Guardian*, 7 December, 4.

Bell, E. (1994) 'The medium and the massage', *Observer*, 2 October, 17.

Bennie, L.G. (1998) 'Brent Spar, Atlantic oil and Greenpeace', *Parliamentary Affairs* 51(3): 397–410.

Blumler, J. (1989) 'Pressure groups and the mass media', in E. Barnouw (ed.) *International Encyclopaedia of Communications*, New York: Oxford University Press.

Brindle, D. (1998) 'Rise of the selfish gene', *Guardian* (*Society*), 21 January, 29.

Bromley, M. (1997) 'The "tabloiding" of Britain: "quality" newspapers in the 1990s', in H. Stephenson and M. Bromley (eds) *Sex, Lies and Democracy: The Press and the Public*, London: Longman.

Bruck, P.A. (1992) 'Discursive moments and social movements; the active negotiation of constraints', in J. Nasko and V. Mosco (eds) *Democratic Communications in the Information Age*, Toronto: Garamond Press.

Burt, E. (1998) 'Charities and political activity: time to rethink the rules', *Political Quarterly* 69(1): 23–30.

Charity Commission (1995) *Political Activities and Campaigning by Charities*, London: HMSO.

—— (1997) *Annual Report*, London: HMSO.

—— (1998) *Income of Registered Charities in England and Wales*, http://www.charity-commission.gov.uk/ccfacts.htm#intro.

Deacon, D. (1996) 'The voluntary sector in a changing communications environment: a case study of non-official news sources', *European Journal of Communication* 11(2): 173–197.

Deacon, D. and Golding, P. (1991) 'The voluntary sector in "the information society"', *Voluntas* 2(2): 69–88.

—— (1994) *Taxation and Representation: the Media, Political Communication and the Poll Tax*, London: John Libbey.

Deakin, N. (1987) *The Politics of Welfare*, London: Methuen.

—— (ed.) (1996) *Report of the Commission on the Future of the Voluntary Sector*, London: HMSO.

Eastwood, M. (1998) 'Charities: defining issues', *Guardian* (*Society*), 19.

Ericson, R., Baranek, J.B. and Chan, J.B. (1987) *Visualising Deviance: a Study of News Organisations*, Milton Keynes: Open University Press.

—— (1989) *Negotiating Control: A Study of News Sources*, Milton Keynes: Open University Press.

Fenton, N., Golding, P. and Radley, A. (1993) *Charities, Media and Public Opinion: A*

Research Report, Loughborough: Department of Social Sciences, Loughborough University.

Franklin, B. (1997) *Newszak and News Media*, London: Arnold.

Gaskin, K., Vlaeminke, M. and Fenton, N. (1996) *Young People's Attitudes to the Voluntary Sector: A Report for the Commission on the Future of the Voluntary Sector*, Loughborough: Loughborough University.

Golding, P. (1992) 'Communicating capitalism: resisting and restructuring state ideology – the case of "Thatcherism"', *Media, Culture and Society* 14(4): 503–522.

Hunt, M. (1993) 'Uncuddly charities – out in the cold?', *The Third Sector*, 16 December, 8–9.

Jones, M. (1984), *Voluntary Organisations and the Media: a NCVO Practical Guide*, London: Bedford Square Press/NCVO.

Kuhnle, S. and Selle, P. (1992) 'Governments and voluntary organisations: a relational perspective', in S. Kuhnle and P. Selle *Governments and Voluntary Organisations*, Aldershot: Avebury.

Langer, J. (1997) *Tabloid Television: Popular Journalism and the Other News*, London: Routledge.

McNair, B. (1998) *The Sociology of Journalism*, London: Arnold.

Major, J. (1992) Introductory address, in *Enough of the Rhetoric! An Action Plan for the 1990s*, Tonbridge: CAF.

Morrison, E. (1997) 'Odd jobs: disability programme producer', *Guardian*, 19 February, 23.

NCVO (National Council for Voluntary Organisations) (1989) *Broadcasting and the Voluntary Sector*, London: NCVO.

—— (1990) 'Effectiveness and the Voluntary Sector', *Report of a Working Party Established by NCVO*, London: NCVO.

—— (1998) *UK Voluntary Sector Almanac*, London: NCVO.

Noble, L. (1997) 'Partners 2000: marriage of convenience', *Guardian*, 5 November, 32.

Pharoah, C. and Welchman, R. (1997) *Keeping Posted: Current Approaches to Communication in the Voluntary Sector*, London: Charities Aid Foundation.

Qaiyoom, R. (1992) *From Crisis to Consensus: A Strategic Approach for Local Government and the Black Voluntary Sector*, London: Sia.

Rose, R. (1989) *Politics in England: Change and Persistence*, Basingstoke: Macmillan.

Rowe, M. and Thorpe, V. (1998) 'Cinderella charities feel the pinch', *Independent on Sunday*, 14 June.

Seymour-Ure, C. (1987) 'Leaders', in B. Pimlott and J. Seaton (eds) *The Mass Media in British Politics*, Aldershot: Avebury.

Taylor, M. (1992) 'The changing role of the non-profit sector in Britain: moving towards the market', in B. Gidron, R. Kramer and L. Salamon (eds) *Government and the Third Sector: Emerging Relationships in Welfare States*, San Francisco: Jossey Bass.

Thatcher, M. (1985) 'Facing the new challenge', in C. Ungerson (ed.) *Women and Social Policy*, Basingstoke: Macmillan.

Tuchman, G. (1972) 'Objectivity as strategic ritual', *American Journal of Sociology* 77: 660–679.

Wolfenden Committee (1978) *The Future of Voluntary Organisations*, London: Croom Helm.

Chapter 4

Dying of ignorance?

Journalists, news sources and the media reporting of HIV/AIDS

Kevin Williams

The media are judged to have played a crucial role in determining successive governments' response to AIDS. Berridge (1992) points out that the media have always played a role in the construction and presentation of disease, but AIDS figured prominently in media coverage throughout the 1980s: AIDS was the first 'media disease' (Street 1988). It was widely reported in news broadcasts, newspapers, television documentaries as well as soap operas and people identified television and the press as their most important source of information about the disease. Many people living with HIV and AIDS have testified to the impact of media coverage on their lives. Norman Fowler, Secretary of State for Health during the height of the crisis, has spoken of the 'magnificent' efforts of the media as part of the government's campaign to educate the public about AIDS. For Berridge there is an evident correlation between the media treatment of the disease and the development of AIDS policy (1992: 16). In particular, the media played a 'critical role in generating a growing sense of crisis and in focussing on issues with which the government and their advisors had to deal' (Strong and Berridge 1990: 247). But this assessment has proved contentious. Fox, Day and Klein (1989) argue that the influence of the media on policy makers was minimal. Ministers and civil servants were able to make policy on the basis of rational needs and professional advice in the face of the growing hysteria of the mass media.

This chapter explores two related aspects of the media's role in shaping policy on AIDS – and in helping people to learn about the disease. First, the media response to AIDS is examined; this response was not homogeneous. There were obvious differences between particular media, but even within the press and television it is possible to identify a number of agendas and attitudes. A struggle took place inside media organisations, between editors and reporters and crucially between specialist correspondents and general reporters, about rival ways in which to frame the understanding of the disease. The outcome of this struggle assumed different forms in the various news organisations. Consequently, public understanding and policy makers' perceptions of AIDS were shaped by a range of media accounts of the disease.

A second aspect of the connection between the media and policy concerns the variable relationships enjoyed by news media with their sources of information. The different accounts of AIDS in the media reflected the competition between sources to shape the coverage of issues. Activists and policy makers identify the media as central actors in the political process which no organisation from the central institutions of the State to the smallest campaigning group can ignore. AIDS was a new disease. It came from nowhere. The role of sources was crucial in determining the media's coverage. Karpf (1988) has discussed the power of a small number of medical experts to exert a disproportionate influence over the reporting of health matters. The media's treatment of AIDS to some extent followed the existing pattern of health reporting in that powerful and official sources were dominant. The coverage, however, also provides insights into the conditions, opportunities and situations under which alternative or non-official sources can intervene successfully to shape media accounts and influence the policy process. The complex process of competition between sources to influence the media, what has been described as 'promotional politics', raises questions about the role of the media in the policy process. The media do not report in a vacuum. They do not simply report events, opinions and issues to which policy makers have to respond. They are an integral, ever present and deeply enmeshed part of the policy-formation process.

AIDS and the media – the story

The development of government policy on AIDS has been the subject of a number of studies which identify several distinctive stages through which policy has evolved (see Berridge 1996; Strong and Berridge 1990; Greenway *et al.* 1992; Street 1988, 1993; Fox, Day and Klein 1989; Day and Klein 1989; Weeks 1988; Miller *et al.* 1998; Garfield 1994). The initial phase of the disease in the early 1980s is characterised as one of official neglect. AIDS was seen as an illness[1] confined to marginal groups in society, drug users, haemophiliacs and, above all, gay men. After a period of indifference and resistance to what was happening to people with AIDS, a growing climate of panic culminated in calls for urgent action to counter what was seen as a growing threat to all of society. In 1986 official reaction to AIDS entered into what has been described as a 'period of wartime emergency' (Berridge 1996). The fight against AIDS became a political priority for the government as a consequence of the growing public fears about contagion. This period witnessed the Department of Health (DoH) take the lead in efforts to educate the public about the disease and prevent the spread of the virus. Central to the department's work was an unprecedented public-health education campaign. The state of crisis around AIDS subsided in 1988 when predictions about the spread of the disease in Britain were judged to have been overestimated. Since 1988 the illness has undergone a process of 'normalisation' which has meant it has been treated just like any other illness. Occasional flare-ups have seen the disease come to the fore of health concerns and policy. The 1990s have also been characterised by what Berridge (1996) has described as the 're-gaying' of the disease, with this 're-politicising' of AIDS being the result of the efforts of a number of AIDS groups and organisations.

AIDS arrived in the midst of a huge increase in the attention and resources devoted to the reporting of health and medicine by television and the press. Entwistle and Beaulieu-Hancock (1992) found that health and medical articles in the British press 'had dramatically increased between 1981 and 1990'.[2] Most national newspapers during this period established designated health pages or sections which provided regular features on health and medicine which go beyond the news reporting of these issues. Consequently there was increased editorial space for more detailed discussion of health issues as well as the provision of practical advice. The growth in newspaper attention was matched by the amount of coverage television devoted to health and medicine. British television in the 1980s launched a number of series of a direct educational nature (see Whitehead 1989; Karpf 1988). In recognition of the importance of the media in the provision of health information the *British Medical Journal* since 1978 has carried a regular 'Medicine and the Media' page (Karpf 1988: 2). Increased attention was matched by a growth in the resources devoted to health reporting. In the 1980s every paper had a medical or health reporter or correspondent. As early as 1967 medical reporters had founded the Medical Journalists' Association 'to improve the quality and practice of medical journalism and to improve relationships and understanding between medical journalists and the medical profession' (Miller *et al.* 1998). This relationship was important in understanding how AIDS was reported.

Disease has always been a large part of the output of the mass media on health and medical matters. According to content analyses made of the British press, disease constitutes one in four stories on health-related matters (Entwistle and Beaulieu-Hancock 1992). This reflects the importance attached to the news value of sex and death which have long been staple features of good copy. When AIDS appeared it fitted the bill. But reporting AIDS was also a challenge to the professional competence of health and medical correspondents. Journalists faced the intellectual task of making sense of a completely new disease. They had to do this in the context of increased competition. The provision of information and understanding had to be balanced by the growing pressures to sell newspapers and build audiences for programmes (Franklin 1997).

Reporting AIDS

There is a tendency in discussing the response to AIDS to assume that policy makers acted on or reacted to a particular line from the 'media'. This view of the conformity in the media's approach to the disease is reinforced by analysis which utilises an ideological approach to explain the limitations of media coverage. Simon Watney in his pioneering work on the media and AIDS argues that the media's coverage was substantively structured by institutional homophobia. He identifies the media as being 'locked into an agenda which blocks out any approach to the subject which does not conform in advance to the values and language of a profoundly homophobic culture' (1987: 52). He makes no distinction between the tabloid and quality press nor between 'popular and serious television'. He stresses that the focus in the media reporting of AIDS was as a 'gay plague' with gay men represented as guilty victims. It cannot be denied that Britain's deeply homophobic culture provided the context in which all media had to report AIDS. There were many examples of prejudicial and anti-gay stories in the press and on television, particularly in the early phase of the disease when Watney's study was conducted.[3] But such an analysis neglects other factors which shaped how the media reported AIDS. It fails to account for the variations which were apparent in the reporting of AIDS between and within different media.

Newspaper reporting of AIDS

The range and diversity of the debate over AIDS in the media was more varied than many have assumed (see Miller *et al.* 1998). Distinctions that have been made are usually on the basis of the difference between the tabloid and the broadsheet papers. The former are often characterised as 'gay bashing' or hostile to the government's campaign to warn of the dangers of the disease while the latter are seen as being more socially responsible and supportive of the attempts to educate people about HIV and AIDS. But it was only a section of the tabloid press that adopted an openly hostile position to the government's official campaign and its message that we were all at risk. The *Sun*, the *Daily Mail* and the *Daily Express* promoted a political agenda that committed them editorially to oppose government policy. The Health Education Authority which was responsible for the campaigns was accused of not telling the truth that AIDS was 'overwhelmingly a homosexual disease' (*Sun*, 3 March 1988). While some tabloid newspapers expressed their editorial view on AIDS with some vehemence, it was also a view that could change. The *Sun*, for example, emphasised heterosexual transmission: 'Despite the smirks, AIDS is not a joke. It does not affect only homosexuals. It can be transmitted through normal heterosexual relations with carriers' (10 November 1986). Within the broadsheet press there were also different accounts of AIDS. The *Sunday Telegraph* and the *Sunday Times* were notably critical of the campaign and its message. The *Sunday Telegraph* was more closely associated with the moralism of New Right groups such as Family and Youth Concern and their defence of family values, while the *Sunday Times*, under the editorship of Andrew Neil, was motivated by personal and political agendas to challenge the medical and scientific orthodoxy about heterosexual transmission.

Differences between the editorial line of newspapers were accompanied by differences within newspapers in their coverage. Newspapers' contents comprise a mixture of stories, features, columns, cartoons, letters to the editor as well as editorials. Each of these formats have different conventions or rules regarding their composition and treatment (Bruck 1989 quoted in Miller *et al.* 1998: 55–56). News stories, for example, rely on facts, 'hard news' and authoritative sources and are usually produced within the daily news cycle, while features rely on a longer production time, focus on 'soft news', encourage analysis and draw on a wider range of opinion. The result is that different formats can produce different accounts and interpretations of an issue or an event. The editorial line of a newspaper could be challenged or contradicted within the pages of the same newspaper. The *Daily Express*, for example, carried within a relatively short period articles which emphasised other perspectives than those conforming to its editorial line, including a lengthy feature on the global crisis of heterosexual transmission of AIDS (1 August 1990), an investigation of unsafe sex on Club 18–30 holidays (23 August 1990) and news stories on 'AIDS fear for women' (13 November 1990) and 'Shock rise in AIDS cases' (20 November 1990) (quoted in Miller *et al.* 1998: 59).

The extent to which divergences in accounts exist within newspapers reflects the nature of editorial control. AIDS was covered by general reporters and freelance writers as well as regular medical or health correspondents. Much of the material on health pages is contributed by freelance writers with varying degrees of experience and knowledge. News stories, however, are the realm of the specialist correspondents. Most newspapers employ specialist medical and health reporters, with the exception of some of the tabloid papers and much of the reporting of AIDS was undertaken by them. Tension developed between these correspondents and general news reporters who began to report more and more about AIDS as the illness became a big, front-page story. Health and medical correspondents were appalled at some of the antics of general reporters or national press stringers (see Meldrum 1990). They believed that the general reporters, particularly those on tabloid papers, were responsible for much of the 'shoddy journalism', that is, the gay bashing, victim blaming sensational copy.

The different approaches of these two groups of reporters results from the distinctive ways in which they define their journalistic roles. General reporters adhere to the conventional role of 'getting the story'. For them it is the 'news value' of the story which is important. Central to the culture of journalism is an obsession with the 'story' which pulls away from the need to inform and educate people about issues. This obsession manifests itself in its most pure form at the tabloid end of the market. Health and medical reporting, on the other hand, has always included an element of proselytising about how people should best look after themselves and avoid illness and disease. AIDS appealed to this sense of social responsibility which was reinforced in 1987 when the government defined the AIDS crisis as similar to a wartime emergency. Prior to this campaign, when AIDS was seen as a disease affecting deviant and marginal groups, reporting was often initiated by specialist correspondents who saw it as 'our duty and our responsibility' to cover the disease. This often was in the face of the indifference and hostility of news editors. Many specialist correspondents believed their role was to convince their news organisations of the need to report the disease. In some cases this led some correspondents to play a more active part in the issue of AIDS than the professional ideology of neutrality would anticipate. Thus when Lord Kilbracken was reported by the *Sun* as confirming that 'Normal sex is safe' (17 December 1989) some of the more concerned correspondents, especially those working for newspapers that might be expected to follow the Kilbracken line, sought to identify ways in which they could best counter the message that heterosexual sex was safe. One tabloid correspondent said that her strategy was to 'try and get as many experts on the phone to rubbish it. You can't just sit there rubbishing it yourself, you're a reporter of other people, but you're selective about who you're picking up the phone to get ' (quoted in Miller *et al.* 1998: 151).

Negotiation between reporters and the editorial hierarchy, in particular the news desk, ranged across a number of aspects of the story. There were struggles over the amount of time and space accorded to AIDS news, over who should cover the story, over the political line of the news organisation and the attitudes of the news desk to the issues involved. The outcome of these negotiations differed from news outlet to news outlet – the matter of space in tabloid papers differs from that of quality papers – but they were shaped by a number of common determinants: the personality of the specialist medical and health correspondent, his or her position within the news organisation, the organisation's understanding of its audience and the degree of editorial and proprietorial interest in the story. The *Mirror's* more liberal line, for example, is associated with the newspaper's proprietor, Robert Maxwell's, involvement with the National AIDS Trust. Newspapers, however, which have a strong specialist correspondent – or a strong team of such reporters – attach more importance to health and medical matters and as a result allowed their correspondents more say in determining the coverage of AIDS.

The identification of AIDS with gay men made initial reporting of the story difficult. According to the medical correspondent of one tabloid newspaper, 'as it was nicknamed the gay plague the bosses weren't that interested'. Some correspondents reported that 'too much talk about gay sexual behaviour' did not go down well in their newspaper. One reporter confided her difficulties in getting stories past her news desk because the attitude was 'who cares about gays?' For Andrew Veitch, the *Guardian*'s medical correspondent in the 1980s, the poor performance of much of the press on AIDS was a product of the failure to 'get through to the people who really make the papers – the editors, the sub-editors, the guys who decide what goes in the pages, the guys who write the headlines you hate so much' (Milbank Foundation 1986). This assessment is echoed by many AIDS educators who admit they made a mistake in always talking to and about journalists, neglecting the people who control what actually is printed, the news desk and editors which one described as 'the almost shadowy group we don't get to in the normal course of events' (quoted in Miller and Williams 1993: 137).

It is the job of sub-editors to write the headlines and to cut a journalist's copy so that it fits in the space available in the paper, a process which often generates headlines markedly different from the text beneath them. The reporter's copy can sometimes be changed radically to suit the needs of the paper and match the news desk's perception of the issue. Medical correspondents were often aggrieved at the way in which the news desk chopped, changed and edited their copy. The power of the news desk and subs is greater on tabloid newspapers. The smaller amount of space devoted to news coverage means that the subs tend to be more interventionist in news stories. This intervention was seen as being responsible for much of the more sensational and prurient reporting on AIDS. One reporter working on a gay newspaper believes that 'a lot of the shit was fed in from the subs; from sub editors who got the story and fed in the crap, fed in the gay plague, fed in the hatred, fed in the contempt' (quoted in Miller *et al.* 1998: 158).

With papers such as the *Mail* and the *Express* the tension between the efforts of the medical reporter and the editorial process was accentuated by the political line taken by the newspapers on AIDS. Correspondents on these papers came under considerable pressure, which occasionally obliged them to suspend their professional judgement. In response to a complaint made by a health educator about a story by a medical reporter from one of these newspapers which was described as 'one of the worse pieces of gay bashing and junkie bashing that you can imagine' the reporter claimed 'it was that or my mortgage because the editor . . . said, "I am not having any more of your gay loving, junkie loving pieces. We are going to tell it like it is"' (quoted in Miller *et al.* 1998: 159). Some reporters were able to stand up to their news desk or editors, mostly on broadsheet newspapers where specialist reporters have much more influence.

Television reporting of AIDS

While there was debate in sections of the British press about AIDS and whether it posed a threat to heterosexuals, television news was more uniform and consistent in its reporting (Miller *et al.* 1998). Television news reporting embraced the scientific and medical consensus established between late 1986 and 1990. It supported government policy that AIDS was a threat to everyone and public education was the only means to combat its spread. As ITN's *News at Ten* stated in 1986, 'The experts agree that everyone is at risk and it is vital to find out about AIDS and how to protect ourselves from it' (ITN 2200, 1 December 1986). Television news shared the concerns of the medical and scientific community about the government's initial reluctance to address the disease. Correspondents often endorsed the pressure on government to act. The

BBC's science correspondent, for example, in reporting the establishment of the government's AIDS Committee in 1986, stated that 'since the early 1980s specialists in the disease have been pleading for more to be done to stop it from spreading. Now it seems at last they are being listened to' (BBC1 1800 10, November 1986). All the major television channels supported the government's health education campaign and participated in AIDS Week when it was launched in the Spring of 1987. This ten-day blitz of health education programmes on AIDS represented an unprecedented degree of co-operation between broadcasters and the government in peacetime. The main messages were that the disease posed a threat to everyone and not just gay men and drug users. To prevent the transmission of the virus 'safer sex' was promoted, particularly the use of condoms. The campaign offered no overt moral messages, although 'sticking to one partner' was recommended. Compulsory testing for the virus was rejected. Criticisms of the campaign were reported but tended to centre on the lack of explicitness in dealing with sexual matters which was the major concern of the medical, scientific and health education professions. Other kinds of criticisms were marginalised. Consequently the questioning by some voluntary organisations of the government's information-giving approach was downplayed and, more significantly, there were few reports of opposition to the campaign on moral grounds. Even when spokespersons for this perspective were interviewed their argument was usually set in a critical context.

Elsewhere on television more critical voices were heard. Channel 4 commissioned a number of documentaries and current affairs programmes which challenged policy on both medical and moral grounds. The current affairs series *Dispatches* broadcast two programmes – *The Unheard Voices* (13 November 1987) and *The AIDS Catch* (13 June 1990) – which reported the views which challenged the scientific orthodoxy on how HIV was transmitted. The access series *Diverse Reports* accessed the moral views of the New Right in the programme, 'AIDS is a four letter word' (17 September 1987). There were also voices critical of the liberal medical approach raised in talk programmes (see Miller *et al.* 1998: Chapter 7). Much of the television coverage in the 1980s, however, focused on providing education and information to help people avoid contracting HIV based on the advice of the government and medical establishment. Even soap operas with their commitment to entertainment used story lines about AIDS to educate their viewers.

The presentation and construction of AIDS in the British media was varied, although the early years witnessed a focus in many newspapers on AIDS as a 'gay plague'. But reporting changed over time with particular approaches to AIDS becoming identified with specific sections of the press and certain newspapers. The focus on AIDS as a contagious disease was central to the output of sections of the tabloid press and some quality newspapers in the early 1980s. The climate of fear that developed around AIDS in the mid-1980s can be justifiably associated with this kind of reporting. The media are seen as responsible for creating a panic amongst the public on AIDS which shaped the government's unprecedented response to the disease.

Television, on the other hand, was supportive of the liberal medical approach with its focus on professional responses to combat the spread of the virus through education and minimising the stigmatisation of those with AIDS. In terms of the policy process the liberal medical agenda of television appears to have had more impact than the New Right views of some of the press. As Berridge (1992: 23) points out 'different sections of the media appear to have had a different impact on the policy process'. The role of the media in shaping popular beliefs about AIDS and determining policy must be qualified by the diversity of the reporting of AIDS. This diversity reflected struggles inside newsrooms and the media. But the difference within the media was also the outcome of competition between different sources of information to use the media to shape the policy agenda on AIDS as well as to construct public opinion on the disease.

Sources of AIDS information and the media agenda

Most news is not observed by reporters. Sigal (1973: 69) points out 'news is not what happened but what some one says has happened or will happen'. Thus the source of information plays a vital role in the news production process. What appears in TV news or in the press is the outcome of a process of negotiation between the reporter and his or her source of information. Gans (1979: 80) defines sources 'as actors whom journalists observe or interview, including interviewees who appear on air or who are quoted in articles'. Some academics believe it is the sources who take the lead in the 'dance' between sources and reporters (see Chapter 1). In particular official sources, that is those that represent powerful social institutions, dominate the content of the news media. Alternative sources of information – marginal or resource poor groups – are regarded as disadvantaged. The contours of the media's coverage of AIDS can be seen as the outcome of the struggle for definitional advantage between organisations with distinctive financial, institutional and cultural capital.

Official sources were able to exert considerable influence over media accounts of AIDS. The government, the medical and scientific community figured prominently in the media's attempt to report, understand and explain the new disease. Specialist correspondents, by the nature of their jobs, tend to develop a close relationship with a relatively small number of news sources and become dependent on them (Ericson *et al.* 1987 and 1989). The close ties between the medical and health specialist correspondents and the medical profession were important in explaining that the bulk of the health and medical specialists in the press and on television news followed the 'liberal medical approach' to AIDS, particularly in emphasising the spread of HIV amongst heterosexuals and against the stigmatising of people living with the virus (see Miller *et al.* 1998: Chapters 3 and 4). In this sense they were acting as a conduit for growing concerns within the medical community about the official response to AIDS.[4] General reporters, on the other hand, are less able to build up a list of regular contacts in any particular area and are thus less dependent and more resistant to the views of their sources.

Specialists were critical of general reporters in their reporting of AIDS primarily on the basis that they did not check with the right sources. One health correspondent on a Sunday newspaper sums up the views of many of his colleagues when he describes general reporters as journalists who 'tend to get things wrong because they don't check adequately or they don't talk to the right people'. He believes they 'just talk to dubious characters who have theories that, you know, AIDS came from outer space or something' and 'they don't want to spoil a good story by checking it with somebody who might know better . . . ruin it by discovering it is untrue' (Miller *et al.* 1998: 149).

The close co-operation between television and official sources explains their rejection of the arguments from the New Right and decision to embrace the scientific-medical consensus developed around AIDS in the mid-1980s. The extent to which broadcasters came on board is shown by the co-operation between the BBC, ITV and the government during AIDS Week. Competition between the broadcasters was suspended as common scheduling of AIDS programmes took place and some of the previously accepted conventions concerning the portrayal of sex were ignored. The broadcasters decided to embrace the campaign because it was presented to them as a national health emergency. British broadcasting with its tradition of public service has a history of 'speaking for the nation' at times of crisis and, as Berridge (1992: 23–24) notes, the AIDS emergency of 1987 was defined as a national crisis. It is also the case, however, that the broadcasters welcomed the return to closer co-operation with government after their prolonged buffeting from the Thatcher administration.

Television news was dominated by official voices in the period between 1987 and 1990. In a study of British TV News during this period the most common type of 'AIDS story' concerned the government's AIDS campaign (Miller *et al.* 1998). This constituted the largest group of news stories ranging from items on the latest phase of the advertising campaign to announcements of policy on anonymous testing. The most common group of interviewees were medical and scientific experts. Other experts and professionals were also well represented: nursing staff, lawyers, counsellors and carers. The people who appeared most regularly across the whole range of AIDS stories were government ministers. Nearly 50 per cent of the interviews were conducted with the different Ministers of Health. These were the central figures in the AIDS story on TV news. The regularity of appearance of government ministers indicates the orientation of television news to the rhythms of political life and government activity. Television news reporting of AIDS conforms to the way in which other diseases have been covered. On health matters doctors and scientists have a higher credibility with journalists than other sources of information. Within the official perspective on AIDS there were differences and these were reflected in the television news coverage. It follows that in the coverage of AIDS there were criticisms of the government's campaign but they were limited by the parameters of the official perspective on the disease. Consequently television news reported differences of opinion about the AIDS campaign but the disagreements aired were confined within the boundaries of appropriate and responsible debate: that is the debate between official sources.

The decision of television to embrace the official line on AIDS was important in combating the impact of the 'gay plague' and 'moral agenda' prevalent in certain sections of the British press. One area in which this was important was in reporting about people living with AIDS. Issues such as discrimination, prejudice, ignorance and fear as well as medical and financial problems were reported. In contrast to the press coverage many TV news reports attempted to inform and educate about the situation of people living with HIV or AIDS who featured prominently on TV news (see Miller *et al.* 1998). Spokespersons of organisations for PWA, for example the Terrence Higgins Trust (THT), Britain's biggest AIDS charity, Body Positive and Frontliners were well represented. This coverage did vary. Few of the interviews were with people who were introduced as gay. Interviews with haemophiliacs were much more common; a dramatic reversal of the actual proportion of gay men and haemophiliacs with HIV or AIDS. Interviews with the children, wives, families and friends of people with AIDS were also broadcast. In a three-and-a-half-years study of television news, however, there were no interviews with partners or lovers of gay men nor any members of their families (Miller *et al.* 1998). Domestic settings were used in this period only for heterosexuals. Television news also made distinctions between 'guilty' and 'innocent' victims. This surfaced explicitly in the coverage of HIV-positive haemophiliacs. One ITN headline referred to this group as the 'innocent victims of AIDS' (ITN 1745, 12 October 1987). Meanwhile the BBC reported on the 'plea from people who got the AIDS virus by accident'. The newsreader explained that haemophiliacs face the threat of AIDS 'through no fault of their own' (BBC 1 1800, 12 October 1987). Such reporting implied that gay men and drug users were to blame if they contracted the virus. Pressure from groups such as the Terrence Higgins Trust (THT), however, made such judgemental reporting less common. In fact, the labelling of innocent and guilty victims was taken up as a news story.

The closeness of co-operation between the broadcasting institutions and the government over AIDS had consequences at a later stage. Some broadcasters were uncomfortable at the degree to which they co-operated with the government. Regrets were expressed by some ITV executives who believed they were compromised by 'trying to sell a point of view' during AIDS Week (quoted in Miller *et al.* 1998: 95). Such feelings led some broadcasters to respond by commissioning programmes that were critical of the science of AIDS. It was in this context that programmes such as those in the *Dispatches* series which challenged the medical orthodoxy over the transmission of HIV were aired. These critical voices, however, were the exception rather than the rule.

The ability of official sources to exert influence over how medical correspondents and television reported and represented AIDS, reflected their success in the competition for definitional advantage between sources of information: this is an unequal struggle in which organisations rich in financial, institutional and cultural resources prevail. Bodies such as the Department of Health, the Health Education Authority, the British Medical Association and the scientific community have more money, human resources and credibility with the media to promote their message. Smaller organisations such as the Terrence Higgins Trust and the Conservative Family Campaign lack financial and institutional resources and are obliged to work much harder to achieve a reputation for the provision of reliable, regular and credible information. The struggle around the provision of AIDS information to the British public, however, illustrates the practical problems that influence the ability of official and non-official sources to shape media accounts of the disease.

The failure of an official source

The Health Education Authority (HEA) was responsible for running the government's AIDS campaign when it was established in 1987. The body placed great emphasis on using the mass media as part of its education efforts. The HEA recognised the importance of targeting specific media outlets, editors and reporters to create a positive climate to support its advertising campaign. This was spelt out in the 'Total public communication strategy' drawn up for the HEA by the advertising agency Boase, Massimi, Pollit (BMP). A proactive public relations campaign was envisaged which sought to 'brand' the HEA the 'most useful source of AIDS information'. The implementation of this strategy, however, was influenced by several factors, including health educators' distrust of the mass media, the HEA's relationship with the Department of Health (DoH) and the low status of health education in the eyes of the mass media.

Health educators have always had a certain reluctance in their dealings with journalists. They have regarded the media as 'untrustworthy' and 'sources of conflict and misinformation' (Holmes 1985: 18). The press and public affairs officers at the HEA found it difficult to get health educators to talk to journalists. Many health educators saw journalists as 'always pestering us and finding things out and blowing them up . . .' (quoted in Miller and Williams 1993: 128). As a result there was a resistance from HEA staff to the efforts of the public affairs division to educate them on the need to be open and accessible to journalists. The reticence of many HEA staff influenced journalists' perceptions of the HEA's usefulness as a source of AIDS information. The ability to get information from the HEA was also hampered by the complex bureaucracy developed in the organisation. This had the effect of drawing out the decision making procedures so that the simplest piece of information could take a very long time to emerge. This was a reflection of the environment in which the HEA had to operate with government caution over the campaign. But the effect for the media was that it could 'take a long time to get the simplest piece of information . . . a long time to get hold of people . . . to have the HEA view put across' (HEA public affairs official quoted in Miller *et al.* 1998: 141). The problem was compounded by the low status of health education as a profession. Health educators are near the bottom of the journalists' 'hierarchy of credibility'. Doctors and scientists have much greater authority and therefore credibility for journalists. In spite of the particular problems the news media face in sorting out the disputes or uncertainties around HIV/AIDS, health educators have difficulty in being included in news accounts.

Another factor influencing the HEA press and PR strategy was its relationship with the Department of Health. The department did not look favourably on the HEA trying to establish itself as the 'most useful source' of AIDS information and got 'shirty' at what it saw as efforts to encroach on its functions. These concerns were formalised in a Memorandum of Understanding drawn up between the Department of Health and the HEA in 1990. While accepting that the HEA has a right to give advice in public and private where appropriate, the document circumscribes the conditions under which public statements can be made. Press releases had to be checked by administrative civil servants and clearance was often delayed. Quite often a 'terribly straightforward and anodyne press release' would 'disappear down a black hole in the Department of Health'. Sometimes, 'press releases didn't get out at all'. Such delays discouraged the issuing of statements by the HEA press office. The pithy quote wanted by journalists to bolster a good story was not always forthcoming. The lack of quotable material and the restrictions placed on the HEA made it difficult for the organisation to establish effective relations with journalists who despaired of what they saw as the authority's 'fence sitting'.

The success of an alternative source

The Terrence Higgins Trust was formed in 1983 to provide information on HIV/AIDS. By the late 1980s the Trust had established itself as the leading AIDS voluntary agency and had established itself as a credible source of AIDS information regularly consulted by journalists. No other voluntary organisation was as widely quoted and widely used as a resource – even *EastEnders* relied on the trust in the development of their story lines which featured AIDS (see Miller *et al.* 1998: 113). Analysis of press coverage of AIDS between April and July 1993 found that 'The Terrence Higgins Trust is easily the most visible organisation amongst [those] we looked at' (McKeone 1993: 4). The ability of the trust to overcome its lack of authoritativeness was due in part to the quality of information it provided. But it can also be explained by the media friendly approach and the strategies used to manage the media. Its main spokesperson was particularly successful in conforming to the needs of television. Some people inside the gay community have argued that these efforts compromised the trust message. But by 1988 the success of the trust's information strategy meant that any discussion of HIV and AIDS on television and the radio would not be a typical exchange between a doctor and interviewer but would be a three-way debate in which someone affected by HIV/AIDS would be involved. This helped to change media representation of disease.

The role of the Terrence Higgins Trust in pressing for more open discussions of safer sex played an important part in the broadening of discussion in the media about sex, sexuality and sexual practices. The trust 'managed to do things that had never happened on television or radio before'. This included spokespersons talking about masturbation on *Women's Hour* and fist fucking on BBC1. Since 1987 the ability to talk about sex and sexuality on television and radio has expanded. For another THT spokesperson 'things like Sex Talk would never have been possible without the kinds of things that I did on Open Air, and others have done' (quoted in Miller *et al.* 1998: 143). The success of the trust was not, however, even. It was able to establish its presence far more in television and the quality media where the sense of 'social responsibility' is more developed.

It was also the case that the trust was able to exert more influence during certain periods. It was able to gain most access during the period of 'wartime emergency' in 1987 when there was greater pressure for more open programming and information. There was more opportunity for pressure groups to influence policy in the early years of the disease at a time where policy making was relatively open. Members of the gay community and concerned clinicians were able to access the policy arena as confusion existed over the science of AIDS and what to do about the new disease. There was close relationship between activists, scientists and clinicians and sections of the policy-making community inside government. They all used the media to promote their agendas and positions to affect government policy. The overwhelming aim in the early and mid-1980s was to get the government to act. The routinisation of the disease saw the decline of the access and influence of the trust. As the pressure on the policy community subsided and policy making became more routine – which coincided with a cutback in grants to the trust in 1991 and the closing of the AIDS division of the HEA in 1990 – the involvement and media profile of the trust and other pressure groups diminished.

Media and the policy process – conclusions

The policy formation process around AIDS highlights a number of factors concerning the role of the media in the making of policy. The media played an important role in shaping the development of AIDS policy, especially in establishing a climate of opinion in the mid-1980s which demanded government action. But there were substantial variations in the approach of different sectors of the media to the disease which reflected agendas inside specific media but also the efforts of external news sources intent on shaping the reporting and representation of AIDS. The media were at the centre of the efforts of the policy community around AIDS to promote their agendas and achieve their aims. A particularly significant feature here was the close relationship between activists, including gay organisations, doctors and scientists, and key sections of the media in promoting the need for action and a non-punitive response. This relationship has been described as a 'symbiotic and sometimes tense one' in which the media 'were not always receptive to the advances of the AIDS policy community' (Berridge 1992: 20). The degree of receptivity, however, varied within the media.

Some parts of the media were in more than close harmony with conservative, reactionary and dissenting voices over AIDS. These voices did not prevail – although they did play a part in the policy formation process. The success of the liberal medical approach to the disease was not a triumph of professionalism over irrationality and prejudice. The framing of policy was constantly compromised by the varying abilities of a range of interests to exert pressure at different times, often through the media. The lack of clarity and explicitness, the confused and contradictory messages of the 1987 AIDS education campaign attest to this (see Miller *et al.* 1998: Chapter 2). In the process, government sources of information despite their advantages were not always able to 'set the agenda'. Conversely non-official or 'resource poor' sources exerted more influence in the media than would be expected at certain stages of the development of the disease. Finally – although the case of AIDS might not be typical – it does indicate that the media's relationship with policy makers and their sources of information is more complex than that of two dance partners (Gans 1979). Both partners are closely intertwined and the media are an integral part of the struggle to make policy.

Notes

1 Acquired Immune Deficiency Syndrome (AIDS) is not an illness. It refers to the infections and disease that result from the breakdown of the immune system which can be brought about by the virus, HIV. In this chapter AIDS is used as a shorthand to cover the range of clinical conditions from infection with the virus to the development of the syndrome.
2 Their study of the content of the tabloid and broadsheet newspapers over a two-month period in 1990 recorded a total of 2959 articles from eight newspapers. This showed a marked increased when compared with an earlier content analysis undertaken in 1981 which recorded 1397 articles on health and medical matters from seven newspapers for a similar period.
3 Watney's argument should be read in conjunction with some of his later writing which appears to modify his position on the media representation of AIDS. See S.

Watney (1992) 'Short term companions: AIDS as popular entertainment', in A. Klusacek and K. Morrison (eds) *A Leap in the Dark: AIDS, Art and Contemporary Cultures*. Montreal: Vehicle Press.

4 This is not to say that the reporting of AIDS by specialist correspondents was always 'liberal'. Their close proximity to medical sources reinforced the view of AIDS as a gay disease before 1985. Naylor (1985) has pointed out that the treatment of AIDS as a gay disease at this time was a consequence of reliance on the medical profession which first misidentified AIDS as a gay disease and sought explanations for the aetiology of the disease in the lifestyles and behaviour of homosexual men.

References

Berridge, V. (1992) 'AIDS, the media and health policy', in P. Aggelton, P. Davies and G. Hart (eds) *AIDS: Rights, Risk and Reason*, London: Falmer, 13–27.

—— (1996) *AIDS in the UK: the Making of Policy 1981–94*, Oxford: Oxford University Press.

Christiansen, C. and Harding, C. (1984) 'Mobilization of health behaviour by the British press', *Journalism Quarterly* 61: 364–370.

Day, P. and Klein, R. (1989) 'Interpreting the unexpected: the case of AIDS policy making in Britain', *Journal of Public Policy* 9(3): 337–353.

Entwistle, V. and Beaulieu-Hancock, M. (1992) 'Health and medical coverage in the UK national press', *Public Understanding of Science* 1: 367–382.

Ericson, R., Baranek, P. and Chan, J. (1987) *Visualizing Deviance*, Milton Keynes: Open University Press.

—— (1989) *Negotiating Control: a Study of News Sources*, Milton Keynes: Open University Press.

Fox, D., Day, P. and Klein, R. (1989) 'The power of professionalism: policies for AIDS in Britain, Sweden and the United States', *Daedalus*, Spring, 93–112.

Franklin, B. (1997) *Newszak and News Media*, London: Arnold.

Garfield, S. (1994) *The End of Innocence: Britain in the Time of AIDS*, London: Faber & Faber.

Gans, H. (1979) *Deciding What's News: a Study of CBS Evening News, NBC Nightly News, Newsweek* and *Time*, New York: Vintage.

Greenway, J., Smith, S. and Street, J. (eds) (1992) *Deciding Factors in British Politics*, London: Routledge.

Holmes, P. (1985) 'How health hit the headlines', *Nursing Times*, 10 April, 18–19.

Karpf, A. (1988) *Doctoring the Media*, London: Routledge.

McKeone, D. (1993) *Impact: Impact Media Analysis Trend Report for the Health Education Authority (AIDS and HIV Coverage) April 1993–July 1993*, London: Infopress.

Meldrum, J. (1990) 'The role of the media in reporting AIDS', in B. Almond (ed.) *AIDS – A Moral Issue: the Ethical, Legal and Social Aspects*, Basingstoke: Macmillan.

Milbank Foundation (1986) *AIDS: Impact on Public Policy: Proceedings of a Conference 28–30 May*, New York: New York State Department of Public Health and Milbank Foundation.

Miller, D., Kitzinger, J., Williams, K. and Beharrell, P. (1998) *The Circuit of Mass Communication*, London: Sage.

Miller, D. and Williams, K. (1993) 'Negotiating HIV/AIDS Information: Agendas, Media Strategies and the News', in J. Eldridge (ed.) *Getting the Message: News, Truth and Power*, London: Routledge.

Naylor, W. (1985) 'Walking time bombs: AIDS and the press', *Medicine in Society* 2(3): 5–11.

Sigal, L. (1973) *Reporters and Officials*, Lexington: D.C. Heath.

Street, J. (1988) 'British government policy on AIDS: learning not to die of ignorance', *Parliamentary Affairs* 41(4): 490–507.

—— (1993) 'A fall in interest? British AIDS policy', in V. Berridge and P. Strong (eds) *AIDS and Contemporary History*, Cambridge: Cambridge University Press.

Strong, P. and Berridge, V. (1990) 'No one knew anything: some issues in British AIDS policy', in P. Aggelton, P. Davies and G. Hart (eds) *AIDS: Individual, Cultural and Policy Dimensions*, Basingstoke: Falmer Press.

Watney, S. (1987) *Policing Desire: Pornography, AIDS and the Media*, London: Comedia.

—— (1992) 'Short term companions: AIDS as popular entertainment', in A. Klusacek and K. Morrison (eds) *A Leap In The Dark: AIDS, Art and Contemporary Cultures*, Montreal: Vehicle Press.

Weeks, J. (1988) 'Love in a cold climate', in P. Aggelton and H. Homans (eds) *Social Aspects of AIDS*, Lewes: Falmer Press.

Whitehead, M. (1989) *Swimming Upstream: Trends and Prospects in Education for Health*, London: Kings Fund.

Part 2

The Media Reporting of Social Policy

Chapter 5

Poor relations

State social work and the press in the UK

Meryl Aldridge

A legacy of fear and suspicion

Many occupations are unhappy with their coverage in the news media. In the past, most complaints alleged superficiality or distortion. Now the demands of promotional culture (Wernick 1991; Fairclough 1991) can make no news even worse than bad news. A high 'corporate profile', often used by government as a key indicator of effectiveness in the quasi-market competition for public funds, has become crucial for public sector agencies and organisations. While high-visibility groups like the police try to improve their image, low-visibility players like HM Customs and Excise work to establish their social importance through 'fly-on-the-wall' documentaries (Schlesinger, Tumber and Murdock 1991).

Few occupations, however, have had their sense of grievance about media treatment given official endorsement. The Inquiry Panel on the death of Kimberley Carlile made a 'Reasoned Decision' to meet in private on the basis of hostile press coverage (Blom 1987: 273); and the government Command Paper reporting the Butler Sloss inquiry into allegations of widespread familial child sexual abuse in County Cleveland contains a specific section on the role of the news media in the crisis (Cm. 412 1988: 168–171). During the mid-1980s articles in social work trade journals frequently reflected the preoccupation of both managers and frontline staff in local authority social services departments with media responses to their work. Since 1990 this kind of semi-public anxiety has diminished, though the private concerns of social workers and departments may not have done. A review of *Community Care* for the period January 1997 to August 1998 produced only one major article on the news media, and that related to the possible damage caused by the portrayal of people with a mental illness (*Community Care*, 28 August–3 September 1998). Nevertheless, 1998 research into reader attitudes still showed that 'The majority of those surveyed felt that the way the media covers social work issues makes their jobs more difficult to do' (*Community Care*, 30 April–6 May 1998).

Social workers' fears about the impact of hostile reporting on public attitudes may be exaggerated since few areas of social research are as hotly contested and inconclusive as studies of media effects. As we shall see, the episodes engraved in the social work collective memory are of press coverage, while survey data regularly report that most people regard television as their primary source of news (ITC 1996). But television and radio are fugitive. Archives of news and documentary are few and are not accessible to the public. In contrast, dramatic or distressing press coverage can be retained and referred to both by consumers and producers. A key aspect of media routines when dealing with new events is to interpret them through previous, similar events, often by looking back to earlier news coverage ('going to the cuttings'). Nor do news media operate independently; in conditions of intense competition other media are a cheap and accessible source of news (Keeble 1994: Chapter 3). Once established, therefore, interpretive frames tend to persist.

Even more importantly the UK press, unlike broadcasting, is free to be politically partisan. Dealing with family breakdown, young people in trouble with the law, elderly people struggling to maintain an independent household, or people in poverty: social workers and their employing agencies are always operating on the terrain of political conflict. When social work becomes news, it is unlikely to be bland and in the intensely reflexive world of news media, even impartial broadcast media can reinforce and amplify the interpretive frame placed on an event by reporting its press treatment as a topic in its own right. Empirically, then, social workers' concerns about press reporting should not be dismissed as of no consequence. More sociologically, their belief that it is important is, as W.I. Thomas classically formulated it, 'real in its consequences'. To put the 'problem' of social work in the press into perspective we must deconstruct it: this prompts a number of questions. Are we talking about local as well as national newspapers? Are we taking into consideration all national newspapers? Local authority social services have a range of responsibilities: for child protection, for the care of adults who need support because of disability, mental illness or the consequences of aging. Is there a difference in the press response to these different facets of state social work? Do we take into account the wider politico-historic context?

Although social workers have come to fear that any controversy will cause a cascade of press abuse the reality is more complex. There are even circumstances in which social work gets a 'good press', for instance, when doing 'griefwork' in situations of loss and bereavement. Social workers' support for survivors and those bereaved in the Clapham rail crash of 1988 and the Hillsborough football stadium disaster of 1989 was reported[1] briefly but approvingly in the press (Aldridge 1994: Chapter 6).

Social services in the press: case studies

When social workers recount their adversarial relationship with the news media, the critical precipitating event is usually said to be the 1973 criminal trial and official inquiry that followed the death of Maria Colwell and the subsequent official enquiry. Maria, aged seven years, was killed by her stepfather while she was in the care of the local authority.[2] The case attracted very extensive publicity both nationally and locally and established a template of news coverage which was applied again when three similar cases occurred over a short period in the mid-1980s. Essentially the deaths of Jasmine Beckford, Tyra Henry and Kimberley Carlile were represented as preventable, if only the departments concerned had been better managed and co-ordinated and the workers involved had been more expert, more experienced and better supervised. In short, social services should have intervened more. Yet the Cleveland crisis of 1987 (when suspicions of sexual abuse within families led to large numbers of children being taken into care) and similar events in Rochdale (1990) and the Orkney Islands (1991) resulted in the excoriation of social services for taking children into care by intervening too much.

In none of these cases was there any suggestion that the staff or departments had acted in other than good faith. By contrast, during the 1990s there has been real scandal: a series of court cases in which social services staff have been accused of serious, long-term, sexual abuse of young people in their care. Surely the combination of breach of trust, policy failure and sexual wrongdoing would attract the most vitriolic press coverage? In fact these dreadful events have been downplayed or ignored, particularly in those papers which social workers fear most, the mass tabloids. This may, at least in part, reflect the legal prohibition against naming either the perpetrators or survivors of abuse, but this neglect also suggests that it is not simply the intrinsic characteristics of an event that determine whether and how the news media will take it up. The explanation lies in the economics and politics of newspapers themselves.

Not low profile but no profile

The fact that all the instances mentioned above relate to social work with children is not haphazard, but fundamental. Social work becomes news because it is about the politics of the family as we can see from a major aspect of social services work that is almost entirely ignored by the press, even when mistakes are made, like the care of elderly people. For instance, when the local government ombudsman criticised the London Borough of Hammersmith and Fulham for failing to meet the needs of a confused elderly resident, only the *Guardian* (8 June 1992) covered the story. After a resident had lain dead for six weeks in her Wirral Borough Council sheltered home, the council ordered an inquiry but only the *Daily Telegraph* (9 July 1991) reported it. An 'important test case' (*Community Care*, 16 July 1992) in the High Court in which a group of residents in local authority homes tried to establish their rights seems to have been entirely ignored by the national press (Aldridge 1994: 105–107).

Why then, was the possible closure of several local authority elderly persons' homes the subject of a very high-profile campaign in the Nottingham *Evening*

Post from late 1991 to mid-1992? Two aspects of the news treatment provide the key. First, that it was never placed within a 'social work' frame. The dispute was reported as a matter of local politics, while the staff were portrayed as quasi-family 'carers'. (Social services management hardly got a mention.) Second, the elderly people at the centre of the furore were rendered almost entirely passive in the construction of stories, the use of language and in pictures: '"Tearful pleas from Beattie, 99"; "Why can't they leave us alone?"' (1 November 1991) – a resource to trigger an emotional response. The 'address' was not to readers in the same situation but to younger people in their capacity as voters, employees or family members. When the issue re-emerged during the summer of 1998 the *Evening Post*'s focus was on closure as an employment dispute. This time residents were almost invisible.

'He let her die'

Social workers dread that, whatever the complex actuality, the death of a child in care will lead to sensational press coverage organised round 'the search for blame'. This belief has some foundation. Between 1985 and 1987 some of the newspaper treatment at the conclusions of three very highly-publicised trials represented the supposed errors of social workers as almost equivalent to the guilt of the convicted person. Martin Ruddock (1991), as the child's social worker, gives a paradigmatic account of being a key witness in the Kimberley Carlile case: massed photographers outside the court, the 'door-stepping' of his family, 'fishing expeditions' for background information at his local pub. At the end of the trial, he writes, the *Daily Star* published a seven-page shock issue in which his picture was placed alongside those of her stepfather and her mother with the caption 'He let her die'.

Reports on the earlier death of Tyra Henry had attributed supposed blame in less personal terms, but nevertheless all sectors of the press assumed that there had been avoidable errors: 'Life sentence for Tyra's father' was the front page-lead in the *Daily Telegraph* (26 July 1985) with a subsidiary story headed 'Row over who was to blame'. The *Daily Express* (26 July 1985) devoted its first three pages and entire editorial to the trial outcome, including an item headlined 'Probe reveals basic blunders'. The editorial talks of 'bumbling amateurism' and workers being 'fobbed off or fooled' while the *Sun* had a banner across pages two and three in white-on-black: 'Our deadly blunders'.

Like the Kimberley Carlile case, the interpretive frame in the Tyra Henry coverage closely matched that of the Jasmine Beckford trial in early 1985. This is not, however, to be understood simply in terms of lazy journalism or unimaginative editorial mind-sets. The intensity and tone of the coverage was crucially linked to the political context of the mid-1980s, when the Conservative government under Margaret Thatcher was at its most confident and radical. Local government was the crucial terrain of conflict as a number of very vocal Labour-led local authorities were pursuing left-wing policies around issues of 'race', gender and sexual orientation. These 'loony left' councils provided a perfect ideological target to mask the more prosaic central government goal of reducing central government contributions to local authority spending in order that direct taxation could be reduced. All three cases referred to above took place in left-wing London boroughs; in two of them the local politics of 'race' was central. Both Jasmine Beckford and Tyra Henry were African-Caribbean. The professional and organisational conflicts and confusions surrounding their lives and deaths reflected intense controversy over how child protection practice should adapt to a multi-ethnic and multi-cultural population. Antagonisms between elected members, senior officers and staff in the London Borough of Lambeth, culminating in a strike by frontline staff, enlarged the news value of the Tyra Henry case well beyond the trial, particularly in the broadsheets. In the tabloid sector the racialisation of the case took a variety of forms from the pseudo-analytical 'Are black power politics costing the lives of children?' *(Daily Express*, 27 July 1985) to the crude 'Animal gets life' (the *Sun*, 26 July 1985), simultaneously illustrating the discourses of otherness and dangerousness then being mobilised to legitimate the reconstruction of local government and social policy (Parton 1991; Smith 1994).

If professional 'failure' was the sole driver of newsworthiness, condemnatory press treatment similar to that recounted above might be anticipated every time a child in care comes to harm. The pivotal importance of the political context is demonstrated by cases where, though they were apparently similar to those discussed above, media attention was low-key, short-lived, or even non-existent. (For more detail see Aldridge 1994: 51–62.) Charlene Salt died in Oldham, Lancashire (rather than London) despite multi-agency involvement. After the trial verdict in October 1985, although there was extensive coverage in 'how could this happen?' mode, responsibility was placed firmly at the door of Charlene's parents. Later that year, the parents of an African-Caribbean boy were tried for manslaughter at Nottingham Crown Court. It was reported that his mother had unsuccessfully approached social services for help, but despite the potential 'race' angle, national press coverage consisted of small factual items on inside pages. Sudio Rouse was in the care of the Conservative-held (rather than Labour-held) London Borough of Croydon when she died. The subsequent murder trial in 1991 was covered extensively in the national press (perhaps because of its geographical accessibility and some of the grim details of the child's death) but with no editorial comment and general acceptance of the director of social services' assurances that an internal inquiry had resolved any problems of practice.

'Simply a terrible botch'

Between March and September 1990 Rochdale (Lancashire) Social Services took legal measures to protect seventeen children from suspected ritual abuse. In mid-September it was announced that there would be no prosecutions, for lack of criminal evidence. The social services committee asked for a report on practice from the central government Social Services Inspectorate (SSI). In March 1991, after a case in the High Court lasting three months, ten of the fifteen children still in care were returned to their parents. The court judgment contained very adverse comments on aspects of the social work intervention.

Nearly a decade later, many of the positions taken up during the Rochdale events seem less secure. While Jean La Fontaine (1998) found no evidence of links between Satanism and child abuse, the uncovering of the systematic sexual abuse of children and young people has occurred with ghastly regularity. (See, for example, Davies 1998). As Kitzinger claims, however, the contemporary hysteria about paedophilia has constructed it as 'stranger danger' rather than involving family members (Chapter 13). In Rochdale (as in Cleveland and the Orkneys) parental rights were being challenged.

The Rochdale events raised very complex issues of law and evidence. What is particularly notable about the press coverage is the drive to simplify and to accept 'common sense' attitudes and explanations, even in newspapers addressing a sophisticated professional audience, like the *Guardian*. The coverage in the *Daily Telegraph* was more even-handed, providing a very detailed account of the legal judgment and allowing a 'voice' not only to aggrieved parents but also to members of the social work agencies involved. Two factors may account for this curious reversal. First, the *Guardian* was originally based in Manchester and still has a strong presence (and source of intelligence) in the north west through its sister the *Manchester Evening News*. Over Rochdale, it adopted the style of a local paper, identifying with the local community. Consequently, second, it may have responded more sympathetically to several pressure groups representing parents which pursued a well-organised media relations strategy, possibly including the leaking of the SSI report. Its response to the High Court judgment was harsh and unequivocal 'Rochdale: simply a terrible botch' (*Guardian*, 8 March 1991). The paper interprets the judgment as establishing that there had been no abuse. In fact social services were criticised for their failure to produce an evidentially sound basis for their actions in most (but not all) cases – hardly the same thing (see Chapter 2 for a different explanation of the *Guardian*'s coverage).

The *Daily Mail* had no problems with complexity. From the start its accounts were inscribed with support for the parents and scorn of the local authority's actions: '"Satan case"' parents in clear, say police' (*Daily Mail*, 14 September 1990), another instance of treating lack of robust proof as equivalent to disproof. The SSI report was represented as having been demanded by central government and being utterly condemnatory, whereas it was neither. On 8 March 1991 the High Court judgment was given most of the front page, supported by an editorial drawing parallels with the 'scandalous oppression of innocent parents' which had previously occurred in Cleveland. Alongside the editorial was a feature about allegedly Trotskyite councillors in the London Borough of Lambeth.

Neither the *Sun* nor the *Daily Mirror* covered the case as extensively as the broadsheets and mid-market tabloids, nor in such partisan terms.

'Four pages of utterly compelling reading'

After several separate police investigations over more than a decade, in 1991 Frank Beck was tried (with two other defendants) on sixty charges of rape, buggery and sexual assault against young people resident in the local authority homes that he had worked in and managed. His victims included staff as well as residents, women and men. Beck was sentenced to life imprisonment (and died of a heart attack in prison). Leicestershire County Council had already set up an independent internal inquiry. At the end of the trial the Secretary of State ordered a national inquiry and a further internal investigation. The matter was also referred to the Police Complaints Authority.

The Beck case demonstrated that social workers could be not merely 'amateurish' but criminal wrong-doers and that their managers might have failed to stop them. Given previous denunciations of state social work in the press, the logical inference would be that the trial and its aftermath would be – literally – front-page news. Moreover, earlier the same year investigative journalism for a television documentary and by the *Independent* had uncovered inhumane (but not criminally deviant) practices in Staffordshire children's homes, also accompanied by ignorance or tolerance on the part of managers and elected members (Aldridge 1994: 81–89). News of Alan Levy and Barbara Kahan's report (1991) on the 'pindown' affair had been extensive and, in a well-established pattern of news media operation, had 'sensitised' newspapers to similar controversies elsewhere in the UK. Residential social work was on the news agenda.

In fact, the press treatment of the Frank Beck trial was relatively low-key in relation to its implications. While the ten-week case was in progress, national press interest was sporadic, triggered by Beck himself giving evidence and by allegations about a local MP. Despite the sensational nature of the charges, there was more consistent reporting of the trial in the broadsheets than either mid- or mass-market tabloid newspapers.

At the beginning of the Beck trial there had been legal restraints on reporting (as there had in Rochdale) the lifting of which was news in itself. As far as can be established, however, after the verdict and sentencing there was no reason not to print the kind of background and 'colour' stories typical of other major trials, like the cases of Charlene Salt and Rikki Neave. In the Leicestershire scandal, moreover, much useful material was presented ready-made to the news media by the publication of the Newell internal inquiry report, a detailed saga of management incompetence. The *Leicester Mercury*, which had covered the case extensively almost every day under a linking logo, produced a pull-out supplement (30 November 1991): 'Today we publish the secret report on the Beck years of evil; four pages of utterly compelling reading'. In the national newspapers sampled, however, only the *Independent* put the case on page one, where it appeared as a descriptive 'hard news' item, without editorial comment. Nor did the *Daily Mail* make any explicit comment, although its page-two coverage gave more space to 'Blunders over Beck' (30 November 1991) than to the case itself. The *Daily Mirror*'s presentation was dramatic, but on page nine, while the *Sun* provided extensive text but also in hard news format only and on page seven.

Ten years on probation

During the mid-1980s, when other agencies of state social work found themselves with a high and very unwelcome media profile, the probation service in England and Wales was almost invisible. In two of the instances of the death of a child in care referred to above (Tyra Henry and Charlene Salt) the accused man was under the supervision of the service, but neither the work done, nor the effectiveness of probation itself were questioned. Only once has a probation officer been subjected to media accusations of personal responsibility for an avoidable tragedy. The conviction of Colin Evans, in December 1984, for the sexual assault and murder of Marie Payne (aged four years) was given very extensive coverage in all the national newspapers. At the end of the trial the *Sun* devoted five pages to it and the *Daily Star* nearly six. At the trial it emerged that Colin Evans had a very long record of sexual offences yet his supervising probation officer had introduced him to a Christian voluntary organisation without informing them of his record. This conferred respectability with other social work agencies and users which allowed Evans to set up a babysitting organisation (unconnected, however, with Marie Payne's death). All the newspapers criticised the probation officer in trenchant and personal terms; all but three printed a photograph of him. The case also reverberated politically, with members of parliament demanding that a register of sex offenders be set up.

While most of the national press followed up the policy and politics of the case, only the *Daily Mail* news and editorial treatment questioned the *idea* of probation work. It located the issue in a much wider frame: the 'scandalous leniency' of the whole apparatus of social control: 'Our courts, our probation and social services, our schools and education authorities cannot toy tolerantly with violators and corrupters of youth'. In a classic example of the *Mail*'s technique of imputing guilt by juxtaposition this editorial (18 December 1984) shared the page with a feature claiming that London supply (temporary replacement) teachers were left-wing failures and misfits. Condemning the probation service as practitioners of social work has been a unique theme in the *Daily Mail* which has been pursued relentlessly ever since. The paper is the most loyal in its support of the Conservative Party and a consistent advocate of conventional values, notably the patriarchal family and the strong state. According to the *Mail* almost all players in the criminal justice system are 'soft' and/or 'out of touch' (Aldridge and Eadie 1997).

Given the high political salience of law and order, the probation service's quiet life could not continue. Despite the Thatcher administration's well-cultivated reputation for toughness in relation to crime, Home Secretaries of the period favoured relatively liberal policies, including the wider use of 'community disposals'. Consonant with the party's traditional position, however, a series of government policy documents and speeches from 1988 onwards required that probation work be more focused on concepts of punishment and control. No more 'clients', but 'offenders' (Aldridge 1994: 122–124). Both locally and nationally the probation service was directed simultaneously to toughen its image and to increase its visibility in the local community. The Association of Chief Officers of Probation (ACOP) and the National Association of Probation Officers (NAPO) both responded by developing their media relations work (Aldridge 1994: 130–134; Schlesinger, Tumber and Murdock 1991). Given its greater financial resources and structural freedom as a trade union, NAPO had more success.

Among local probation areas the importance attached to promoting the service's work was very variable (and remains so). When it was actively pursued, though, it could generate just the kind of 'good news' in local media that had been demanded. In a three-month period of 1991, for example, a probation public relations officer working in the south west of England collected thirty-six items about his area, of which thirty-three were neutral or positive (Aldridge 1994: 131). When Michael Howard became Home Secretary, however, priorities changed dramatically. From 1993 he played a key role in trying to re-establish Conservative credibility over law and order, under the slogan 'Prison works'. Clearly a policy centred on imprisonment has profound implications for the probation service, but Michael Howard's strategy was much more radical, not just uncoupling the probation service from social work, but eroding its autonomy by dismantling its training. Inevitably his attempt to discursively reconstruct probation training and practice as flawed and the profession's response were pursued in part through the news media (Aldridge and Eadie 1997; Aldridge 1999). Neither the Home Secretary nor probation professionals, ironically, gained the extent or type of press attention that they desired.

'More former soldiers and police officers are to be recruited to the probation service to dilute its "liberal do-gooding ethos"', reported the *Guardian* (27 June 1994) in response to a Home Office briefing, as the future tense construction clearly indicates. An announcement about the new form of professional training was expected by the autumn but did not appear. As subsequent events showed, the Home Secretary was finding that few interested parties shared his views about the probation service, so classic techniques of news management were deployed. In the 'slow news' hiatus between Christmas 1994 and the New Year, the *Daily Mail* (29 December 1994) printed, across two pages, an 'exclusive' by the political editor headed 'Howard calls up the probation troops'. Doubts as to whether his proposals would gain public endorsement seem to have persisted. As the *Guardian* pointed out (25 February 1995) the announcement was 'buried' by appearing on the same day (22 February) as the publication of a major policy document on Northern Ireland. Apart from the faithful *Daily Mail*, the only papers that reported the issue were *The Times* and the *Daily Express*, both in neutral hard news style, and the *Guardian* in a report dominated by dissenting voices.

Unfortunately for those in the probation service, this lack of press response continued during their campaign against the dismantling of their training system. Like the Home Secretary, NAPO and other stakeholders were attempting mobilise support. Their hope was that the broadsheets would take up the issue and stimulate a response from politicians and other sections of the 'policy community'. Though unlikely, coverage in the tabloid press would be very welcome as it would confirm that probation training was a public issue that might result in political embarrassment. Even NAPO did not expect active support from the real 'public': as so often the press reaction was being used as a surrogate for public opinion. The campaign lasted for most of 1995, but neither a major House of Lords debate featuring three former Home Secretaries, and expressing almost unanimous hostility to the training proposals, nor a mass lobby of parliament by probation staff attracted significant national press coverage (Aldridge and Eadie 1997; Aldridge 1999). The demonstration was widely reported in local media which, though important for morale, is not significant in terms of national policy and politics. NAPO's final tactic was to challenge the Home Secretary's proposals through judicial review but it lost the case in February 1996. As this deviated from a run of defeats for Michael Howard in UK and EU courts, it had a certain novelty value and was reported in all the broadsheets.

The probation training saga was arcane, protracted – lasting over three years – and appeared to affect directly only a very small number of people. It was never going to be newsworthy for mass tabloid papers. According to NAPO, even the broadsheets seemed to find it 'dry', despite its significance for other professional groups in a close relationship to the state (Aldridge 1999). Looking back, it is likely that the real problem for the defenders of probation training was that it remained an abstract policy matter. It was never transformed into party politics, a domain deeply incorporated into the structures and daily routines of newspapers where, vitally, issues can be dramatised and personalised.

The Labour party, then in opposition, resisted the Home Secretary's attempts to dismantle probation training without a House of Commons debate, but it maintained an ominous silence on the substance. In government Labour, far from reversing the training changes, carried out a review of the whole probation service. The resulting consultation document appeared in August 1998 proposing far more swingeing changes than those pursued by Michael Howard, including making probation officers into civil servants and thus directly answerable to central government. The preoccupation with corporate profile persisted: a key part of the review process had been the search for a new, 'tougher' name for the service. Apparently Jack Straw had thought better of his earlier enthusiasm for 'reviving the old-fashioned title "corrections service"' (*Guardian*, 27 December 1997). Instead, finding a name formed part of the public consultation process. It appears, however, that the probation service remains stubbornly lacking in news value. Of the papers sampled on 7 August 1998 the government's announcement of the policy and consultation process was covered by the *Guardian* with a news items and adverse opinion piece, only as straight news by the *Daily Telegraph* (page 2) and the *Daily Mail* (page 26), not at all in the *Sun,* and on page 15 of the *Mirror* where a two-sentence box headed 'Name is on probation' opens 'Ministers are asking the public to think up a new name for the Probation Service, because they can't'. Even the *Daily Mail*, under the heading 'Probation service gets a macho makeover' expresses an uncharacteristic mix of irony and scepticism. In the reflexive world of post-modern promotional politics, even senior ministers cannot guarantee a result.

Understanding social work news

National and local newspapers in the UK are run for profit and are free to be politically partisan. Indeed, the political sympathies of national daily papers are a crucial aspect of their identity and position in the market. The interplay of these two factors explains nearly everything about the press treatment of state social work.

Obviously a newspaper needs readers. They pay directly for the product; the size and spending power of the readership determines advertising revenue. No newspaper, therefore, can address itself primarily to sections of the population with little to spend. Even the mass tabloids, specifically pitched at 'ordinary folk' (a code for working class) are filled with news of and for people between young adulthood and middle age. They may not be well off but, typically, they are setting up households and having children. Money is being earned and spent. Newspapers, in other words, have a powerful commercial interest in the family-based household which, by itself, explains their greater responsiveness to child protection work than to social work with elderly people or those with a mental illness.

As well as being economically crucial – and ever more so in a society driven more by consumption than production – the family is a key site of political cleavage, over the potentially competing rights of women and men, children and adults. This is the terrain on which state social work operates, so it is inevitable that professional practice will often be newsworthy, justified or not and skilful or not. The *Independent* is positioned as supporting children's rights and addresses a professional audience, hence the very extensive resources invested in the 'pindown' affair. While the *Daily Mirror* concentrated only on the personal experience of those involved, it, too, implicitly supported a welfare system in which children are seen as having rights as well as needs.

Conversely, the *Daily Mail* powerfully and consistently promotes the conventional, patriarchal family where parents' (particularly fathers') rights prevail. The parents of the children subject to pindown did not feature as an organised voice in the controversy (unlike Rochdale) so the *Mail* showed little interest in this instance of social work failure.

If state social work were as accessible to families in difficulties as the NHS is intended to be for the sick, the cost would be commensurately huge. Most of the Conservative changes to the welfare state in the 1980s were intended to reconstruct welfare services as a minimal system of containment for failure and deviance, in which resources were concentrated on the 'dangerous'. Apart from the struggles over local government and the politics of difference, already referred to, the cases of Jasmine Beckford, Tyra Henry and Kimberley Carlile were also politicised in this sense. Social workers were being accused of lack of expertise in identifying and controlling the 'other/them' on behalf of 'us'. Taken together with the very real drama and tragedy at the centre of the cases, extensive and melodramatic media coverage was not merely likely, but overdetermined.

So social work with children will always be contested, but in recent years its significance as a political symbol and metonym has diminished. Cambridgeshire Social Services was heavily criticised during and after the trial in 1996 of Ruth Neave for the murder of her son Rikki (of which she was acquitted). It could not have been otherwise: social work's alleged failings were part of the defence case; the department had itself declared its practice as falling short; and further inquiries into its operation were ordered by central government. Most press comment, however, did not target individual social workers, nor enlarge the issue any more than might be the case where, say, a health authority's failings were in the news. The *Daily Mail* devoted most of its two-page coverage to the allegedly obvious 'dangerousness' of Neave, including the curious accusation that 'By 16 she was having sex with men' (31 October 1996). Arguably, however, the Neave trial was big news because of other features of the case, notably allegations of drug use, witchcraft, threats and intimidation. At the conclusion of a much more brutal child murder case, the judge said 'The social services [Northeast Lincolnshire] have already instigated a wide-ranging internal inquiry into these matters – I don't think they are thorough enough' (*Guardian*, 30 July 1998). Although all the papers sampled reported the verdict and sentence in the case, only the *Daily Mail* – 'Boy of 4 taken off "at risk" roll killed by couple' (30 July 1998) – gave the social work and 'preventable death' motive prominence in its report.

The Rikki Neave trial also illustrates the different interpretive frame applied by local newspapers. While the national papers all reported the first and last day, there were only occasional reports during the intervening four weeks, ranging from six in the *Daily Mirror* to none in the *Daily Mail*. The Peterborough *Evening Telegraph* covered the story every day, sometimes prominently and in detail. The outcome took up all of the front page and seven inside pages. A local paper, however, must appeal to the whole population, not a section defined by age, class and politics. Accordingly, the editorial comment emphasises not individual blame but community responsibility for the events and for recovery: '. . . a shadow hangs over our city' (*Evening Telegraph*, 31 October 1996). Everyone is given space to justify themselves, including social services. It is clear that Ruth Neave was a controversial figure: she pleaded guilty to five cruelty charges and was sentenced to seven years' imprisonment. Nevertheless, the background features on her life and behaviour are complex and sympathetic. Similarly the material on Rikki Neave resists the 'tragic tot' reflex in favour of an account of a sad little boy from a difficult background.

Frank Beck's wrongdoing extended over many years beforehand, so the case failed to provide the staple materials for constructing satisfactory news stories (Aldridge 1995). His victims had grown up and dispersed, making it very difficult to produce 'background' and 'colour' featuring either them or their parents. Nor did the young people comfortably fit the frame of innocent 'tragic tot'. One reason that it took so long for Beck to be challenged, according to the Police Complaints Authority report (1993), was that his victims had already been written off as deviants. In the last analysis, however, the key to the mysterious silence over the Frank Beck case is that he raised too many questions about the solidity of the social and institutional order. This applied as much to the *Guardian*, with its investment in the possibility of professional trust and rational policy-making, as to the *Sun*. Cheeky irreverence cannot work without stable authority structures as both butt and boundary. Deviance and conflict are central to news but newspapers' place in parliamentary democracy – to say nothing of their capitalist rationale – relies on social stability. That a well-respected local authority manager, local councillor and consultant on childcare methods could be behaving as Frank Beck did was too chaotic to be contained within conventional press narratives which, among other things, require a reassuring 'closure'.

Recent events have, unfortunately, simply verified this interpretation of the press response to the Frank Beck trial. A succession of similar cases, involving men working both in local authority and voluntary agency homes, has gone almost unreported in the national press, even though the Conservative government was worried enough to set up a tribunal chaired by a retired High Court judge. The Waterhouse enquiry began on 21 January 1997 (and heard evidence for a year and a half). As the *Independent* reported (22 January 1997) on its front page it was 'Britain's biggest child abuse enquiry: 650 cases, up to 80 staff involved at 30 homes'. The other broadsheet reports were relatively low-key accounts of opening speeches, placed on inside pages. The *Sun* ignored it while the *Mirror* gave it three paragraphs and the *Daily Star* two. The *Daily Mail* devoted most of page 12 to the tribunal, foregrounding the possible culpability of social services management even though the remit covered the role of the Welsh Office and other agencies.

The outcome of the Waterhouse enquiry will undoubtedly be a matter of profound public interest. As we have seen, though, this does not help us predict how the press will treat it. That will be determined by a judgement as to whether it will interest their public. Politically and commercially it is safer to entertain and titillate, even to make readers indignant, than to take risks with their ontological security.

Notes

1 The discussion of press coverage is based on all the national weekday newspapers except the *Financial Times* which does not routinely cover social work and welfare issues. Where a sample has been drawn it usually consists of the *Guardian* (the principal centre-left broadsheet), the *Daily Telegraph* (a right-wing broadsheet), the *Daily Mail*, which dominates the mid-market sector, the *(Daily) Mirror* and the *Sun*. Since the 1997 election neither of these mass tabloids have been easy to place politically. In general, however, the *Mirror* is more sympathetic to collective welfare provision and those that work in the sector.

2 Children may be 'in care' but still living with parent(s). 'Care' is a legal process giving local authority social services (and the NSPCC) the right to take action to protect children who are thought to be at risk of harm.

References

Aldridge, M. (1994) *Making Social Work News*, London: Routledge.

—— (1995) 'Contemplating the monster: UK national press treatment of the Frank Beck affair', *The Sociological Review* 43(4): 658–674.

—— (1999) 'Probation officer training, promotional culture and the public sphere', *Public Administration* 77(1): 73–90.

Aldridge, M. and Eadie, T. (1997) 'Manufacturing an issue: the case of probation officer training', *Critical Social Policy* 17(1): 111–124.

Blom Cooper, L. (1987) *A Child in Mind: Protection of Children in a Responsible Society: The Report into the Circumstances Surrounding the Death of Kimberley Carlile*, London: London Borough of Greenwich.

Cm 412 (1988) *Report of the Inquiry into Child Abuse in Cleveland 1987*, London: HMSO.

Davies, N. (1998) 'The most secret crime' – a series of four articles, *Guardian* 2–5 June 1998.

Fairclough, N. (1991) 'What might we mean by "enterprise culture"?', in R. Keat and N. Abercrombie (eds) *Enterprise Culture*, London: Routledge.

ITC (1996) 'Revealing sources', *Spectrum* (Independent Television Commission magazine), Winter: 23.

Keeble, R. (1994) *The Newspapers Handbook*, London: Routledge.

La Fontaine, J. (1998) *Speak of the Devil: Tales of Satanic Abuse in Contemporary England*, Cambridge: Cambridge University Press.

Levy, A. and Kahan, B. (1991) *The Pindown Experience and the Protection of Children*, Stafford: Staffordshire County Council.

Parton, N. (1991) *Governing the Family*, London: Macmillan.

Police Complaints Authority (1993) *Inquiry into Police Complaints Authority Report of*

Police Investigation of Complaints of Child and Sexual Abuse in Leicestershire Children's Homes, London: Police Complaints Authority.

Ruddock, M. (1991) 'A receptacle for public anger', in B. Franklin and N. Parton (eds) *Social Work, the Media and Public Relations*, London: Routledge.

Schlesinger, P., Tumber, H. and Murdock, G. (1991) 'The media politics of crime and criminal justice', *British Journal of Sociology* 42(3): 397–420.

Smith, A.M. (1994) *New Right Discourse on Race and Sexuality; Britain 1968–1990*, Cambridge: Cambridge University Press.

Wernick, A. (1991) *Promotional Culture: Advertising, Ideology and Symbolic Expression*, London: Sage.

Chapter 6

Home truths

Media representations of homelessness

Steve Platt

On the evening of 16 November 1966, an emotional, black-and-white television drama captivated viewing audiences across Britain and shattered the postwar complacency which held that problems of bad housing and homelessness, if not already things of the past, soon would be. *The Wednesday Play* that evening, on prime time BBC1, was *Cathy Come Home*. Directed by Ken Loach and produced by Tony Garnett, who had made their names collaborating on a previous social-realist dramatic success, *Up the Junction*, the play had an impact that would be unimaginable in later, more media-saturated years. At the time, with television still a novelty and just three terrestrial channels (one of them the fledgling BBC2, then barely two years old) to choose from, it seemed as if virtually the whole nation had turned on to watch Carol White's heart-rending performance as Cathy: and that virtually everyone in the country was talking about the issues raised by the drama the next day.

Cathy Come Home told the story of an ordinary young couple, whose love for each other became strained and finally stretched to breaking point by their inability to find a decent home in which to live and bring up their children. Having been reduced to homelessness, the couple were forced to turn to the state for assistance, whereupon they found themselves compulsorily separated by the rules of the social services hostel in which Cathy and her children were accommodated. Homeless families' accommodation at the time often made no provision for husbands and fathers, who were expected to make their own arrangements elsewhere. Indeed, the 'no husbands' rule was so strictly enforced that, on two occasions in 1965, Kent County Council actually had men jailed for breaking court injunctions prohibiting them from staying with their families at one of its hostels.

Ultimately, as the play's depressing downward spiral developed, Cathy's children were forcibly separated from her and taken into care. The traumatic railway-station scene involving a hysterical Cathy, her screaming children and stony-faced social services personnel as they prised her young baby from her arms, capped a televisual *tour de force* that laid bare the inadequacies of the British welfare state just a few months after Harold Wilson's Labour Party had been returned to power with a massively increased majority and commensurately high expectations. Newspapers the next day spoke of 'the play that shamed the nation'. Ken Loach and the play's author, Jeremy Sandford, were summoned to meet the housing minister to discuss what should be done.

'Deserving' and 'undeserving' homeless people

Cathy Come Home helped to create fertile conditions for the formation of the housing charity Shelter, which was launched within barely a fortnight of the play's first screening. Describing itself as 'a rescue operation', backed by five national bodies in the housing association field, the charity picked up where the television play had left off. Its launch, on 1 December, was marked by the publication of a quarter-page advertisement in the *Guardian* ('provided by a friend of Shelter'). Appearing in a 22-page newspaper in which the most exciting visual image was a picture of Harold Wilson on board the RAF Transport Command Comet *en route* to meet the rebel Rhodesian leader, Ian Smith, the advert was both bold and dramatic. Aimed unashamedly at the social conscience of *Guardian* readers, it used the sort of grainy, black-and-white image of a mother, baby and young child in squalid surroundings that could have been taken straight out of *Cathy Come Home*. Under the heading 'Home Sweet Hell', the text told how:

> Mrs T and her five children live in one room and a cubby hole, in an overcrowded, crumbling house. The room is their kitchen, bathroom, living room and bedroom. Sixteen people use the lavatory . . . Look again at the family above. You hold its happiness in the palm of your hand. Will you pick up a pen and return the coupon now?
>
> (*Guardian*, 1 December 1966)

For its part, the *Guardian* welcomed the formation of Shelter in an editorial that day as 'alms-giving made businesslike'. This was based on the fact that housing associations (to which Shelter proposed to give the bulk of the money that it raised) could 'raise £5 in local authority grants for every £1 subscribed by the public'. '£80,' the *Guardian* noted approvingly, 'matched by a council loan, will rehouse a homeless Londoner' (ibid.).

The response to *Cathy Come Home* and the launch of Shelter contained many of the elements that were to become recurrent themes in the media's treatment of homelessness over the next three decades. First, although Loach and Garnett's treatment of the play had been anything but a liberal appeal for charitable intervention *on behalf of* the homeless, the notion of homeless people as 'victims' – persons for whom things are done rather than who get to do things for themselves – was to prove notoriously difficult to shift. Second, the idea that 'alms-giving' is only a good thing if in some way it is made 'businesslike' or conditional has shaded into countless stories about 'scroungers' and 'waste' in publications less sympathetic towards the homeless than the *Guardian*.

Third, following on from these two approaches, which have their antecedents in Victorian (and earlier) attitudes towards social welfare, there has been a consistent attempt on the part of the media to divide homeless people into 'deserving' and 'undeserving' cases. The 'deserving' homeless, almost invariably in this view, tend to fall into the category of 'victims', while the 'undeserving', as well as being portrayed as the authors of their own misfortunes, fall into the category of 'scroungers' (Rose 1993: 171). And fourth, even in the context of the huge public concern about homelessness raised by the showing of *Cathy Come Home*, there were clear signs of the seasonal, transient and superficial interest in the subject that has so plagued housing campaigners' attempts to raise media coverage and public awareness in subsequent years.

It is notable, for example, that just two weeks after *Cathy Come Home* had stormed the nation's consciences, only the *Guardian* gave serious coverage to the launch of Shelter. Even the *Daily Mirror*, then still in its campaigning heyday (it even sent off the young journalist, John Pilger, to write at length about homelessness among aborigines in Australia), could spare only two paragraphs for the charity's launch. Other papers ignored it altogether.

The seasonal nature of the media interest is notable, too. *Cathy Come Home* relied for some of its impact on the fact that it was screened at the beginning of winter, in the run up to Christmas. Shelter made more of a mark on people's purses than it might have done for the same reason. Stories of homelessness, of people without roofs over their heads or living in cold, damp, substandard housing, don't have the same impact on a balmy summer's day as they do when the nights are closing in and the weather is getting colder. As a journalist specialising in housing and social affairs stories for national newspapers and magazines during the 1980s, I could almost set my calendar by the calls from editors looking for pieces on the plight of the homeless. They'd start when the clocks went back at the end of October, and reach a peak just before Christmas, when almost everyone in publishing seemed to be searching for the classic 'No room at the inn' tale through which to tug at their readers' heartstrings during the lean news periods of the festive season. Housing campaigners, not least among them the media-savvy founders of Shelter, quickly cottoned onto this fact. Soon, too, a new generation of direct action-oriented homeless advocates learnt how to exploit the situation to their own advantage.

The *Evening Standard* 'declares war': newspaper coverage of squatting

Almost two years to the day after its first showing on television, *Cathy Come Home* was repeated for the second time. A few days after that, in direct response to the repeat screening, a group of about fifteen people met in housing campaigner Ron Bailey's house in London, having decided that charitable appeals and expressions of concern about homelessness were insufficient. They set up the London Squatters' Campaign, and after a token occupation of a block of empty luxury flats at the beginning of December, on the Saturday before Christmas they and three homeless people from a nearby council hostel occupied the empty All Saints Vicarage, in Leyton, east London. In his account of this new squatters' movement, Ron Bailey recalls haranguing bystanders outside the vicarage through a megaphone: 'Is there any room at this inn for these homeless people?' and 'Will the church deny families a home, one thousand, nine hundred and sixty-eight years after another family could not find accommodation?' (Bailey 1973: 43).

Squatting was to enjoy a symbiotic – albeit often viciously antagonistic – relationship with the media over the next thirty years. On the one hand, it owed its very existence and growth to the media coverage given to those early – and subsequent – campaigns. Indeed, at one stage during the 1970s it seemed to be impossible to open a local newspaper without finding stories about squatting and homelessness. On the other hand, that coverage could at times be almost unrelievedly hostile. It was one thing when squatting involved 'respectable', self-evidently 'deserving' cases of homeless families occupying empty council properties, often as part of a well-disciplined campaign led by people who were not themselves homeless. It was quite another when the squatters were perceived to be less respectable and deserving – single people, 'outsiders', 'hippies', 'dossers' or drug takers, people without the same steady eye for how their image might play in the media – particularly if they turned their attentions towards empty privately owned properties or were seen to have some sort of wider political agenda.

The initial squatting campaigns organised by the London Squatters' Campaign and other groups carefully cultivated media interest and support. 'Squatters win support of public', 'Canon Collins backs squatters', 'Residents support squatters', 'Ford workers back squatters' – the early headlines helped to reinforce the popular perception of squatting as a legitimate response to the co-existence of empty properties and homelessness. But as squatting moved beyond the tight control of a small, well-organised group of activists, the same papers that had lauded the early squats soon turned on the movement that grew up in their wake.

The occupation of 144 Piccadilly and other central London buildings in September 1969 by a group of primarily young, childless people with often unorthodox lifestyles gave the first indication of just how virulent the press was to become in its opposition to certain categories of homeless. 'Hippie thugs: the sordid truth' declaimed the *People*. 'Hippies' war lords move in' denounced the *Daily Mail*. 'Squatters told: Now it's war' warned the London *Evening Standard*. A *Times* editorial calling for squatting to be made a criminal offence marked the onset of a long press campaign to get the law changed so as to clamp down on not only the 'Hippiedilly' squatters but any homeless people taking direct action to meet their need for housing.

It was a campaign that was as hysterical as it was inaccurate, reaching a crescendo in the summer of 1975, when the proverbial visitor from Mars might have been forgiven for thinking that squatting threatened the very survival of society itself. 'Innumerable houses up and down the country are now in illegal occupation by organised gangs of thugs, layabouts and revolutionary fanatics,' opined the *Daily Telegraph*. 'It has become increasingly clear that the act of squatting is no longer carried out by, or on behalf of, deprived and homeless people,' said *The Times*. 'Many thousands – in all probability the majority – of squatters are freeloaders and layabouts . . . Strong laws are needed to prevent the forces which are undermining the democratic processes of our country,' announced the *Daily Mail*. For the London *Evening News*, in a foretaste of the sort of media attention that was later to be applied to refugees and asylum seekers, squatters were not homeless people but 'the world's waifs and strays', 'foreign scroungers here for the social security and free accommodation'.

Even occupied houses were declared to be in danger from their depredations. *The Times* published a letter from a Miss Elizabeth Harper, who claimed she had just:

> had the appalling experience of turning squatters out of our home in Kensington, left locked and secure three weeks earlier. The squatters arrogantly assumed the right to break in, to live in our home with their dogs, to sleep in our beds in our sheets, to daub crude drawings in black on our walls, to use our food, light, heat and telephone, to steal £300 of antique furniture and above all to dispose of all our treasured possessions.
>
> (*The Times*, 11 July 1975)

According to Miss Harper, the police had refused to take action and she warned that many other *Times* readers could soon return from holiday to find their homes taken over by squatters too.

Reasonably enough, Miss Harper's letter caused outrage. It heralded an open season for squatter bashing in the press. But, almost a month later, another letter was published in *The Times*, this time from the Metropolitan Police Solicitor. Miss Harper's letter 'was not in accordance with the facts', he wrote. 'Miss Harper' was actually a Mrs Such, whose home was in Northumberland, not Kensington, and who had not been on holiday. The telephone the squatters were alleged to have used had been disconnected previously. The house was actually empty awaiting sale, and when police officers had gone there to explain the situation to the squatters, they left 'without any incident occurring'. The Police Solicitor concluded: 'I think you will agree that the facts I have set out . . . present a very different picture from the facts set out in the letter to *The Times* and that the letter is, to say the least, disingenuous' (6 August 1975). From the point of view of the squatting movement, however, the damage had already been done. The press campaign against squatters was to achieve its objective of getting the law tightened (although not in making squatting illegal). It had also succeeded in permanently tarring squatters as politically motivated layabouts and misfits, who jumped local authority waiting lists, moved into people's homes when they were away on holiday, vandalised the houses they occupied – and weren't even really homeless or in need anyway.

Extensive surveys of squatters at the time – including a major national survey carried out for the Department of the Environment – painted a very different picture. Most squatted properties were occupied by people with children; as many as 75 per cent of squatters had no educational or vocational qualifications; they had disproportionately low incomes and savings; and, rather than seeing themselves as part of some ideologically motivated movement against private property rights, the vast majority gave their reason for squatting as an inability to find anywhere else to live at a price they could afford. They represented, in short, a fairly typical cross section of homeless people. Their 'crime', such as it was, had been to take matters into their own hands and seize for themselves the solution to their housing problems. This was sufficient, in the eyes of large sections of the press, to justify one of the most vicious, scurrilous and sustained campaigns of abuse ever mounted against homeless people in Britain.

It was not just squatters who fell victims to the press's desire to distinguish between 'good' homeless people and 'bad', or between the 'deserving' and 'undeserving'. The legislation that clamped down on squatting towards the end of the 1970s coincided with the introduction of the Housing (Homeless Persons) Act in 1977, which imposed a statutory duty upon local authorities to provide assistance to the 'vulnerable' homeless. The principal beneficiaries of this legislation were people with children, who, in the crude media categorisations of the period, fell in the category of 'good' homeless. An amendment to the Act, however, enabled councils to refuse accommodation to anyone who was deemed to be 'intentionally homeless'. It is noteworthy that this was introduced following an intensive, media-supported campaign led by Calderdale Council, in West Yorkshire (it was known as the 'Calderdale Clause' at the time). Among the council's principal targets were squatters, of whom Calderdale's housing committee chairman had declared defiantly: 'There is no way that we are going to rehouse these leeches on society.'

The media, homelessness and policy in the 1980s

By the 1980s, the boundaries of what constituted the 'deserving' homeless were being pushed further back. A reinvigorated right-wing political agenda, which both found expression in and was furthered by the media, began to question whether even some of the Cathys of the day merited the kind of assistance that had been introduced by the 1977 Act. As squatting receded from public view, the 'undeserving' homeless who were most often on the receiving end of media ire were now to be found among the ranks of 'new age travellers', single parents (many of whom were alleged to have become pregnant simply to take advantage of housing and benefit entitlements that don't apply to the childless) and the increasing numbers of homeless beggars on the streets of Britain's major cities (Brynin 1987: 25).

The 1980s were characterised by two major changes in the situation facing homeless people. First, the combination of 'right to buy' council house sales, introduced as one of the first acts of Margaret Thatcher's new administration after her election victory in 1979, together with a virtual halt to new council building to greatly reduce the stock of properties available for letting. Second, an ever tighter benefits regime made it more and more difficult for people on low incomes to find suitable accommodation in the private sector. The result was a big increase in the numbers of homeless people. The figures tell their own story. When *Cathy Come Home* was first screened, local councils were accepting just a few thousand people a year for help as homeless; by 1991, the total had reached 175,171 households. By 1992, meanwhile, the number of new council homes completed in England had slumped to just 2575, compared with 133,000 in 1968 (see Burrows *et al.* 1997: Chapter 1).

The media's approach to this was mixed. While there was a great deal of concerned reporting of the burgeoning homelessness problem in the liberal broadsheets (particularly from 1987 onwards, that year having been the United Nations designated International Year of Shelter for the Homeless), other parts of the press played a different role. Some newspapers were at the forefront both in demanding the benefits changes that so greatly increased the numbers of street homeless (particularly among young people – 16- and 17-year-olds, for example, were stripped of all benefit entitlements) and then in lambasting the begging and 'street culture' that these changes produced. And sometimes the link between press coverage and government policy changes was so close as to be almost umbilical.

In the summer of 1989, for example, the *Daily Mail* ran a story about Ellen Cunningham and her family, who, on 16 July, was reported to be 'settling down with her six children for their 59th night in the Park Lodge Hotel, Tyne and Wear, as the bill for bed and breakfast alone rose to £6785'. The use by hard pressed councils of costly bed-and-breakfast accommodation for homeless families was one of the undoubted absurdities of housing policy in the 1980s. Barred by government edict from the cheaper option of building new homes, councils were instead compelled to put up families in unsuitable (and often substandard) but vastly more expensive private hotels. The waste of public money and the strains it imposed on the families were the subject of much media attention and comment.

In this case, the absurdity of the situation was even greater than usual. Ellen Cunningham had been rehoused in an £805-per-week hotel suite by the same council that had evicted her because she owed £250 in rent arrears. It was a good story – but why had the *Mail* chosen to run it on the fifty-ninth night of her stay at the hotel rather than any other? And why had it chosen to direct public anger towards her as a 'scrounger' rather than towards the council for evicting her over such a small sum? The answer was that the story had been stored up to coincide with the government's announcement that same day of a new plan to cut benefits to people who 'make themselves homeless' by moving away from their home area. So, 'Luxury on the rates' boomed its banner headline about the 'scrounger' Cunninghams, while another highlighted the '£135 million crackdown – Ministers act over homeless'. Again and again, the *Daily Mail* and other papers sympathetic to the government acted as propagandists on its behalf, explaining away the massive rise in homelessness during the 1980s as the product of homeless people's own fecklessness or too liberal housing legislation and benefit regimes that encouraged 'scroungers'.

The same sort of argument was deployed in explanation of the increasing numbers of single parents seeking assistance under the homeless legislation. Young homeless mothers found themselves being stereotyped as sexually promiscuous and morally irresponsible; the myth that large numbers of single young women become pregnant simply in order to get council accommodation grew alongside the sort of newspaper coverage exemplified in headlines such as 'We'll stop the queue jump mums' (*Daily Mail*, 19 January 1994).

One story that repeated itself at various intervals in the press seemed to serve the purpose of demonstrating that people sleeping rough – something that was virtually unheard of until the 1980s apart from a diminishing number of mainly middle-aged or elderly men – didn't have it as hard as it seemed. In 1990, National Sleep-Out Week, in which celebrities such as Esther Rantzen and Paddy Ashdown slept out to draw attention to the plight of the street homeless, served as the catalyst for a whole plague of press 'exposés' of begging. The *Sun*, as ever, had been first in on the act, with a front-page story about a '£200-a-day beggar'. The *News of the World*, *Daily Telegraph* and *Daily Express* all sent out reporters that week to see how much they could panhandle. The fact that none of them managed anything remotely approaching £200 – the *Telegraph*'s reporter collected £6.93 – didn't prevent them from portraying life on the streets as a soft option for people who didn't want to do a proper job. The London *Evening Standard* even found a mother who said her son was being deterred from earning his living by the easy pickings he made as a homeless beggar. 'Please don't give money to my beggar son,' said its front-page story.

These stories were not necessarily untrue; nor were right-wing newspapers and politicians the only sources of concern about dependency on begging. Indeed, it was to provide homeless people with an alternative to begging that the *Big Issue* magazine was set up in 1991. The magazine is sold by homeless people, who retain a proportion of the cover price, and now has a circulation of around 300,000 nationwide. Its founder, John Bird, is uncompromising in his belief that 'begging is bad for you', as he wrote in the *New Statesman*: 'Charity and handouts are no route out of poverty. And those who dole out alms to the needy are doing nothing to help them deal with their problems' (30 September 1994).

'It isn't easy to express such views,' Bird continued, '. . . when newspapers and politicians are waging war on 'welfare scroungers' and blaming the poor for being poor and homeless, rather than the system that made them so. But giving alms to the needy has never changed anything. It may salve the consciences of those who do it, but it does nothing to help those who are the recipients' (ibid.).

But Bird's stand on the subject was not that of the right-wing press. The fact was that as much as these papers might argue that they were merely distinguishing between people in real or self-inflicted need (the distinction between deserving and undeserving homeless once again), or between the 'genuine' homeless and people who were merely taking society for a ride, they were actually helping to create a climate of hostility towards all beggars and all homeless people. Indeed, the *Sun* failed even to acknowledge the difference between begging and *Big Issue* selling, when it returned to the theme of its '£200-a-day beggar' with another front-page story in 1996 'exposing' a '£150-a-day *Big Issue* seller' (*Sun*, 28 October 1996). Sometimes, it seems, homeless people just can't win.

Hostility in the media responded to and reinforced hostility on the part of politicians. In 1994, on a visit to Bristol during the European election campaign, John Major invited citizens 'to "shop" beggars and drive them out of the city' since the sight of beggars was 'an eyesore' and 'begging for cash is inexcusable and unnecessary' (Bristol *Evening Post*, 27 May 1994). A year later, Jack Straw urged a crackdown on 'aggressive beggars, winos and squeegee merchants' as part of a New York-style zero tolerance campaign. In a detailed interview in the *Big Issue* in 1997, Tony Blair seemed to be joining the chorus of disapproval by announcing his support for 'the basic principle' that 'it is right to be intolerant of homeless people on the streets' (*Big Issue*, 6 January 1997). Tory politicians such as the then junior minister, David MacLean, took this as a green light to go ballistic on the issue. MacLean claimed that there were no 'genuine' beggars in Britain because there were plenty of social security benefits (he also added, for good measure, that the majority of beggars were Scottish). Backbencher Terry Dicks threw in his three ha'pence worth by suggesting that beggars should be hosed from the streets (*Guardian*, 11 January 1997).

Again and again, the language used in the press communicated an almost visceral hatred of certain categories of homeless people. By the early 1990s, a new moral panic about squatters, travellers and the emergent 'rave culture' opened the floodgates for a fresh round of scapegoating and abuse. Nor was this limited to the more rabidly right-wing tabloids. The *Sun*'s propensity to overuse of the term 'scum' to describe everyone from IRA terrorists to single-parent squatters was matched by the same sort of dehumanising language elsewhere. Thus, for example, the *Daily Telegraph*, in June 1993, felt no qualms about lumping all squatters and travellers together in an editorial demanding tough government action against this 'swarming tribe of human locusts'.

More recently, asylum seekers, refugees and the disparagingly-titled 'economic migrants' (as if there is something wrong in people migrating in search of a better life for themselves and their families) have been on the receiving end of this sort of thing. Sometimes the language used in the press would not have been out of place in the Nazis' propaganda sheet, *Der Sturmer*. 'While Labour luvvies dribble on at that most historic of northern pleasure outposts, Blackpool,' the *Dover Express* editorialised about Roma and Kosovan asylum seekers in October 1998, for instance, 'we are left with the backdraft of a nation's human sewage and no cash to wash it down the drain. They are parasites who milk the welfare system, shoplift, pickpocket, hang around insulting women and run brothels,' the paper declared.

National newspapers were more circumspect in their choice of words when covering the issue. But the *Daily Mail*'s 'special investigation' into asylum seekers at around the same time ('The good life on asylum alley' as its final headline put it) had much the same inflammatory effect on public opinion. The *Mail* had published the details of properties used to accommodate asylum seekers in Dover. Shortly afterwards the occupants had their windows broken and fireworks thrown inside. 'We will burn you out' threatened a sign left at the scene of the attack.

Homeless people: a 'warts and all' view

It is unsurprising, in the context of such hostility towards people who do not fit the acceptable face of the deserving homeless, that so much media coverage of homelessness shies away from a properly rounded portrayal of its subject matter. A 'warts and all' write-up of homeless people is difficult to attempt, if one's sympathies lie first with the homeless, when the revelation of a single wart is likely to be seized upon as evidence that homeless people are rotten through and through.

Even without such a consideration, there is the problem that the media in general likes to deal in simple stereotypes (Liddiard and Hutson 1998). There is rarely the room here to represent all the complexities of different personalities and human behaviour that mean that the world cannot be divided into straightforward victims and villains, deserving and undeserving. Those sections of the media that start with a more liberal or sympathetic approach to the homeless deal no less in stereotypes than the rest. Reflecting the attitudes of the public at large, they find it difficult to hold onto the fact that someone who is homeless may be both unlikeable and in need at the same time, may be spending too much of their money on drink or drugs and still be worthy of help in getting enough to eat, may have lost their last home in part due to their own actions but still need a roof over their head now. Not all of the homeless are angels, any more than anyone else; not many of them fall into the unambiguously 'deserving' category of that holy family who were forced to sleep in a stable because there was no room at the inn two millennia ago.

In George McKay's compilation, *DIY Culture: Party and Protest in Nineties Britain*, Jim Carey of *Squall* magazine, which has its roots in squatter and traveller communities, tells the story of how the Squall workers were approached in the mid-1990s by a staff feature writer at the *Daily Telegraph*. 'She was keen to write an article on squatting and wanted to know whether we knew any 'middle-class squatters' she could interview. Asked what she meant by the phrase, she replied: 'People who earn a high wage and squat for fun.' She was told that Squall had never heard of a high wage earner who squatted for fun but that we might be able to put her in touch with some real squatters. She replied: 'Well, er, unfortunately, you know how it is, this isn't what the *Telegraph* readers want to read about. Do you know any that earn a wage, are articulate and preferably good-looking?' (McKay 1998).

The other side to this coin is provided by the purveyors of media images of homelessness that have never really gone beyond those grainy, black-and-white Cathy-style pictures from the 1960s. When the short-lived *Sunday Correspondent* turned over an entire issue of its magazine to the subject of homelessness in early 1990, it did so on the back of a specially commissioned series of monochrome pictures of homeless-as-victims by Don McCullin. 'Ignored: Britain's poor and huddled masses' said the headline. The *Observer* and *Sunday Times* colour supplements, the *New Statesman* and other publications that would normally want to maximise the use of colour in their pages, all did likewise around the same time. Just as the homeless are always with us, so too, it seems, are our preferred ways of seeing them.

Nowhere is this better understood than at Shelter. Few people will ever have heard of Anne Saunders, but anyone with any interest in homelessness during the 1970s and 1980s is likely to have come across her picture. Shelter's magazine, *Roof*, described her in 1988 as a 'homeless megastar . . . without doubt the most famous homeless person in the land. Or, rather, her photograph is the most popular *image* of homelessness in circulation' (*Roof*, November–December 1988).

The photo shows Anne, head bowed, with a tatty suitcase in one hand while she pushes a baby buggy with the other, struggling against the wind and rain down some isolated country lane. It was used originally on the cover of a 1974 Shelter report on bed-and-breakfast and then on a Shelter poster under the slogan 'Homelessness is Hell'. Her image cropped up repeatedly over the next decade – with the photo itself being cropped to suit local circumstances. For a leaflet in Liverpool, the council cut out the original rural backdrop and substituted a local terraced street; for a report in Hamilton, the designers added some high-rise blocks. In 1987, she featured as the British representative in International Year of Shelter for the Homeless publicity material, since when she has continued to appear in countless newspaper and articles, the image of first choice out of the many thousands of possibilities in the Shelter photo library, for picture editors around the globe.

Roof described Anne Saunders' continuing appeal as 'a sad comment on people's perceptions of an *acceptable* image of homelessness'. It summarised the key elements in that appeal as follows:

> First, she's seen as *literally homeless* – she's out in the open with no roof over her head. People seeing the image don't know that she's en route to the launderette and actually staying in the farmhouse in the background; they see her as trudging down a desolate country lane with nowhere to stay and all her belongings stuffed into one tatty suitcase. She can be seen as homeless in the way the government wants to define homelessness – as *rooflessness* – which is ironic in that most people using this image are committed to a much wider definition of homelessness.
>
> Second, she's seen as *vulnerable*. She is pictured without a man to support and protect her and with a dependent child in a desolate and lonely spot.
>
> Third, she is seen as obviously *deserving*. She's not pretty and vivacious, she's not a flash piece in miniskirt and leather jacket; she's plump, ordinary and dowdily dressed, as befits her homeless status. As time passes, her clothes look even more dowdy and out of date – so much the better. The buggy is a Mothercare basic rather than a Maclaren GTi model: it looks as though it might be second-hand – more brownie points for thrifty, impoverished, deserving Anne. The child looks well cared-for, which is important, and Anne's not puffing on a cigarette, which is *very* important.
>
> Fourth, she is seen to be *stoical*. She isn't taking it out on the child by battering or neglecting it, she isn't protesting, she isn't giving up, she's plodding on in search of somewhere to stay.
>
> These are the reasons that Anne Saunders remains top of the homelessness pops, and it's a depressing thought. The most popular image of homelessness is a stereotypical Madonna and child without a roof over their heads, an image evoking pity and admiration.
>
> (*Roof*, November–December 1988: 6–7)

As a contrast with this, it is worth examining the response to the Channel 4 documentary *No home for Barry*, first screened in the summer of 1990. This followed Barry from when he first arrived in London at the beginning of that year and charted his experiences sleeping rough, trying to sort out accommodation and money and dealing with the gradual deterioration in his emotional and physical health as his problems mounted. The fact that he seemed to bring many of these problems upon himself – not turning up for an appointment at the Job Centre, getting kicked out of his hostel – meant that he wasn't a natural candidate for public sympathy, and many people felt that someone less 'unattractive' should have been filmed to put across the problems facing the homeless instead. One viewer used the *Right to Reply* programme to put his comments thus:

> 'My concern is not for this individual fortunate enough to have his dilettante dilemma logged by a camera crew. It is for the authentically desperate. Every cliché of prejudice against them – that they're in a situation of their own making, they're workshy, shiftless and idle – will have been confirmed by the use of such an untypical and unappetising example of the homeless.'

Similar qualms were expressed about BBC2's *Video Diaries* at the end of May that same year. This gave two young hostel dwellers the chance to tell their stories free from any consideration of the need to present 'acceptable' images of homelessness. One spoke of blowing almost her entire £29.50 social security allowance for the week on a single night out: '£15 for some ecstasy, £8 to get in, £2 for a drink and then just bunk the tubes 'cos I've got no more money.' As with Barry, it was all but guaranteed to pull the very opposite triggers to that long-popular photo image of Anne Saunders.

Any truthful representation of homelessness would have to acknowledge that the ranks of the homeless include the Barrys of this world as well as the Cathys. But any full – and truly meaningful – consideration of the subject needs to go beyond the individual. Each person's individual circumstances are different; each person individually may have a greater or lesser degree of responsibility for their own situation. But social, economic and political forces override the individual. Homelessness, when it comes down to it, is a social problem, not an individual one.

With the best will in the world, this presents a problem for the popular media, which is always better at telling an individual story rather than providing meaningful social analysis. Whatever the motives of the storyteller, therefore, there is a compelling need to keep things simple, to keep the story line straight, if for no other reason than that this is what the reader wants. For those who deal in straightforward heroes and villains – the deserving and undeserving – there is no dilemma here. For those who would try to represent nuance and complexity, it is much more of a problem.

References

Bailey, R. (1973) *The Squatters*, London: Penguin.

Brynin, M. (1987) 'The young homeless: pressure groups, politics and the press', *Youth and Policy* 20: 24–34.

Burrows, R., Pleace, N. and Quilgars, G. (1997) *Homelessness and Social Policy*, London: Routledge.

Liddiard, M. and Hutson, S. (1998) 'Youth homelessness, the press and public attitudes', *Youth and Policy* 59: 57–70.

McKay, G. (1998) *DiY Culture: Party and Protest in Nineties Britain*, London: Verso.

Platt, S. (1977) *Squatters Myth and Fact*, London: Self Help Housing Resource Library.

—— (1980) 'A decade of squatting: the story of squatting in Britain since 1968', in N. Wates and C. Wolmar (eds) *Squatting, the Real Story* London: Bay Leaf Books.

—— (1993) 'Without walls', in a special issue of *New Statesman* 'Gimme shelter' devoted to issues around homelessness, 2 April 1993.

Rose, L. (1993) *Rogues and Vagabonds: Vagrant Underworld in Britain*, London: Routledge.

Chapter 7

The picture of health?

Media coverage of the health service

Vikki Entwistle and Trevor Sheldon

Introduction

Health and medical stories feature prominently in news and current affairs media, in part reflecting their obvious relevance to many people. We all get sick and we all have some sort of stake in health services. Media coverage of health care reflects and reinforces our hopes, fears and concerns. Analyses of media coverage of health services can provide insights into the political and social dynamics of health care, the media, and social values. This chapter examines the findings of selected studies of news and current affairs reporting of health and medicine. It explores various factors that influence how journalists identify, select and present stories about the health service, and reviews recent developments in health care and the reporting of health care.

Studies of media coverage of health and medicine

Researchers from a range of disciplines have analysed media coverage of health and medicine. Their studies have varied in terms of the media genres they have examined, the scope of their subject matter and the analytic approaches they have used. This section summarises selected studies of UK media coverage of health policy and health care. While much of the discussion is relevant to news reporting of health care issues in other countries, there are international differences in media coverage that reflect social and cultural differences as well as the highly variable ways of financing, organising and regulating both health care and the news media.

Several researchers have identified recurring paradigms in media coverage of health and medicine. Journalists, editors and producers, like the rest of us, view the world through interpretive frameworks – conceptual spectacles that filter information and cause it to be seen and understood in particular ways. 'The use of interpretive frameworks in news and current affairs reporting will mean that a certain pattern of selection of events will appear newsworthy' (Best *et al.* 1977: 23). It also means that events will tend to be presented in particular ways.

An analysis of the nature and range of interpretive frameworks used in health reporting is important because the media have significant potential to shape the ways in which audiences view and understand health policy and health service issues, and the ways in which people interact with health services (the same is true for mental health, see Chapter 8).

The mass media and the National Health Service (1970s)

In 1977, Best *et al.* argued that media reporting of health services was underpinned by three assumptions:

(a) that the aims and practices of modern scientific medicine represent 'excellence' in health care and are central to progress in health;
(b) that the production and consumption of health services are the principal means of promoting better health;
(c) that because the National Health Service (NHS) is part of the public services sector of the economy, better health (more health services) depends on the creation of more 'wealth' in the market sector of the economy.

(Best *et al.* 1977: 23–24)

This analysis had several implications for the types of stories that the media reported. Familiar contemporary story lines included the opening of a new hospital, the discovery of a new 'cure', the latest organ transplant, and statements about the need to curtail health spending because economic growth was inhibited by public-sector borrowing. High technology, institutional-based curing activities received more attention in media reports than community or home-based caring activities, and technical procedures to deal with health problems received more attention than simple measures to prevent health problems. Finally, the increasing level of spending on health care and other public services was reported and framed by news media as a problem (Best *et al.* 1977: 26–27).

Doctoring the media (1980s)

Just over a decade later, the medical news stories that Karpf found familiar were: 'the breakthrough (an operation or new treatment, often connected with hearts or babies, or better still, both); the disaster (health consequences of earthquakes, fires, explosions, accidents); the ethical controversy (currently surrogate mothers, test-tube babies); the scandal (deaths from prescribed drugs, drugs withdrawn from sale, mental hospital stories); the strike (National Health Service dispute); the epidemic (its course and treatment); and the official report or speech – government or medical – on a health problem' (Karpf 1988: 28–29).

Karpf identified four main interpretive frameworks or approaches to the reporting of health and medicine. The medical approach celebrates 'medicine's curative powers'. On television, this approach features white coated male doctors, stethoscopes, ambulances, test tubes, injections, operating theatres and drips. The approach is organised around diseases (particularly acute diseases) that disrupt the body's normal functioning, but it does not investigate the causes of disease. The approach focuses on clinical investigations and operations, emphasising high technology, hospital-based interventions. Medical doctors are considered the legitimate authority on what constitutes disease and how it should be treated. The approach embodies a conviction that doctors will find a cure for disease, and equates health with medicine. It implicitly tells patients and potential patients what medicine could do for them.

The consumer approach – 'criticising the doctor–patient relationship' – presents patients' experiences and views of illness, medical care and the doctor–patient relationship. It focuses on the consultation and suggests that there are conflicts of interest between the doctor exercising power and the patient struggling to empower herself. Programmes (or articles) developed within this approach recommend sources of health information, give information that could help patients make choices and report on self-help groups. They compare treatments and spell out their consequences, sometimes focusing on illness that is itself caused by medical treatments.

The look-after-yourself approach – 'appealing for changes in individual behaviour' – focuses on aspects of individual behaviour and lifestyle that cause or prevent illness. It presents patients as active, though perhaps unwitting self-harmers who have the ability to prevent their illnesses. Programmes (or articles) developed within this approach dispense advice and encourage audiences to stop smoking, eat healthily and get fit. Medical doctors play an important role, but as authoritative health educators rather than providers of cures.

The environmental approach – 'stressing the social origins of illness' – focuses on preventable causes of illness. Rather than blaming individual lifestyles, however, it implicates environmental and social factors as major contributors to ill health. The approach is explicitly political. It also reflects disquiet about science and challenges the notion that technological solutions are always safe and always represent progress (adapted from Karpf 1988: 9–22).

Karpf argued that these four ways of framing health stories were all current in the wider culture and suggested that they did not represent an exhaustive compendium of all medical programming. Rather, they were 'skeletons which individual programmes flesh out in their own way, with cross-breeds and hybrids aplenty' (Karpf 1988: 9). Karpf believed that the medical approach was most deeply embedded in the British media (Karpf 1988: 25), and that this approach was likely to continue to dominate (Karpf 1988: 236–239). Since the publication of Karpf's book, several more narrowly focused analyses of media coverage of health-care issues have supported the existence of the approaches to reporting that she identified. Some, however, have challenged her argument that the medical approach to reporting is dominant.

'Sexy docs and busty blondes'

Bradby, Gabe and Bury (1995) studied tabloid news reports of hearings by the General Medical Council's professional conduct committee in 1990–91. Not surprisingly, given tabloid newspapers' interest in salacious stories, they found that cases of doctors committing sexual offences against patients received prominent coverage. By contrast, relatively few of the cases involving non-sexual offences against patients, colleagues, the medical profession or health authorities were reported as news. There was little overt criticism of doctors' professional conduct. The problem of sexual misconduct by doctors was constructed as one of male 'sexual urges' rather than as an abuse of professional power (Bradby, Gabe and Bury 1995: 468). 'As a result', the authors argued, 'the picture presented has been somewhat ambiguous, both challenging and enhancing medical authority' (Bradby, Gabe and Bury 1995: 473). Reference to Karpf's categories suggests that the cases of sexual misconduct were reported within the consumerist framework, but this was overwritten by the dominant stereotypes that are used in reporting of gender and sexual issues. The lack of criticism of professional conduct appears to reflect a medical approach to reporting.

'Medical dominance or trial by media?'

Bury and Gabe selected three television programmes (an exposé transmitted in 1988, a documentary from 1993 and a drama first televised in 1986) to illustrate their argument that television 'though falling short of putting medicine regularly on trial, now represents health and medicine in a more challenging light than it once did' (Bury and Gabe 1994: 66).

The exposé programme focused on problems associated with lorazepam, a benzodiazapene tranquilliser. Individual users of the drug highlighted its side effects and the difficulties of withdrawing from it once addicted. The programme placed most of the blame for these problems on the company that produced the drug which Bury and Gabe believed was 'an easy target . . . given the pharmaceutical industry's long standing role in contemporary society as a potent symbol of indefensible profit making' (Bury and Gabe 1994: 72). But the programme was also critical of the medical profession, arguing that general practitioners should not have continued so readily to prescribe the drugs and should have given their patients more help to withdraw from them.

The documentary highlighted examples of the poor conditions encountered by patients and staff within a London teaching hospital. It considered resource problems and an ongoing efficiency drive. It exposed competing claims on resources from different departments within the hospital and tensions between medical staff and managers. Bury and Gabe argued that 'in such a context the image of the doctor as hero, saving lives against the odds, now has to compete with a new image of the doctor as a representative of sectional interests' (Bury and Gabe 1994: 77).

The drama studied was an episode of *Casualty* that was first screened in 1992. The episode included a scene in which a manager informed a consultant that his bid for a trauma unit in his department had been unsuccessful. Other scenes involving discussions between characters revealed various opinions about the reasons underlying the decision and the consequences of it. The consultant went to the press and claimed that medical opinion was being overridden, patient care was deteriorating and the failure to win the bid for the trauma unit would make matters worse. Thus among the various sub-plots involving the patients, the drama explored the possibility that doctors can be preoccupied with politics as well as clinical care, that there are tensions among health-care staffs and that financial issues can affect the quality of care provided for patients.

Research in medical journals and newspapers

A study in 1995 analysed a sample of reports published in two prestigious medical journals, the *British Medical Journal* (*BMJ*) and the *Lancet*, and compared them with news articles in broadsheet newspapers, to try to establish the extent to which professional discussions of health issues were reported in the lay press (Entwistle 1995). The five journal-article topics most widely reported as news were: the number of deaths caused by tobacco smoking, a new treatment for people who have had a heart attack, the success rates of assisted conception techniques, evidence that small babies were more likely to develop diabetes, and the problems experienced by people with diabetes who were transferred from human to animal insulin (Entwistle 1995: 921). Of these, the three topics that were about the treatment rather than the cause of health problems were all based on research into the effects of fairly 'new' treatments for common problems. Human insulin was particularly controversial at the time and a legal case was being fought by people who claimed to be adversely affected by it. Some research papers that the journals considered sufficiently important to include in their press releases did not trigger adequate interest among journalists to generate stories in the lay press. Research reporting that many elderly people had visual problems, for example, that had not been recognised by health professionals was not picked up as news. Nor was an article that described the use of questionnaires to help general practitioners target asthma care or an article that argued that the British medical system discriminated against Asian doctors (Entwistle 1995: 921).

The widespread reporting of promising new developments within medicine combined with the relative journalistic neglect of low-technology medicine and the health problems of older people are consistent with Karpf's description of a medical approach to coverage informed by assumptions identified by Best and colleagues. While reports of problems associated with human insulin might at face value be assumed to reflect a consumerist approach to reporting, they originated from a traditional medical source and varied in the credibility they attached to patients' own reports of problems.

These studies suggest that over a period of at least two decades, an approach to reporting that emphasises the benefits of technological medicine has persisted in at least some elements of news reporting of health and medicine, but other interpretive frameworks have also been used. Recent developments in health care and the frameworks used to report them are discussed later in the chapter following a consideration of some of the key influences on media coverage of health care.

Influences on media coverage

A range of actors and other factors influence news and current affairs reporting about health services. The main actors are the journalists, producers and editors on the one hand, and the organisations and individuals who serve as subjects and sources of stories on the other. The other factors that have an impact include the interests and aims of both of these groups, and the norms and constraints of the environments in which they operate.

Journalists

The importance of health and medical topics to the media is illustrated by the fact that most national newspapers and radio and television news programmes have specialist health, health services or medical correspondents. These are mostly experienced journalists who, having secured their specialist positions, tend to remain in post for some time. Consequently, they tend to acquire some subject expertise and come to know their regular sources of news and stories quite well. Like all journalists, however, they are subject to the constraints of news or current affairs reporting and the norms of the media outlets they work for.

The stories that journalists write and the way they are written partly reflect the imperatives and occupational rules of journalism, but they are also influenced by journalists' role perceptions and values. News reporters have deadlines to meet and a limited amount of space or air time to work with. The stories they write about health care have to compete with stories about other topics and will be judged using the same criteria of newsworthiness. Journalists are therefore under pressure to produce stories that are dramatic (perhaps unexpected or controversial), unambiguous, relevant to their audiences, and preferably personalised (Hartley 1982: 75–81).

Journalists who are pressed for time acknowledge that the activities of the press and public relations officers in a wide variety of organisations can influence their selection and development of stories. They make use of press releases that bring events to their attention, present issues as newsworthy, suggest frames or angles for reporting, offer quotable comments and generally make it easier for them to write a story. Journalists, moreover, tend to rely quite heavily on a limited number of regular sources. The specialist health correspondents on national newspapers, for example, routinely look through the *Lancet* and the *British Medical Journal*. They expect to be able to base at least one story each week on a research paper or letter published in those journals (Entwistle 1995: 920).

Journalists develop approaches to help them identify and select stories quickly. Specialist health and medical correspondents interviewed in 1991 and 1992 said there were certain topics that they routinely recognised as potentially newsworthy. These included: common and fatal diseases, rare but interesting or quirky diseases, health problems with a sexual connection, new or improved treatments, and controversial subject matter or research findings (Entwistle 1995: 921). Some topics are newsworthy for a while and then go out of fashion. For example, during the mid-1980s, quarterly statistics about the numbers of people who had died from AIDS were routinely turned into news articles. Now these statistics are rarely reported (see Williams: Chapter 4). In the late 1990s, journalists seem more interested in cases of meningitis and new variant Creuzfeldt Jacob Disease.

Health and medical correspondents often have a complex set of role perceptions. They need to write or produce reports that will interest audiences. They may also be keen to provide information that will benefit readers, for example by alerting them to effective new treatments or problems with existing ones. Some have a sense of responsibility not to unduly raise hopes or cause alarm, but they recognise that this may conflict with the need to present unambiguous and dramatic stories. Some journalists perceive themselves as acting as watchdogs for the public interest. They are thus keen to scrutinise the activities of health-care providers and to report on the availability and effects of treatments. Some journalists will explicitly or implicitly take up a campaigning stance, for example to encourage greater recognition of a debilitating problem, to lobby for provision of a particular service or to raise funds for a local hospice or particular items of hospital equipment.

Journalists' values influence their stories. Their opinions about particular organisations and individuals will influence their decisions about whether or not to report particular events, who to approach or use as sources, and how to package different viewpoints. Their perceptions of the motives, credibility and public authority of information sources are likely to favour some over others. The pharmaceutical industry, for example, may be presented less sympathetically in the media than medical research charities, and medical doctors may be given more credibility than health service managers or health professionals such as nurses who are perceived to be lower in the professional hierarchy.

The NHS and its environment: media subjects and sources

The NHS has diverse and overlapping social roles which means it may be viewed from several perspectives. It is a provider of health care, a social institution for the protection and support of individuals in need and also an employer. Again, the NHS is an arena in which professional groups obtain and use power, it is a user of public and private finance and a cause of household spending and finally the NHS is a purchaser of pharmaceuticals, medical and surgical devices, and other commodities. Consequently, it is a highly politicised institution that embodies many contested values.

The NHS, moreover, interacts with a range of organisations and individuals, including politicians, professional organisations and workers' unions, patient and consumer groups, the pharmaceutical industry and suppliers of diverse types of equipment and consumables. Many of these serve as both subjects and sources of news stories. Some of them see the media as important means of communication and influence, not least because they offer the attractive possibility of influencing public perceptions (and hence of generating pressure for action) without having to go through professional or government channels. In this section we consider some of the motivations and strategies that organisations have for negotiating access to the media and influencing media content.

Media reports of events in the health service are of key importance to politicians as one of the main currencies of success or failure. Politicians with responsibilities in the Department of Health need to be seen to be improving health care or successfully implementing government policies. They also need to avoid publicity that might reduce public confidence in the health service or themselves. For these reasons, they increasingly attempt to secure the kinds of media coverage that serve their interests. The Department of Health has a 'good news unit' that makes regular announcements to promote coverage of favourable news stories and a 'rebuttal unit' that collects material to help press officers respond to criticisms. Spin doctors serving as advisors to ministers also work to ensure that favourable interpretations are placed upon events and that bad news and unfavourable interpretations are stifled (Butler 1998: Chapter 1).

Health service managers also have reasons for using the media. They might want to explain to their local population, for example, why they propose to configure services in a particular way. They might also seek to influence demand for services, either upwards or downwards. They may, for example, want to promote uptake of care among people with conditions for which effective treatments are under utilised, or to discourage people from consulting about trivial conditions that can be appropriately self-medicated (Rogers *et al.* 1998: 1817). Managers might also see the media as a means of encouraging the public to contribute to the NHS, for example in the form of blood or organ donation, first aid training or funds for expensive equipment or services.

Health service managers are often supported by dedicated communication executives or press officers (Lloyd 1998).

Other organisations have different reasons for seeking favourable media coverage. Patient groups, for example, may be keen to secure higher profiles and improved services for their members; professional groups may be looking for support for their pay claims or sectional interests; researchers may seek to raise the profile and impact of their work; charities that provide services or fund research seek public awareness of, and donations to, their cause; and pharmaceutical companies want to encourage sales of their products. In the USA, media reports are also very important to health-care organisations who are competing for a market share (Johnson 1998).

Organisations gear themselves up to engage with the media according to the importance they attach to securing favourable publicity and the resources they are able to dedicate to it. Organisations with sophisticated media relations arrangements are likely to have an advantage over those that are not so well equipped, and patterns of media relations activity may well influence the distribution and nature of media coverage (see Chapters 3 and 4). Over twenty years ago, Best *et al.* suggested that the dominant framework of reporting that they observed was reinforced by the 'well developed public relations activities' of medical equipment manufacturers, pharmaceutical companies and medical professional organisations. These activities drew attention to technological innovations, 'miracle drugs' and professional policies (Best 1977: 28). As organisations representing other interests have developed their media relations activities, there is more competition for the attention of journalists. Journalists are now exposed to, and encouraged to adopt, a wider range of interpretive frameworks. But they still think about their sources and make their own decisions about whether or not to use particular stories and angles.

Media relations activity influences health policy and services

Attempts to secure access to the media and favourable coverage can directly or indirectly influence policy and practice. Pressure on politicians to keep announcing good news, for example, may lead to health policy initiatives or health service developments being launched prematurely, repackaged or relaunched in order to maintain an image of progress. Eventually, this may descend to the level of 'stunts' that have more to do with fuelling publicity than developing effective action to meet considered policy objectives (Maynard and Sheldon 1997). When policy makers are in the thrall of the news media, health policy is likely to become short term, less strategic and more dominated by daily events.

Pressure to suppress or contain bad news, and to be seen to be responding to problems, may also lead to policy makers being over hasty and populist. A Secretary of State for Health, for example, commenting on a judgment passed by the General Medical Council after a lengthy hearing about the performance of heart surgeons in Bristol (see p. 128), said on television that he thought all three doctors (rather than only two of them) should have been struck off the medical register. It was suggested that his statement was influenced by spin doctors' interpretation of public opinion, and that 'in a calmer moment he surely would not advocate judgment by public opinion rather than a judicial process that operates under act of parliament' (Smith 1998: 1917–1918).

Constraints on media relations

Sources within and outside the National Health Service (NHS) may experience constraints on what they can say to journalists because of contractual obligations, legal requirements, or ethical norms. In the 1990s, for example, during the last years of the recent Conservative government, many NHS employees had gagging clauses built into their contracts to prevent them 'blowing the whistle' to journalists about problems in the health service. Until the early 1990s, professional codes of conduct discouraged doctors from reporting incompetent or negligent colleagues (General Medical Council 1987), and peer pressure continues to be a deterrent (Snell 1998). Health-care professionals are ethically obliged to treat patients in confidence and are therefore not able to comment to the media about particular cases unless the patients concerned give their permission.

Recent developments in health care and the media

Journalists' interpretive frameworks are not independent of the paradigms used by other members of society, so changes in the ways in which society looks at health-care policy and services are likely to lead to changes in the types of stories carried in the media.

Over the last few decades there have been some significant shifts in the ways in which people in Britain look at medicine and health services. These shifts often correspond to broader social trends and some are triggered or accelerated by particular events. The media have been 'implicated' in many of the changes, but their precise influence is difficult to establish. Some of the most important changes and how they might be linked to the introduction of new interpretive frameworks and emphases in reporting are discussed below.

The erosion of medical power

The authority and power of medical doctors has been substantially challenged and their mystique has to some extent been deconstructed. Pressure has increased for doctors to be more accountable, and professional self-regulation has become less acceptable. Many factors have influenced these changes, which have also been seen in other professions.

Within health care, growing awareness of variations in medical practice led to the realisation that clinical practice does not always reflect what research evidence has been shown to be most effective at improving health (Smith 1992: 117). A movement promoting 'evidence-based health care', developed largely from within the professions (Evidence-based Working Group 1992), and policy makers and health service managers started to encourage 'clinical effectiveness' (NHS Executive 1996a).

The rise of evidence-based health care and the contesting of the hegemony of the medical profession have strengthened the view that research evidence in the public domain is a sounder basis for decision making than the opinion of senior doctors, however eminent these doctors might be. The traditional sources of medical authority including the Royal Colleges have been challenged by the increasing availability of research evidence, which sometimes contradicts their opinions.

Probably one of the most significant events to affect the standing of the medical profession in Britain in recent years was a case involving surgeons from Bristol who had high mortality rates for their surgery on children with heart problems. An anaesthetist who was concerned about the surgery was unsuccessful in his attempts to get something done about it and the surgeons continued to operate despite the poor outcomes. Eventually, a newspaper article about the surgeons prompted the General Medical Council to initiate an enquiry (Anonymous 1998). The enquiry highlighted many issues relating to the setting and assessment of clinical standards and the training and monitoring of individual professionals (Smith 1998; Treasure 1998) and brought the medical profession to a 'defining moment' (Horton 1998: 1901).

The Bristol case attracted a lot of media interest that in turn accelerated the introduction of, and gave more legitimacy to, several new policies aimed at improving standards of health care. These included the introduction of a performance management framework, including the publication of hospital mortality rates, and clinical governance (Smith 1998: 1917). These policy responses also reflect the greater use of external verification or audit of activity that is typical of the 'new public management' (Power 1977: 10).

Examples of clinicians or health-care organisations making mistakes or achieving poor outcomes from their care now appear quite often in the news. Problems that have been highlighted recently include misdiagnoses, failure to investigate fully the cause of symptoms, delays in the initiation of appropriate treatment, and overtreatment. Problems with particular medical techniques and with the technology that supports screening and treatment systems are also reported. The following selection of headlines is typical of articles critical of doctors and medical systems: 'Patients claim they woke during surgery' (*Guardian*, 17 February 1998); 'E.-coli victims "suffered from delays"' (*Independent*, 22 April 1998); '"Misdiagnosis" claim doctor had earlier missed boy's rare illness' (*Scotsman*, 7 May 1998); 'Therapy error in cancer cases' (*Press and Journal*, 8 May 1998); 'Danger doc put women at risk' (*Scottish Mirror*, 17 July 1998); 'Surgeon is suspended over breast operations' (*Scotsman*, 17 July 1998), and 'Disease could be spread by surgical tools' (*Daily Telegraph*, 28 August 1998).

In addition to the 'naming and shaming' of apparently poorly performing or negligent doctors the institutions of medicine have recently been examined critically in the public domain. *The Citadel*, a programme screened by Channel 4, featured the editor of the *Lancet* challenging the medical establishment as it is represented by the Royal Colleges of Surgeons and Physicians, the British Medical Association and the General Medical Council. Articles in broadsheet newspapers have also criticised professional institutions. A recent feature claimed that 'Although they call themselves "guardians" of clinical standards, the 14 medical royal colleges and three faculties of Britain and Ireland do not boast an enviable record in encouraging medical progress' (Moore 1998: 2).

The rise of consumerism

The decrease in professional power and authority has been accompanied by increasing attention to the views of patients, the public and organisations representing their interests. The NHS 'patient partnership' strategy professes a commitment to promoting the involvement of individual patients in decisions about their care, and to enabling service users to influence NHS policy and planning (NHS Executive 1996b: 4). Although implementation of this policy is far from complete, activities to promote consumer participation in various aspects of health care are becoming more widespread.

In keeping with government policy, news reports no longer always assume that doctors should decide what is best for patients. Several cases of people who have been treated contrary to their wishes have been reported as news stories and the right to choose to refuse treatment or to opt for active euthanasia has also been debated in the pages of the press. Respect for individual patients' preferences is embedded in the framing of some reports.

The promotion of patient involvement in health-care decision making has highlighted the need to give people information about the effects of health-care interventions (Entwistle *et al.* 1998). The importance of information has also been highlighted in the courts, where patients have sought redress because they believe that companies selling products or doctors delivering interventions have given inadequate or misleading information on their risks and benefits. These cases tend to be widely reported.

Technological innovation continues

New drugs, devices and techniques are continually being developed in attempts to improve health care and generate profits. The recent emphasis on evidence-based health care and clinical effectiveness, however, has stressed the need to assess health technologies and evaluate the benefits and harms of new developments.

Promising new drugs and technical developments are still enthusiastically reported as news and the media do not seem to have lost their appetite for stories of progress towards a cure for cancer. There have been changes, however, in the types of development that are reported within the framework of technical progress in medicine. Some of the transplants that were once reported as news, for example, are now a relatively routine part of medical practice. Today only complex multi-organ transplants or those carried out on very young babies make the news. The Human Genome project has attracted much interest in recent years and the identification of genes associated with particular diseases is now fairly regularly reported (sometimes prematurely) as progress on the way to a cure. The following represents a typical crop of headlines triggered by technological developments: 'Drug found to cut the risk of breast cancer by half' (*Daily Telegraph*, 7 April 1998); 'Gene holds key to beat lung cancer' (*Daily Mail*, 28 April 1998); 'Cancer: is this finally a cure? New drug can destroy tumours' (*Express*, 5 May 1998); 'British team leads race for cancer "cure"' (*Independent*, 6 May 1998); 'New drug to fight obesity "epidemic"' (*Daily Telegraph*, 17 July 1998); 'Hereditary cancer link discovered' (*Guardian*, 22 July 1998), and 'Ultrasound used in new test for risk of Down's syndrome' (*Scotsman*, 31 July 1998).

Another departure in 'new medical technology' reporting is that more attention is now paid to treatments primarily for older people. Hormone replacement therapy for menopausal women, for example, prostate cancer screening for older men, new but as yet poorly evaluated treatments for dementia, and Viagra, a drug for erectile dysfunction have attracted considerable media interest. The proportion of older people in the population is growing and they have become a more politically and economically significant constituency.

If side effects are mentioned in news articles about the introduction of new treatments, they tend to be downplayed and given little attention. Other news articles, however, focus on the problems of treatments and emphasise what is wrong with them, saying little about their benefits. The frameworks used in news reports appear to vary along the 'career' of a health technology (McKinlay 1981). For example, a contraceptive implant, Norplant, received a lot of favourable publicity when it was launched in 1993. Early articles highlighted its contraceptive effectiveness, convenience, long-term action and reversibility. Although some articles mentioned side effects, these tended to be dismissed as minor. A few years later, it emerged that some women experienced heavy and prolonged menstrual bleeding while using the contraceptive implant and difficulties when they tried to have it removed. Media coverage of Norplant in 1995 and 1996 was almost entirely negative, focusing on the problems experienced by some users and losing sight of the usefulness and acceptability of the product to others (Entwistle *et al.* forthcoming).

Concern with social solidarity and fairness in the NHS

Although it is now recognised that some forms of care have always been rationed within the NHS (Sheldon and Maynard 1993), rationing was rarely publicly discussed until the media started to report the case of Jaymee Bowen referred to initially in media reports as Child B.

Jaymee had an aggressive form of leukaemia and her doctors thought there was only a slim chance of her being cured. The treatment that offered the chance of a cure had such distressing side effects that the doctors thought it was not in her best interests. Jaymee's father disagreed and found a doctor who was willing to treat her privately. However, Jaymee's health authority refused to fund this treatment on the NHS. Jaymee's father took the health authority to court and his story to the news media. Jaymee was treated privately with an unevaluated new treatment and survived for almost a year. She became a celebrity as the media followed her progress. When she died, little attention was paid to the adverse effects of the treatment she received, and she was remembered as the plucky little girl whose case brought rationing to public attention (Entwistle *et al.* 1996a: 587 and 1996b: 87–88 and 158–170).

Jaymee's story was widely heralded as a landmark case. Although the contested treatment decision was not primarily about rationing, it was often presented as such in the media (Price 1996). The case triggered debate about what forms of health care should be rationed, whose treatment should be prioritised, and how such decisions should be made. Media reports introduced the concept of opportunity costs and pointed out that difficult choices have to be made about how money for health care is spent. Other issues raised by the case, such as the uncertainties of medicine and the difficulties of decisions about how to treat seriously ill children were not emphasised in newspaper coverage of the case (Entwistle *et al.* 1996b: 130–131). In a climate in which the NHS was highly politicised, many media outlets framed a case that was primarily about clinical effectiveness and a patient's best interests as an example of rationing (Entwistle *et al.* 1996a: 1591).

News articles about new treatments sometimes report concern that these treatments might not be made available on the NHS. In the last few years, treatments for multiple sclerosis, dementia, erectile dysfunction and obesity have all been launched amid debates about their availability. Some news reports express indignation on behalf of the people who are apparently to be 'denied' even when there is little evidence that the treatments will be beneficial. Others concede that the NHS cannot fund all possible treatments and consider strategies for restricting the treatments for those in most need or highlight examples of other treatments that could be funded for similar costs.

Awareness has grown of inequalities in access to health care. Geographical variations in the availability and quality of particular services have been debated at a political level, and research highlighting such variations has been picked up by the news media. The media also gave a clear voice to critics of the internal market that the Conservative government introduced into the NHS. They repeatedly pointed out that the market created a two-tier service, with patients of fundholding general practitioners getting a better service than those of non-fundholders.

Thus various stories in the news media reflect a concern to see the NHS treat everyone well and fairly according to their need and regardless of their ability to pay, the status of their general practitioner, or the area of the country in which they live. Reports constructed using these frames reflect the deep seated notions of social solidarity on which the NHS is based.

The effects of media coverage

The precise impact of media coverage on health policy is difficult to establish because the media are not the only arena in which issues are debated and are only one influence on policy. But publicity in the media can create pressure that significantly influences policy makers. Concerns, for example, that the Conservative government were not fully implementing the results of research which would improve the equity of resource allocation in the NHS (Smith *et al.* 1994) led to extensive media coverage, a Select Committee of inquiry and subsequent commitments by the Secretary of State to act on the evidence. Highly publicised increases in the numbers of patients waiting for hospital procedures led a government with an (arguably ill-considered) focus on the size of waiting lists (Smith 1997) to significantly distort resource allocation for health care.

By imbuing the media with importance as a political arena, politicians give the media power that can in turn influence policy and the fate of politicians.

Media reports and campaigns can shape the way people understand issues. They can influence professional behaviour (Maclure *et al.* 1998) and public demand for particular services (Grilli *et al.* 1998). It is not clear, however, how the characteristics of the messages presented and the context in which they appear interact to produce an impact.

Conclusions

The constraints of news reporting, journalistic routines and journalists' individual role perceptions and values all influence media coverage of health policy and health services. The media relations activities of organisations and individuals with diverse agendas can also influence journalists' decisions about which issues and events to report and how to interpret and present them.

Most of the broad interpretive frameworks that were identified in media coverage of health services from the 1970s and 1980s have persisted to the present day, although they have evolved to some extent and other frameworks can be identified in reports about different aspects of health services.

The interpretive frameworks used in media reporting reflect and in turn reinforce changes in society. Reports in the UK news media of the 1990s suggest that although the medical profession still retains huge authority we are more willing to challenge it and make it more accountable. We continue to be optimistic about developments in health care but are more aware than previously of the need to ensure effectiveness and value for money. We know that there are reasonable limits to public spending on the health service, but remain vigilant against examples of unfairness. We are still passionate about the need for a health service that will treat everyone well and fairly according to clinical need and regardless of ability to pay.

References

Anonymous (1998) 'A serious departure from safe professional standards', *General Medical Council News* 3: 8–10.

Best, G., Dennis, J. and Draper, P. (1977) *Health, the Mass Media and the National Health Service*, London: Unit for the Study of Health Policy.

Bradby, H., Gabe, J. and Bury, M. (1995) '"Sexy docs" and "busty blondes": press coverage of professional misconduct cases brought before the General Medical Council', *Sociology of Health and Illness* 17: 458–476.

Bury, M. and Gabe, J. (1994) 'Television and medicine: medical dominance or trial by media?', in J. Gabe, D. Kelleher and G. Williams (eds) *Challenging Medicine*, London: Routledge, 65–83.

Butler, P. (1998) 'Message in a throttle', *Health Service Journal*, 20 August, 9–10.

Entwistle, V. (1995) 'Reporting research in medical journals and newspapers', *British Medical Journal* 310: 920–923.

Entwistle, V.A., Watt, I.S., Bradbury, R. and Pehl, L.J. (1996a) 'Media coverage of the Child B case', *British Medical Journal* 312: 1587–1591.

—— (1996b) 'The media and the message. How did the media cover the Child B case?', in M. Marinker (ed.) *Sense and Sensibility in Health Care*, London: BMJ: 87–171.

Entwistle, V.A., Sheldon, T.A., Sowden, A.J. and Watt, I.S. (1998) 'Evidence informed patient choice: practical issues of involving patients in decisions about health care technologies', *International Journal of Technology Assessment in Health Care* 14: 212–225.

Entwistle, V.A., Watt, I.S. and Johnson, F. (forthcoming) 'Media coverage of Norplant: the rise and fall of a health technology'.

Evidence-based working group (1992) 'Evidence-based medicine', *JAMA* 268: 2420–2425.

General Medical Council (1987) *Professional Conduct: Fitness to Practise*, London: GMC.

Grilli, R., Freemantle, N., Minozzi, S., Domenighetti, G. and Finer, D. (1998) 'Impact of mass media on health services utilisation (Cochrane Review)', in *The Cochrane Library* 3, Oxford: Update Software.

Hartley, J. (1982) *Understanding News*, London: Methuen.

Horton, R. (1998) 'How should doctors respond to the GMC's judgements on Bristol?', *Lancet* 351: 1900–1901.

Johnson, T. (1998) 'Medicine and the Media', Shattuck Lecture, *New England Journal of Medicine* 339: 87–92.

Karpf, A. (1988) *Doctoring the Media: the Reporting of Health and Medicine*, London: Routledge.

Lloyd, P. (1998) 'Off message', *Health Service Journal*, 7 May, 26–29.

Maclure, M., Dormuth, C., Naumann, T., McCormack, J., Rangno, R., Whiteside, C. and Wright, J.M. (1998) 'Influences of educational interventions and adverse news about calcium channel blockers on first line prescribing of antihypertensive drugs to elderly people in British Columbia', *Lancet* 352: 943–948.

McKinlay, J.B. (1981) 'From "promising report" to "standard procedure": seven stages in the career of a medical innovation', *Millbank Memorial Fund Quarterly* 59: 374–411.

Maynard, A.K. and Sheldon, T.A. (1997) 'Time to turn the tide', *Health Service Journal*, 25 September, 24–26.

Moore, W. (1998) 'Royal flush', *Guardian* (*Society*), 2 September, 2–3.

NHS Executive (1996a) *Promoting Clinical Effectiveness: a Framework for Action in and through the NHS*, Leeds: Department of Health.

—— (1996b) *Patient Partnership: Building a Collaborative Strategy*, Leeds: Department of Health.

Power, M. (1997) *The Audit Society: rituals of verification*, Oxford: Oxford University Press.

Price, D. (1996) 'Lessons for health care rationing from the case of child B', *British Medical Journal* 312: 167–169.

Rogers, A., Entwistle, V. and Pencheon, D. (1998) 'A patient-led NHS: managing demand at the interface between lay and primary care', *British Medical Journal* 316: 1816–1819.

Sheldon, T.A. and Maynard, A.K. (1993) 'Is rationing inevitable?', in R. Smith (ed.) *Rationing in action*, London: BMJ Publications: 3–14.

Smith, R. (1992) 'The ethics of ignorance', *Journal of Medical Ethics* 18: 117–118, 134.

—— (1997) 'New government, same narrow vision', *British Medical Journal* 316: 643.

—— (1998) 'All changed, changed utterly: British medicine will be transformed by the Bristol case', *British Medical Journal* 316: 1917–1918.

Smith, P., Sheldon, T.A., Carr-Hill, R.A., Martin, S., Peacock, S. and Hardman, G. (1994) 'Allocating resources to health authorities: results and policy implications of small area analysis of use of inpatient services', *British Medical Journal* 309: 1050–1054.

Snell, J. (1998) 'Blowing in the wind', *Health Service Journal*, 27 August, 20–23.

Treasure, T. (1998) 'Lessons from the Bristol case', *British Medical Journal* 316: 1685–1686.

Chapter 8

Media and mental health

Greg Philo and Jenny Secker

Introduction

It is difficult to imagine a more appropriate time to consider the impact of the media on British mental health policy. At the time of writing, the doubts increasingly voiced over the past five years about the effectiveness of community-based care for people experiencing mental distress have recently come to a head in the form of a press release from Frank Dobson, the Secretary of State for Health in England and Wales, stating categorically that community care for this group has failed (Dobson 1998). While Mr Dobson's statement makes clear that the government does not intend a return to the previous model of institutional care, it does place emphasis, alongside other measures, on the need for more effective methods of ensuring compliance from those who resist voluntary engagement with the mental health services in order to protect both the public and themselves. At the same time a review of the Mental Health Act was announced to ensure that the proposed changes in practice will be backed up by changes in the law.

This emphasis on protection and compliance backed up by legislation is made more explicit in a speech delivered the following day by the Minister for Mental Health to the External Reference Group charged with developing a new national service framework for mental health (Boateng 1998). Here, the first aim of the government's 'new vision' for mental health is described as 'to protect the public and provide safe and effective care for those with severe and enduring mental illness'. In his conclusion, the Minister re-emphasised the need to win public confidence by making society 'a place of greater safety for those living with mental illness, be they patients, their carers or *neighbours in the wider community*' (our italics).

In the view of many people involved in the field of mental health, this emphasis on protection and public confidence, and indeed the revision of a policy which had historically received broad cross-party support since publication of the watershed White Paper *Better Services for the Mentally Ill* in 1975, is due in large part to the way in which the British mass media have reported and represented mental health issues since publication of the NHS and

Community Care Act in 1990. Only two years after implementation of the Act, for example, the policy director of the National Association for Mental Health (MIND) highlighted the prominence given to the reporting of violent incidents involving people labelled mentally ill and pointed to the danger that the impact on public opinion could well lead to new, more coercive policies based not on a proper examination of the risks but on a 'knee-jerk response' to ill-considered fears (Sayce 1995).

Despite the high level of concern about media reporting expressed by Sayce and earlier commentators (e.g. Vousden 1989 and Birch 1991), few studies have systematically examined the part played by the media in shaping public attitudes to mental health issues. Although North American research has revealed a predominance of negative stereotypes in the press and on television (Day and Page 1986; Signorelli 1989), until recently no equivalent research had been undertaken in Britain. Similarly, although there have been attempts to relate audience attitudes to viewing specific programmes and films (Domino 1983; Wahl and Lefkowits 1989; Wober 1989), or to coverage of particular incidents (Appleby and Wessely 1988), the design of these studies has limited their capacity to explore the complexities of attitude formation and media influences. (For a critical review of these studies see Secker and Platt 1996.)

To meet the need for greater understanding of these issues the Glasgow Media Group carried out a series of studies, between 1993 and 1995, examining how mental illness is portrayed by the British media and exploring the impact of media coverage on public attitudes and beliefs. In the following two sections of this chapter we discuss the main findings of this research: we conclude by considering the implications for community care and other relevant policy initiatives.

Media representations of mental illness

In order to assess how the British media portray mental illness, we surveyed and analysed the content of local Scottish and national media output during the month of April 1993, including factual and fictional formats aimed at both adults and children.[1] The purpose of the content analysis was to identify the dominant messages about mental health issues. The analysis of news stories focused on the use of headlines and different types of news language, the ways in which characters in stories were labelled as 'mentally ill', as well as the types of actions with which they were associated. In the fictional material, key story lines relating to mental illness and the structure of plots and dramatic action were examined.

The survey yielded 562 relevant items which were allocated to one of five categories of coverage: violence to others, sympathetic coverage, harm to self, 'comic' images, and criticisms of accepted definitions of mental illness. Table 8.1 reveals that media coverage linking mental illness with violence to others

Table 8.1 Media coverage of mental health/illness, April 1993

Output category	*Number of items*	*Percentage of total*
Violence to others	373	66
Prescriptions for treatment/advice/ recovery	102	18
Harm to self	71	13
'Comic' images	12	2
Criticism of accepted definitions	4	1
Total	562	100

formed by far the most common category, two-thirds of all items analysed. The great majority of these items were news reports of violent crimes in which the perpetrators were labelled as mentally ill through the use of terms like 'mad', 'maniac' and 'psycho'. Reports of an incident involving an attack on a woman and her daughter as they played bingo, for example, described the attacker variously as 'a knife maniac' and 'a madman' (*Sun*, 5 April 1993), as 'a crazed knife killer' and 'a maniac' (*Daily Star*, 5 April 1993), and as 'a crazed knifeman' who 'went berserk' (*Daily Sport*, 5 April 1993).

This association between mental illness and violence, which predominated in newspaper reports, was reinforced by fictional portrayals in films shown on television. Richard Dreyfus, for example, pursued a 'crazed killer' in *Stakeout* (ITV, 27 April 1993), while Kurt Russell played a reporter involved with a 'psycho killer' in *The Mean Season* (BBC1, 30 April 1993). Film reviews in newspapers and magazines provided further reinforcement of these themes. The teenage magazine *Big* gave its highest rating of '7 out of 10' to a new release, *A Taste of Killing*, in which students were said to be befriended by 'a complete nutter' and 'twisted psychopath' (21 April 1993).

In forging the link with violence, films of this genre also connected mental illness with 'split personality'; during the sample period, this theme was featured in most of the popular soap operas. *Coronation Street*, for example, from early 1993, had been developing a story line concerning a young nanny, Carmel, who was portrayed initially as a 'fresh-faced, home-loving Irish girl' but, in later episodes, it emerged that behind this angelic front lurked an intensely manipulative character who would clearly stop at nothing to win the married man with whom she had become obsessed.

These items linking violence and mental illness outweighed the second most common category (advice for prescriptions for treatment) by a ratio of almost four to one. But even these figures risk understating the relative coverage of the two categories, since items portraying violence tended to enjoy a high media prominence, whereas 'advice' was typically confined to back-page material in newspapers and magazines such as problem pages and health columns.

The majority of items in the third category, 'harm to self', were non-fictional reports of suicide or attempted suicide. For the most part these reports portrayed the events concerned as tragedies by focusing on their human context of depression and anxiety. The *Sun*, for example, reported the death of a model under the headline 'Death leap a cry for help' (4 April 1993), while the death of a Conservative Party worker was reported by the *Daily Record* under 'Secret pain of suicide Tory' (8 April 1993).

In some cases, however, reports of self-harm emphasised a 'bizarre' aspect of the events described. Extensive coverage of this type was given, for example, to the story of a man who had apparently jumped from a high-rise block and survived by landing on a car: 'Nissan impressed as man falls 200 ft' (*Guardian*, 3 April 1993). In similar vein, some newspapers focused on sexual angles which could be linked to self-harm: 'Suicide of sex slave nutter' (*Sunday Sport*, 24 April 1993); 'Tragic patient had sex fantasy' (*Sun*, 20 April 1993).

There were only a few items which fell into the category of 'comic' images, but, in one very striking example from television, Ruby Wax again evoked the violent images which characterised other media coverage when she introduced Joanna Lumley with these words:

> 'We have someone here with us tonight who recently joined the ranks of the chronically barking – the good news is that she has been rehabilitated via the miracle of 450 volts of electromagnetic current zapping through your brain . . . I know you are going to be kind because if you are not she may pull a knife . . .'
>
> (*The Full Wax*, BBC1, 22 April 1993)

The final category, 'criticisms of accepted definitions', also received very little coverage. The definitive fictional account in this category, *One Flew Over The Cuckoo's Nest*, was not shown during the sample period and there was very little similar material, despite ongoing debate about the validity of diagnostic categories such as schizophrenia amongst both service users and mental health professionals (Johnstone 1989). Although one episode of *Casualty* (BBC1) did explore the way in which behaviour is socially defined as 'irrational' or 'unbalanced', this programme was not typical and it was unusual to find material which went beyond the bounds of sympathy.

In summary, while the survey did reveal examples of more positive or questioning coverage (see Philo 1996), the great majority of the coverage contrasted starkly with the emphasis of the relevant regulatory bodies, and of journalists and broadcasters themselves, on fair and accurate reporting (e.g. Broadcasting Standards Council 1994). Two points are significant here. First, although the diagnosis of schizophrenia may be disputed, the experiences of distress, withdrawal, voice-hearing and troubled thoughts with which it is associated are far removed from the 'split personality' so prevalent in media images. As Wahl

(1995) points out, a diagnosis of 'multiple personality disorder' does exist, but this bears no relation to schizophrenia and is extremely rare. Equally, as Wahl also points out, the confusion of the terms psychopath and psychotic, encapsulated most vividly in the use of the term 'psycho', represents a confusion of two discrete, incompatible diagnoses.

Second, but more significant, the media association of mental illness with violence is undermined by the available empirical research evidence. In the United States, for example, a large scale epidemiological study found that 90 per cent of respondents who were diagnosed mentally ill had never been involved in violence (Swanson *et al.* 1990), leading one commentator to conclude:

> None of the data give any support to the sensationalised caricature of the mentally disordered served up by the media, the shunning of former mental patients, or regressive 'lock 'em all up' laws proposed by politicians pandering to public fears . . . Clearly, mental health status makes at best a trivial contribution to the overall level of violence in society.
>
> (Monahan 1992)

Similarly, an official inquiry in the UK found that, of the 2000 homicides recorded in England and Wales between 1991 and 1993, only thirty-four were committed by people who had been in contact with mental health services (Steering Committee of the Confidential Inquiry 1996). Detailed examination of 22 of the 34 cases, moreover, calls into question the 'stranger danger' implied by much media coverage. In more than 90 per cent of these cases, the victim was known to the assailant, with a quarter of cases involving the murder of children by their mothers. Ironically, even this evidence was inaccurately reported by much of the British media in ways which were more likely to fuel than allay public fears (Crepaz-Keay 1996). The thirty-four homicides identified in media reports, moreover, contrast sharply with the 5000 suicides associated with mental illness in 1991 alone (Department of Health 1993a); deaths which received only scant media attention during the sample period.

The following section examines the impact of media misrepresentations on public beliefs about mental illness.

Media impact on attitudes and beliefs

Research conducted since publication of the NHS and Community Care Act has revealed consistent and considerable ambivalence in public attitudes towards people experiencing mental distress. Despite expressing high levels of sympathy for this group, respondents to the studies have been markedly reluctant to accept mental health service users as full members of society: for many this reluctance reflected their belief in a strong association between mental illness and violence (Department of Health 1993b; Brockington *et al.* 1993; Huxley 1993). This study of audience responses to the type of media coverage revealed by the above survey suggests that the media play a significant part in shaping these public attitudes and perceptions.

In order to assess the impact of media representations on beliefs and attitudes, seventy people were recruited to take part in focus groups and were asked to complete a programme of exercises and interviews. In the exercises, sub-groups of two or three people were invited to write news reports based around copies of original headlines from newspapers. They were also asked to write dialogue for an episode of ITV's *Coronation Street* prompted by still photographs from the programme. Finally, each member of the group gave individual written replies to a number of open questions.

In writing their own stories, the audience groups demonstrated a remarkable ability to reproduce the style and language of television and the press. Some group members could reproduce detailed and accurate scripts from *Coronation Street*, months after the relevant scenes had been transmitted. The photographs they were given related to the 'Carmel' story line outlined on p. 137 and the scenes depicted had apparently generated an intense hostility towards this character among the majority of the group members who had seen them. Invited to say how they would have reacted to Carmel, many group members responded with phrases such as 'killed her', 'battered her bloody mouth in', 'kicked hell out of her' and 'I would have killed the cow'. A much smaller number suggested that she needed psychiatric help – a judgement which was made mostly on the basis of their own professional or personal experience in the area. But even here, the judgement could be accompanied by a list of other things which had to be 'done' to a women first:

> '(I would have) thrown her out of the house, denounced her in public and with Martin [the husband] by my side, let the whole world know what she was up to. Then suggested to her that she needed psychiatric help.'

Media presentations were also a powerful influence on beliefs about the nature of mental illness. For example, the character Trevor Jordache in the soap opera *Brookside* was presented as alternating between being an amiable loving family man and making violent threats to his wife: 'you won't tell anyone, because if you do I'll kill you, do you understand?' (17 April 1993). In the popular press, he was referred to as 'psycho Trevor' (*Daily Star*, 19 April 1993) and in our group interviews, he was spontaneously referred to as being 'what a mentally ill person was like'. As one female interviewee commented:

> '. . . in *Brookside*, that man who is the child-abuser and the wife-beater, he looks like a schizophrenic – he's like a split personality, like two different people.'

Of greatest significance here is the extent to which beliefs derived from *fictional* media accounts clearly affected attitudes in *real life*. One interviewee, for example, claimed that mentally ill people:

> 'Could be alright one minute and then just snap – I'm kind of wary of them . . . That *Fatal Attraction* she was as nice as nine pence and then . . .'

Such comments can reveal very deep levels of fear. Another interviewee wrote in her reply that mentally ill people were 'quite likely to be violent – split personalities usually tend to be violent'. She went on to write: 'I would tend to be more wary as some mentally ill people can be very clever and devious'. The source of her views was given as 'probably from TV and newspapers, I think!' And she went on in her interview to comment that: 'Hungerford, that type of thing – anything you see on the news, it's likely to be violent when it is connected with mentally ill people', thus illustrating that 'factual' accounts could also influence attitudes considerably.

Overall, 40 per cent of the people who took part in the study believed mental illness is associated with violence and gave the media as the source of their beliefs. Indeed, the depth of anxiety experienced and expressed was so considerable that some media accounts appeared to exert substantial influence on beliefs about mental health. Other research studies, however, exploring different areas of media content, have generally found that personal experience is a much stronger influence on belief than the messages which are given by media (Philo 1990). But this research revealed that this pattern could be reversed. In a significant number of cases (21 per cent of the sample) the people concerned had non-violent experience of mental illness which was apparently 'overlaid' by media influences. These people traced their beliefs mostly to violent portrayals in fiction or to news reporting. This influence for media representations was illustrated by a young women who lived near Woodilee Hospital just outside Glasgow. She wrote that she had worked there at a jumble sale and mixed with patients. Yet she associated mental illness with violence and wrote of 'split/double personalities, one side violent'. She then went on to explain:

> 'The actual people I met weren't violent – that I think they are violent, that comes from television, from plays and things. That's the strange thing – the people were mainly geriatric – it wasn't the people you hear of on television. Not all of them were old, some of them were younger. None of them were violent – but I remember being scared of them, because it was a mental hospital – it's not a very good attitude to have but it is the way things come across on TV, and films – you know, mental axe murders and plays and things – the people I met weren't like that, but that is what I associated them with.'

In a further example, one interviewee had visited a hospital in Glasgow many times to see a relative who had been a patient there for twenty-five years. She associated mental illness with violence and cited 'TV films' as the source of her beliefs: '*Texas Chainsaw Massacre*, *Freddy's Revenge*, *Nightmare on Elm Street*, *Psycho* – I watch a lot of them, I like all those ones'. She was asked specifically if the feeling about violence came from the films rather than what she had seen when visiting. She replied: 'Oh aye – every day I was up visiting, I never saw any violence and he was in a big open ward'.

Implications for mental health policy

While many commentators have pointed out that the success of community care policy depends in large part on the adequacy of the resources made available (Scottish Affairs Committee 1995; Mental Health Act Commission 1993), it is also clear that the co-operation of the communities concerned is equally essential. Although research has demonstrated that, in favourable circumstances, community care initiatives can achieve their aim of improving the quality of life of people diagnosed mentally ill (e.g. Thornicroft *et al.* 1992), other studies have revealed the extent of local opposition in many areas to the development of community-based services (Wahl and Kaye 1992; Scottish Mental Health Forum 1992).

It seems likely that the media messages revealed by this survey have played some part in fuelling opposition and indeed the research established clear links between media representations and public attitudes to community care among the audience sample. One participant, for example, related her own beliefs about violence and mental illness to 'Hollywood film and television drama', then commented: 'I feel that government policies in Britain of putting mentally ill people in the "care of the community" is dangerous'. In turn, in an era when politicians of all political hues profess to take serious account of public opinion in developing their policy agenda, it seems likely that the beliefs expressed by our audience groups have had some influence on the revision of community care mental health policy recently announced by the Secretary of State. Nor is community care the only policy area likely to be affected by adverse public attitudes. In common with the policies of the previous Conservative government, the public health Green Paper recently published by the Labour government identifies mental health as a priority, proposing in particular the creation of job opportunities for people with mental illness, alongside measures aimed at reducing the incidence of mental illness and the prevention of suicide (HMSO 1998).

That the public fears which have jeopardised community care also pose a threat to these proposals is illustrated by studies which have consistently demonstrated that people who have experienced mental illness are likely to face obstacles in obtaining employment as a result of negative attitudes on the part of employers (Farina and Felner 1973; Oppenheimer and Miller 1988).

There is a further extremely significant consequence of media portrayals of mental illness. Previous research has suggested that the stigma associated with mental illness may prevent people from seeking help with mental health problems before these become more serious (Wahl 1995; Royal College of Psychiatrists 1995). In turn, this may undermine attempts to reduce suicide rates, since the incidence of suicide has been shown to be closely associated with depression (Wilkinson 1994).

Our own follow-up research with thirty-two mental health service users (Philo 1996) both supports these conclusions and illustrates the part played by media misrepresentations in deterring people from seeking help. As one participant explained:

> 'I'd been quite ill at the beginning of the eighties and I was referred to the clinic and I wouldn't go because I was frightened because I had all these pictures in my head because I had been watching *Maybury* [a drama series about a psychiatrist].'
>
> (ibid.)

A final extract from the study illustrates how media portrayals can seriously undermine service users' own confidence and self-esteem, with clear implications for public health policy goals:

> 'When I was told I was schizophrenic, I was very intimidated by it – I thought I was some sort of monster. I didn't actually feel like a monster, but when they said I was schizophrenic, I just couldn't believe it . . . It's just such a hell of a word, you know, and it has got a hell of a stigma . . . I just thought it was Jekyll and Hyde. I was just one of those people I'm characterising this morning [for having incorrect beliefs about mental illness] . . . but you're really more likely to hurt yourself – what was blasting through my head was you'll never get a job, you'll never get a sick line, you'll have nowhere to live. It was just going through my head, kill yourself.'
>
> (ibid.)

Although there is little doubt, then, that the mass media can exert considerable influence over audiences, it would be wrong to assert that the media alone are responsible for forming our beliefs and shaping the social policy agenda. The media exist within and are part of developing social cultures. Where mental health is concerned it seems likely, as Wahl (1995) has also suggested, that the media both reflect and fuel deeply held fears. Some messages on violence and mental illness are located within and exploit deep anxieties about the unknown and unpredictable in what we perceive to be a very frightening world. But the fear and stigmatising effects produced by media accounts are problems in their own right and the implications for social policy require to be addressed if policy is not to be made, as Sayce (1995) prophesied, on a knee-jerk response to ill-considered fears.

Note

1 The media sample analysed embraced a comprehensive review of UK national newspapers, radio and television programmes (including films broadcast on television), as well as Scottish local papers (such as the *Edinburgh Evening News*), national papers like the *Scotsman* and Scottish television programming, for a period of one month – April 1993.

References

Appleby, L. and Wessely, S. (1988) 'Public attitudes to mental illness: the influence of the Hungerford massacre', *Medicine, Science and the Law* 28(4): 291–295.

Birch, J. (1991) 'Towards the restoration of traditional values in the psychiatry of schizophrenia', *Context*, Spring (8): 21–26.

Boateng, P. (1998) 'A place of greater safety: safe, sound and supportive mental health services for the new millennium', *Speech for the first meeting of the External Reference Group for the mental health National Service Framework*, 29 July.

Broadcasting Standards Council (1994) *A Code of Practice*, second edition, London: Broadcasting Standards Council.

Brockington, I., Hall, P., Levings, J. and Murphy, C. (1993) 'The community's tolerance of the mentally ill', *British Journal of Psychiatry* 162: 93–99.

Crepaz-Keay, D. (1996) 'A sense of perspective: the media and the Boyd Inquiry', in G. Philo (ed.) *Media and Mental Distress*, London: Longman.

Day, D. and Page, S. (1986) 'Portrayal of mental illness in Canadian newspapers', *Canadian Journal of Psychiatry* 31 (December): 813–817.

Department of Health (1993a) *The Health of the Nation Key Area Handbook: Mental Illness*, London: Department of Health.

—— (1993b) *Attitudes to Mental Illness*, London: Department of Health.

Dobson, F. (1998) 'Frank Dobson outlines third way for mental health', *Press Release 98/311*, 29 July, London: Department of Health.

Domino, G. (1983) 'Impact of the film *One Flew Over the Cuckoo's Nest* on attitudes to mental illness', *Psychological Reports* 53: 179–182.

Farina, A. and Felner, D. (1973) 'Employment interviewer reactions to former mental patients', *Journal of Abnormal Psychology* 82: 268–272.

Huxley, P. (1993) 'Location and stigma: a survey of community attitudes to mental illness – part 1, enlightenment and stigma', *Journal of Mental Health* (2): 73–80.

Johnstone, L. (1989) *Users and Abusers of Psychiatry*, London: Routledge.

Mental Health Act Commission (1993) *Fifth Biennial Report*, London: HMSO.

Monahan, J. (1992) 'Mental disorder and violent behaviour – perceptions and evidence', *American Psychologist* 41(4): 511–521.

Oppenheimer, K. and Miller, M. (1988) 'Stereotypic views of medical educators toward students with a history of psychological counselling', *Journal of Counselling Psychology* 35: 311–314.

Philo, G. (1990) *Seeing and Believing: the Influence of Television*, London: Routledge.

—— (1996) *Media and Mental Distress*, London: Longmans.

Royal College of Psychiatrists (1995) *Attitudes Towards Depression*, London: Royal College of Psychiatrists.

Sayce, L. (1995) 'An ill wind in a climate of fear', *Guardian (Society)*, January 18: 6–7.

Scottish Affairs Committee (1995) *Closure of Psychiatric Hospitals in Scotland, vol. 1*, London: HMSO.

Scottish Mental Health Forum (1992) *Community Care and Consultation*, Edinburgh: Scottish Association for Mental Health.

Secker, J. and Platt, S. (1996) 'Why media images matter', in G. Philo (ed.) *Media and Mental Distress*, London: Longmans.

Signorelli, N. (1989) 'The stigma of mental illness on television', *Journal of Broadcasting and Electronic Media* 33(3): 325–331.

HMSO (1998) *Our Healthier Nation: a Contract for Health*, London: HMSO.

Steering Committee of the Confidential Inquiry (1996) *Report of the Confidential Inquiry into Homicides and Suicides by Mentally Ill People*, London: Royal College of Psychiatrists.

Swanson, J., Holzer, C., Ganju, V. and Jono, R. (1990) 'Violence and psychiatric disorder in the community: evidence from the epidemiological catchment area surveys', *Hospital and Community Psychiatry* 41: 761–770.

Thornicroft, G., Gooch, C. and Dayson, D. (1992) 'The TAPS project 17: readmissions to hospital for long term psychiatric patients after discharge in the community', *British Medical Journal* 305: 996–998.

Vousden, M. (1989) 'Loony lefties and mad mullahs', *Nursing Times* 85(28): 16–17.

Wahl, O. (1995) *Media Madness: Public Images of Mental Illness*, New Brunswick NJ: Rutgers University Press.

Wahl, O. and Kaye, A. (1992) 'Mental illness topics in popular periodicals', *Community Mental Health Journal* 28: 21–28.

Wahl, O. and Lefkowits, J. (1989) 'Impact of a television film on attitudes towards mental illness', *American Journal of Community Psychology* 17(4): 521–528.

Wilkinson, G. (1994) 'Can suicide be prevented?' *British Medical Journal* 309: 860–861.

Wober, J.M. (1989) *Healthy Minds on Healthy Airwaves: Effects of Channel 4's 1986 Mental Health Programme Campaign*, London: Independent Broadcasting Authority Research Department.

Chapter 9

Thinking the unthinkable

Welfare reform and the media

Peter Golding

When the United Nations *Human Development Report 1998* appeared, it revealed a somewhat damning picture of the UK as one of the most impoverished nations of the developed world: the UK was ranked fifteenth out of the seventeen countries included in the poverty index used by the report. In the UK one in seven of the population was below the poverty line, and the country contained about 30 per cent of Europe's children in poverty (UNDP 1998: 28). This was not the image conjured by the sparkling glitter of new Labour's 'cool Britannia', its millennium dome ascending symbolically skyward from reclaimed London mudflats, and consumer spending running riot on digital television sets in the homes of a population who were now all middle class.

Something was amiss, and as ever it was in the working and reworking of popular cultural narratives provided by the news media that explanations could be forged and framed. When the 'new Labour' government of Tony Blair came to power in 1997, one of its primary targets in the battle to 'modernise' the British state was the social security budget. Social security minister Frank Field, with a reputation for an independent and tough approach in this area after an early career as a 'poverty lobbyist', and several years chairing the Commons Social Services Select Committee, was charged with 'thinking the unthinkable'. But this task, as always, had to draw on public and deeply rooted mythology and understanding. In this chapter I briefly review how this process was worked out in the 1990s by examining news coverage of poverty and social security, and its consequences for public beliefs and policy.

Welfare to work: shifting gear in the rhetorical battle

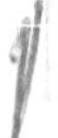

In earlier work I have argued that contemporary understanding of welfare is drawn from three roots – 'efficiency, morality, and pathology: efficiency of the labour market and the economy; morality of the work ethic and self-sufficiency; and the pathology of individual inadequacy as the cause of poverty' (Golding and Middleton 1982: 48). These three vary in intensity as conditions change. With rising structural unemployment (growing from 1 million in 1979 to 1.9

million in 1996), awareness of and familiarity with the circumstances and causes of unemployment became more diffuse through the population. But the increasing moralism of work as the only route out of poverty, and as the best cure for residual idleness, increasingly formed the core of a hardening set of political axioms arguing that duties as much as rights were the key to modern citizenship. This rhetoric became pivotal to the Blairite agenda, and to the welfare reforms the new Labour government began to pursue in office. Samuel Smiles was back in favour. While the worthy toiled, 'Most wretched and ignoble lot, indeed, is the lot of the idlers' (Smiles 1908 [1875]: 7).

The intense 'scroungerphobia' evident in both press and public attitudes in the 1970s abates somewhat in this later period. But the rhetoric and vocabulary are by now set. Drawing on this three-part framework, news about social security now becomes merely a variant on the earlier period. Within that a predictable and familiar set of motifs recur. First, the economic burden posed by social security expenditure, a restraint on growth and a punitive impost on the hard-working tax paying majority. Second, the need for control and punishment for illicit dependency on benefits, and especially for fraud. Third, the clear and necessary boundary to be drawn between the deserving and undeserving poor, with single parents moving into greater prominence in the 1990s alongside the unemployed (see Chapter 15). Both receive vituperation as external to the social system, in association with the foreign or alien claimant. Fourth, the new moralism draws attention to the unduly pleasant 'lot of the idlers', when there is work to be done.

Tory Social Security Secretary Peter Lilley had the headline writers drooling in 1992 when yet another 'biggest crackdown ever against social security fraud' was launched at the party's annual conference. His gruesome adaptation of a Gilbert and Sullivan ditty ('I've got a little list/Of benefit offenders who I'll soon be rooting out/And who never would be missed . . .') had them rolling in the aisles and across the front pages. As the *Mirror* warned of 'Dole scroungers facing new blitz', more simply in the *Daily Star* it was 'Stuff the spongers'. War was yet again declared on this outgroup of wasters, idlers, and loafers, a group set apart from the rest of society. The language of warfare underlines this imagery in two ways. First, battle is declared (as in the *Daily Mail* front-page spread, '£2bn blitz on dole cheats' (10 July 1995). Welfare claimants have endured more 'blitzes' than the Luftwaffe could ever have imagined possible. Second, readers are constantly reminded of their outgroup status by the recurrent and exemplary reporting of foreign spongers. In one brief period for example, from the *Mail* stable, we had 'A one man fraud factory', about a 'baby-faced 37-year-old' Nigerian who 'used Britain's benefits system like his own private bank' (*Mail on Sunday*, 21 September 1997); 'Thieving refugee sent benefit cash back home', about a Vietnamese caught shoplifting (*Daily Mail*, 25 July 1997); 'Irish fiddler takes British tax-payer for £1 million' (*Mail on Sunday*, 20 July 1997); 'First family of fraud' about a Pakistani family being tried for social security fraud in a Dutch court (*Daily Mail*, 20 April 1998); and an 'exclusive' exposé of the 'scandal of the illegal immigrant benefits industry' (*Daily Mail*, 30 June 1997). Scorned for this scandalous exploitation of our softness and generosity as a nation, scroungers are as excoriated as other objects of social contempt, as hinted at by headlines like 'Fraud-busters make a dawn swoop on welfare scroungers' (*Sunday Mirror*, 29 March 1998), the comparison with drug dealers or child abusers not far from the surface.

Social security fraud, as I demonstrate below, remains a staple of reporting of the benefits system. Yet the arithmetic of this area of criminal activity remains riddled with anomalies. Calculations of annual fraud figures depend on presumptions that short-term fraud would have continued if undetected. This indeterminacy gets played out in media reporting by the eternal refrain that '£1.4 bn benefit fraud is tip of iceberg' (*Daily Telegraph*, 10 July 1995). Dee Cook has carefully contrasted the policy and ideological response to social security fraud with tax evasion, which, as she points out, is equally a cost to the public purse resulting from criminal fraud. By 1995/96 the Department of Social Security was undertaking over 10,000 prosecutions annually, compared with 192 by the Inland Revenue. In the same year, even assumed benefit 'savings' (which include payment 'irregularities') arising from this action amounted to £1.2 billion, compared with £5.2 billion actually accrued from imposing 'compliance' on would-be tax evaders (Cook 1997: 102,105). Yet the latter remains veiled behind either total invisibility or humorous disregard for what is seen to be a victimless and innocent piece of mischief we would all engage in, given the opportunity.

Blurring the dividing line between welfare dependency and criminality fuels the sense that an unnecessary burden is being placed on the public purse by all this largesse. The day after disabled activists chained themselves to the railings at Number 10 in protest at threatened benefit cuts, that voice of middle England, the decade's most successful newspaper the *Daily Mail*, in its new conditional Blairite pose, argued that 'while those in genuine need will not be abandoned' the reforms would 'make sense of a welfare structure which creates a culture of dependency, fails to eradicate poverty, and yet imposes an ever-increasing burden on the economy' (23 December 1997, see Chapter 13). This was the welfare structure, as an earlier *Mail* lead article had pointed out, that 'has spawned a debilitating culture of welfare dependency, fecklessness, and fraud' (15 August 1997). The result, warned the *Sunday Times*, is that 'Benefit fraud is a way of life in Britain's sign-on society' (31 October 1993), a diagnosis echoed in the double page spread in the *Daily Mail* headed 'Sign up here for sick-note Britain' (14 April 1998).

This fecklessness arises from the alleged luxury of the lifestyles endowed by social security benefits, and from the indolence and ease with which the system is exploited. My clippings files bulge with annual examples of the, invariably misleading, summertime accounts of social security enriched holiday-makers. The *Daily Express* front-page lead 'Dole cheat's sun holiday' ('A dole cheat soaked up the Caribbean sunshine while still claiming benefit in Britain'), catches the flavour (16 August 1995). But towering over all such narratives are those of the 'super-scroungers' (compare Golding and Middleton 1982: 60–64). Among the more prominent such bogey figures recently was 47-year-old former pig worker and invalidity beneficiary Paul Booth, who in 1998 found himself getting more column inches than the resigning social security minister Frank Field. The *Daily Mirror* gave a double-page spread to Mr Booth and his two-family, eleven-children household (8 April 1998). By the following week further investigation enabled the headline 'Scrounger and a liar' to be printed (14 April 1998). Not to be outdone the *Sun* topped its story with a mock-up medal, 'S.O.B. Order of Scroungers of Britain', and invited its readers to submit details if they knew 'a bigger parasite than Paul Booth? We're looking for one to win our Scroungers of Britain gong' (8 April 1998). As the paper editorialised, 'Wasters like Booth are a huge millstone round our necks . . . layabouts who do nothing but breed should be cut off without a penny.' And it added archly, and none too elliptically, 'Perhaps we should cut something else off too'. The same allusion had informed the paper's front-page lead a month earlier that 'Blair snips Jack the dads' as absentee dads were to find that 'Their pay packets or benefits will be slashed in a massive crackdown on scroungers and cheats' (*Sun*, 27 March 1998).

The notion that social security was a drag of enormous proportions on the motor of economic growth had become prominent in political orthodoxy again by the advent of the new Labour government. The 1998 Green Paper on Social Security in which Frank Field unveiled his unthinkable thoughts was rapidly distilled by the press into two congruent themes. First it was another 'War on cheats' (*Sun*, 27 March 1998), in which 'Welfare cheats face spot fines' (*Express*) as the 'Shake-up in welfare hits the workshy' (*The Times*). To help this policy along the *Sun* invited us to 'Shop a bad dad – Field war on spongers who cost us a fortune' (30 March 1998). In fact criticised from left and right the Green Paper soon saw its two principal begetters, Field and Social Services Secretary Harriet Harman, both out of office, victims of hubris and the charge that 'Ministers fire welfare blanks' (*Guardian*, 27 March 1998). But the central message of modern welfare reform was well and truly forged. In a forceful front-page spread the *Express* shows a bewhiskered Field as Moses coming down from the burning bush, tablets in hand, alongside the divine full page headline 'Thou shalt not shirk' (27 March 1998).

The second theme continued to be the welfare burden which made all this necessary. As the *Mail* had explained a year earlier, 'Labour's radical social security reformer Frank Field yesterday pledged to cut the Government's £90 billion a year welfare bill' ('Field sharpens the axe for a purge on welfare' – 5 May 1997). In fact, as many commentators have noted, UK welfare expenditure is relatively low by international standards. By 1995/96 UK expenditure on 'social protection' ranked ninth out of eleven in European comparisons, with only Italy and Portugal lower (ONS 1998: 140). Equally, as Hills points out, '. . . the UK is not a high tax country. Over the last twenty years the UK has moved from being slightly above the mid-point of the international range of tax as a share of national income to being clearly well below the international average' (Hills 1997: 240).

Nevertheless, the public rhetoric tells another story. Behind these 'unbearable' cost levels lies, of course, the excessive allocation of welfare generosity, not merely to too many recipients, but to quite clearly the wrong people. Maintaining a necessary cultural distinction between the deserving and undeserving poor remains one of the cardinal boundary sustaining functions of the public media, even though there are occasional shifts in the demographics of those two groups. In the early 1990s, and occasionally thereafter, periodic outbursts of puritanical outrage at single parents placed that large and rapidly growing group firmly in the firing line. Eventually the conclusion was clear: 'Lone parents are the biggest cheats: single mothers may be lying their way to £1 billion' (*Daily Mail*, 6 August 1998, see Chapter 15). Not surprisingly, given both the popular and policy onslaught, we then find 'Fewer single mothers claiming benefit' (*Daily Mail*, 28 May 1998). In contrast was the poignant tale of former legendary Liverpool soccer hard-man Tommy Smith, given a sympathetic treatment in his battle to regain his cancelled disability living allowance ('Soccer star's penalty is £120 a week', *Express*, 8 May 1998). Equally sympathetic treatment is received by the 'genuinely' disabled, as in the case of an unambiguously 'deserving' woman whose plight was headlined in the *Sun* as 'No arms, no legs . . . but you're not disabled' (13 April 1998), in a story about a thalidomide victim whose Severe Disablement Allowance was stopped when the DSS found evidence of her selling puppies five years previously. By contrast our attention was drawn to the naivety and absurdity of Oxfam's venture into poverty in the UK. Real poverty is of course to be seen in the fly-encrusted faces of children lying helpless and starving on the dusty sun-baked ground of a far-away disaster zone. As a *Daily Mail* feature, headlined 'Can you spot the difference', pointed out, 'generous people who wish to give to Oxfam are encouraged to do so by pictures of skeletal mothers and children in Africa'. To help us understand the point, an accompanying photo of 'an African famine victim' is juxtaposed with a family snap of Paul Booth, the 'superscrounger', and his apparently rudely well-fed and voluminous family. This is not 'the poverty that means wearing rags or having no roof at night' (9 April 1998).

The durability of the deserving poor and the deeply-held foundational myths that sustain them enables a proud tradition of campaigning journalism to surface periodically. In December 1997 the *Mail on Sunday* claimed a success in its 'campaign' on the much-maligned Benefits Integrity Project, with 'Benefits U-turn ends disabled mother's order' (28 December 1997) in a story about a woman crippled by multiple sclerosis whose Income Support had been withdrawn. Even more emotively signalling a nostalgic search for its heroic campaigning past, the *Daily Mirror* produced a three-page 'Poverty – shock report' feature on the 'virus' which is 'spreading at an alarming rate . . . The name of this virus is poverty' (30 October 1998), with a two-column photo spread of a three-year-old girl clutching her doll in the bleak passage of a 'grim Liverpool estate'. Only the relegation of the feature to pages 33–35 signalled a very different set of priorities from the barnstorming polemics of the *Mirror* under Bartholomew and Cudlipp half a century earlier.

Powerful myths about poverty, public expenditure, and the moral economy of welfare remain immovably planted at the core of public understanding of policies related to social security. Since the 1980s some of these myths have been severely tested by changing economic conditions, yet their potency seems largely undiminished. These exemplars, however, should not disguise the very limited nature of news coverage of pertinent areas of public policy, and it is to that wider, and more calculated picture, that I now turn.

Small but imperfectly formed: a measure of social security news

To obtain a measure of social security coverage in the media this section extracts relevant data from a larger study of policy news undertaken at the Communication Research Centre at Loughborough University.[1] The data summarised here cover all national UK news media throughout the year October 1996 to September 1997. The first and most obvious finding is how little coverage social security gets. In that period there were just twenty-four stories primarily about social security on the BBC's main evening television bulletin, eleven on ITN, and in broadsheet newspapers not many more (twenty-six in the *Guardian*, twelve in *The Times*). Social Security is not big news, even compared with other social policy areas such as education, housing and health. Figure 9.1 shows the percentage of news coverage devoted to social policy as a proportion of all 'non-foreign' news across different types of media. Health

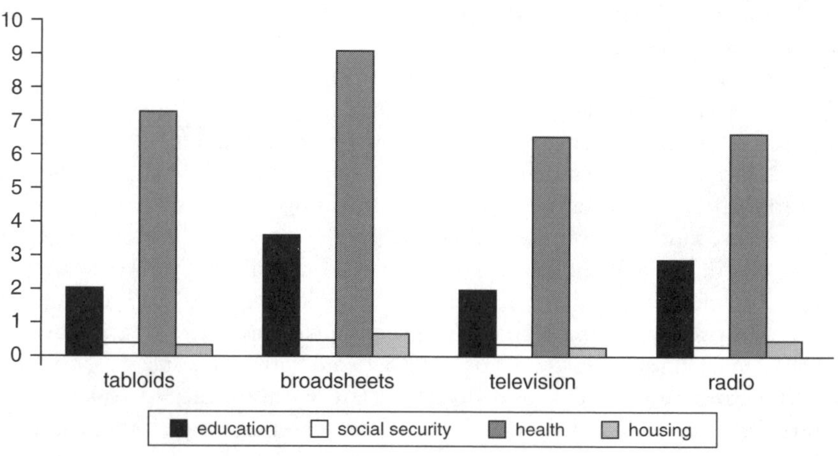

Figure 9.1 Types of policy news in all media over one year

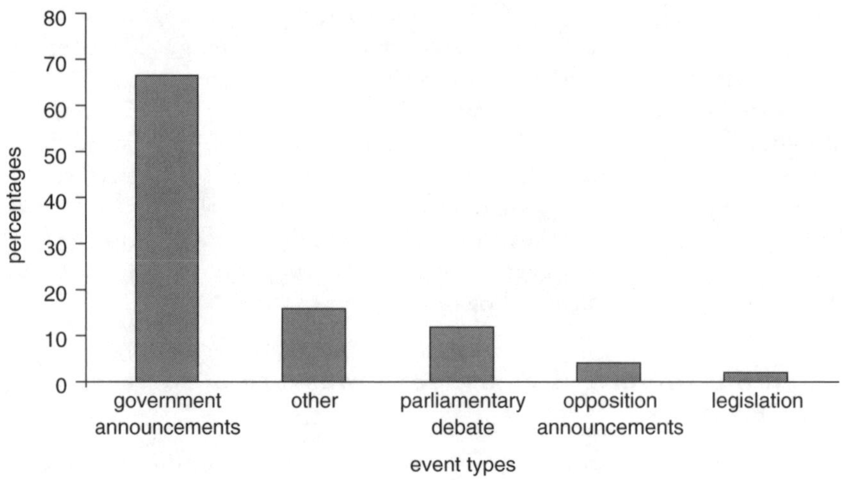

Figure 9.2 Types of social security stories in TV bulletins

is by far the most regularly reported, even dwarfing education in a period when all the main parties were ostensibly committed to that field as a priority.

Social security, like other areas of social policy, is first and foremost about politics. Poverty, benefits, and welfare are refracted through the legislative cycle and the machinery of government, or at least that fraction of it which surfaces in media exposure. Figure 9.2 shows the extent to which government announcements dominate the field of social security television news.

During the same period (October 1996 to September 1997) the Prime Minister appeared in roughly 15 per cent of all such social security news items and other government ministers in 60 per cent. Claimants and non-political actors of any kind made up just 12 per cent of the total actors appearing in these stories. When social security minister Frank Field published his Green Paper it received high-profile coverage, but nothing so extended and close focused as his ill-tempered resignation saga some weeks later.

One facet of this less than comprehensive account of social security and poverty in the major news media is a diminishing attention to social policy news of any kind. In recent years frequent charges of 'tabloidisation', not least from within journalism, have argued that the major news media, most especially broadcasting and the serious newspapers 'of record' had abandoned their traditional and honourable role of serving citizens with the essential diet of information required to perform their democratic role, and were instead moving to a more diverse and diverting fare with aspirations to entertain more than inform (Franklin 1997). I have examined the empirical foundation of this claim elsewhere (Golding *et al.* forthcoming). Figure 9.3, however, shows the preliminary findings of a long term analysis of social policy news

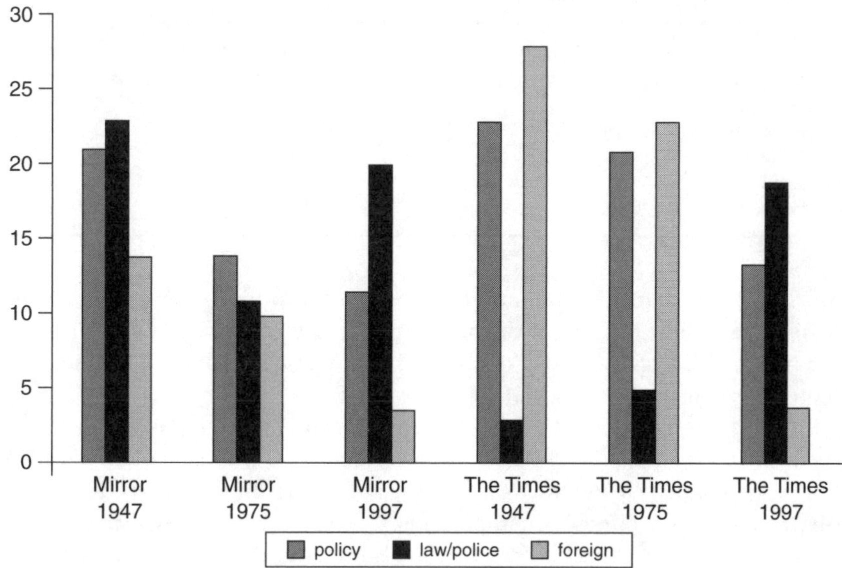

Figure 9.3 Policy news in the press, 1947, 1975 and 1997

(defined as news about social security, health, housing, and education) in the *Daily Mirror* and *The Times* in 1947, 1975, and 1997. It shows a clear trend in both titles towards a much greater proportion of crime stories, and a rapidly diminishing proportion of both social policy stories and indeed of foreign news.

With such a diminishing scope for news about poverty and social security it matters more than ever what aspects of these issues are given prominence or attention. It is not altogether surprising, given the historic confusion in the British psyche between the iniquities of the criminally indigent and the life-styles of the merely impoverished, that social security and crime news occupy close quarters in the journalistic corpus. In the period of our content analysis we examined both crime and social security stories. Of all stories that were primarily about one or other of these topics, 27.1 per cent (in the tabloid press), 16.6 per cent (in the broadsheet press), and 11.7 per cent (in broadcast news) were about both – that is were about criminal activity associated with social security. As I have noted above, it would be difficult to attribute this to the prevalence or scale of social security abuse, but it does certainly register a consistent association between the two areas of activity in the public mind, as we shall see shortly.

My concern throughout this chapter has been, of course, primarily with the news media. Nonetheless it would be remiss not to recognise that the welfare state in its various guises forms a luminous backcloth for the fictional lives of

Table 9.1 Claimants in TV fiction: the main soaps

	EastEnders	*Brookside*	*Coronation Street*	*Emmerdale*
Unemployed	2	3	1	4
Single parents	4			3
Pensioners	1	1	1	3
Disabled			1	1
Other claimants	1		1	

much popular drama, and no more so than in the working class sagas of the soap operas. Table 9.1 shows the number of characters regularly appearing in the major UK television soap operas in 1998 whose livelihood was evidently rooted in their use of the social security system.

In the lives and doings of these twenty-seven characters, and others like them, are embodied powerful and rich evocations of the understandings which imbue public perception of issues like social security. In *EastEnders,* for example, Irene (who claimed unemployment benefit despite living with her boyfriend Terry), fell foul of Susan (who also lives in the square but works for the Department of Social Security), leading to an inevitable showdown in the Queen Vic pub. There can be little doubt, though evidence awaits, that in such constructions lie the source of much of the imagery and explication deployed by people in responding to news and experience of major social issues like poverty and social security.

Responding to the 'wretched and ignoble': public attitudes

There is some evidence that public attitudes have, in recent years, softened and extended to suggest a broader understanding of the ways in which sections of the population are being cut adrift from 'comfortable Britain' (see Golding 1991). Despite that, the more severe responses which lie deep-rooted in our culture, and on which much of the media coverage illustrated here is based, seem entrenched. Table 9.2 shows data from the British Social Attitudes surveys using items initially developed in the 1970s (Golding and Middleton 1982: 183).

If anything the same surveys show that hostile attitudes to those who do not avoid dependency on the state have hardened. Although such attitudes soften in periods of recession, animosity to presumed fraudsters remains consistent, a pattern that offers circumstantial evidence, though no more, for a contrast between the fluctuating direct experience of people in the wider economy and their more constant exposure to the punitive odium attached to social security 'abuse' in the mainstream media. The sturdy beggar and his cousins, the 'wretched and ignoble', live on in pre-millennial Britain.

Table 9.2 Attitudes towards social security claimants

% Agree	*1987*	*1989*	*1991*	*1993*	*1994*	*1995*	*1996*
Many people who get social security benefit don't really deserve any help	31	29	26	24	26	30	28
Around here most unemployed people could find a job if they really wanted one	41	52	38	27	32	38	39
Most people on the dole are fiddling in one way or another	32	33	28	31	34	33	35

Source: Bryson 1997: 77

Conclusion: the 'underclass' and the mythology of welfare

In the 1990s, theories popularised by writers like Charles Murray (1984, 1994) argued that a section of the population in the USA, and in other countries like it, notably in the UK, had become detached from the mainstream of society, primarily by virtue of its distinct culture. What separated this group from the majority was its 'deplorable behaviour', making them a quite separate 'underclass'. The term, and the imagery and mythology on which it drew, became deeply rooted in the policy aspirations of social security reformers across the political spectrum. It was, of course, but a renaming of that multitude whose 'vicious habits and destitute circumstances make it certain that . . . they must hunger and sin, sin and hunger' till death in the 'darkest England' where General William Booth took his Salvation Army a century ago (Booth 1890: 3). While an alternative and more recent language of 'social exclusion' expressed the structural forces preventing the entry of large numbers into the benefits and delights of late-twentieth century society, both rhetorics established symbolic barriers between the consumers of the social security and benefits system and the larger majority whose labours and diligence provided that system's resources.

The discursive battle to understand and encapsulate the mystery of severe and extensive poverty within the affluent communities of late-twentieth century society takes place in the pages of the daily press, and on the screens of the nation's living rooms, as much as on the floor of the House of Commons. That battle seems as flourishing and as critical as it was in General Booth's time, and no less is at stake.

Note

1 The data in this section draw on research undertaken as part of the ESRC-supported project Information and Democracy (ESRC ref: L126251016). I am grateful to Shelley McLachlan for assistance with data analysis and collation, and to Liz Sutton for the graphics.

References

Booth, W. (1890) *In Darkest England and the Way Out*, London: International Headquarters of the Salvation Army.

Bryson, C. (1997) 'Benefit claimants: villains or victims?', in R. Jowell *et al.* (eds) *British Social Attitudes: the 14th Report*, London: Social and Community Planning Research.

Cook, D. (1997) *Poverty, Crime and Punishment*, London: Child Poverty Action Group.

Franklin, B. (1997) *Newszak and News Media*, London: Arnold.

Golding, P. (1991) 'Poor Attitudes', in S. Becker (ed.) *Windows of Opportunity: Public Policy and the Poor*, London: Child Poverty Action Group.

Golding, P. and McLachlan, S. (forthcoming) 'Tabloidisation and the British media', in C. Sparks and S. Splichal (eds) *Tabloidisation and the Media*, Maryland, USA: Hampton Press.

Golding, P. and Middleton, S. (1982) *Images of Welfare: Press and Public Attitudes to Poverty*, Oxford: Martin Robertson.

Hills, J. (1997) 'How will the scissors close? Options for UK social spending', in A. Walker and C. Walker (eds) *Britain Divided: the Growth of Social Exclusion in the 1980s and 1990s*, London: Child Poverty Action Group.

Murray, C. (1984) *Losing Ground*, New York: Basic Books.

Murray, C. (1994) *Underclass: the crisis deepens*, London: Institute for Economic Affairs.

ONS (Office for National Statistics) (1998) *Social Trends* 28, London: HMSO.

Smiles, S. (1908 [1875]) *Thrift*, London: John Murray.

UNDP (United Nations Development Programme) (1998) *Human Development Report 1998*, New York: Oxford University Press.

Chapter 10

Are you paying attention?

Education and the media

Tony Jeffs

Education attracted far less media attention prior to the 1950s. Serious and popular dailies tended to restrict reporting to substantive policy changes such as new examinations or school-leaving ages, perennial disputes relating to teacher pay (too low) and numbers (too few), class sizes (too big) and school buildings (too dilapidated), standards (always declining), plus at irregular intervals, 'scandals' featuring unfortunate schools or teachers.

This relative indifference reflected the political vacuum at the centre, since education was primarily a local government responsibility with central government formulating the legislative framework via Education Acts. Enacting this legislative framework always occasioned acrimonious disputes with church leaders and local politicians so ministers wisely stood aside unless pressure to intervene proved irresistible. Consequently fewer Education Acts were passed between 1870 and 1970 than between 1980 and 1998.

But if national papers showed little interest, local papers offered some recompense. Cub reporters went to record the monthly deliberations of education committees. Local papers also included details of prosecutions for truancy and illegal employment of children, along with reports of speech days, sports days, prize-givings and outings. Dry and tedious perhaps but they usually benefited from being compiled by reporters who attended the committee or event. As one reporter explained then he 'actually got to visit schools, met teachers, even kids . . . [and] . . . learnt an awful lot about education just listening to debates and reading Education Committee minutes' (interview). These provincial journalists played a key role in formulating policy because local control often produced intense controversy. The Bristol *Evening Post* (12 May 1965) even claimed (tongue in cheek?) that it devoted more column inches to the decision to go comprehensive than the Second World War.

Tales of anarchy, terror and depravity

National and local papers at irregular intervals spice up coverage with tales of 'outrage' or 'scandal'. Riots and disorder, plus reports of the sexual peccadilloes and errant behaviour of deviant teachers all periodically bring a twinkle to the eye of beleaguered editors.

Pupil protests always secure extensive media coverage. Protesters aspiring to highlight injustice or abuses of power by teachers or officials seek it and their appearance on the streets makes for lively photos and reportage. Individual schools, however, make Herculean efforts to suppress 'bad' publicity so most demonstrations and 'disturbances' go unreported (Adams 1991). Coverage usually ignores the grievances while accentuating the threat such outbreaks pose to good order. Weak leadership or troublemakers are usually identified as the problem, alongside 'modern teaching methods' and poor parenting. Consequently more control, never less control, is typically advocated: solutions seem to involve the advocacy of less liberal rather than more tolerant regimes in schools.

All coverage relating to pupil rebellion and disruption assumes disorder and disturbance are an aberration in 'normal' schools, thus ignoring the extent to which classrooms, even in the most serene of settings, are cockpits where teachers constantly struggle for control. Collective media amnesia regarding the unbroken history of mutiny and defiance, minor and substantive, against compulsory attendance, inadequate schooling and the use of arbitrary punishments ensures structural causes are set aside and the spotlight focused on naughty children and incompetent teachers (Humphries 1981; Adams 1991).

Juxtaposed in media reporting to normal schools, wherein good behaviour and tranquillity prevail, are progressive schools. Dreadful places where order, decency and respect, for learning and adults, we are told, are wilfully cast aside. Here danger, unlike elsewhere, emanates not from the pupils, typically cast as victims, but staff. The chequered history of progressive education in Britain can be partially viewed as a war between reformers and an unrelentingly hostile media. As early as 1820 the *Glasgow Chronicle* began a campaign to close the first nursery and community schools opened anywhere. Located in New Lanark, visited by over 20,000 people in a decade and replicated throughout Europe and North America, they nevertheless attracted a hostile local press. This demanded closure because Robert Owen and his colleagues, while tolerating others' religious beliefs, did not teach religion or attend church. These dangerous men and women rejected corporal punishment, provided free education to age 12 and included the 'arts of living', music, drawing, dance and nature study in the curriculum. All too much for the *Glasgow Chronicle* which orchestrated a campaign which eventually drove out Owen and his colleagues (Donnachie and Hewitt 1993). It is a story endlessly replicated. While exposure of brutality and neglect in schools has always been left to others, the press has fought like a tiger to protect young people from progressive education. Initially radical independent schools attracted a hostile press which uncovered the presence of 'cranks', bolsheviks, anarchists and radicals of various hues within them. Apart from Summerhill, established by A.S. Neill in 1927, and

Prestolee in the LEA (Local Education Authority) sector where Teddy O'Neill faced-down a vicious press campaign, few survived the onslaught. As Gribble, writing of Dartington Hall's demise following a vitriolic tabloid campaign, notes sadly, those who base their practice on 'respect for the individual' and freedom always within the context of a highly authoritarian and centralised system provide limitless 'ammunition' for critics (1986: also 1987).

Until recently these dangerous redoubts were 'found' within the independent sector. Underfunding and the withdrawal of even a handful of pupils ensured that the institution foundered most quickly. Thus constant threat of 'media exposure' and ridicule has largely domesticated progressive education in Britain by forcing those unhappy with the stultifying uniformity of our education system to retreat into 'home schooling'.

In one key respect the reporting of 'scandals' has changed. The themes of indiscipline, left-wing teachers and implied immorality remain but post-1960 dangerous progressives with 'lunatic' ideas have overwhelmingly been discovered operating in LEA schools. This shift coincided with the demise of grammar schools and the introduction of comprehensives. Places where, for the first time, substantial numbers of children from middle class and upwardly mobile homes shared a playground, classroom and even a desk, with working-class youngsters. Amalgamation between grammar and secondary modern schools meant many 'respectable' parents encountered the alien world of the secondary modern for the first time and were seriously unnerved by the experience. Such concerns and fears have been nimbly exploited by Conservative politicians and the media *ad nauseam*. The implied message was that these reforms were a thinly disguised conspiracy to undermine traditional values and to create a socialist system via classroom indoctrination by those who failed to achieve it through the ballot box. The result was an outpouring of articles reiterating the message that these 'new' schools and methods were failing (Denscombe 1984; Weeks 1986). As Wragg concluded, 'there's no such thing as good news out of comprehensives. You can't get it published. The press just don't want to know' (quoted Fletcher, Caron and Williams: 1985: 3). Disorder and disruption, readers were assured, was commonplace and teachers were ill-equipped or unwilling to teach the basics. Eventually, despite all the accumulated evidence that most comprehensives were a success and educational standards were improving, many politicians fell in line with this analysis. Recounting alarmist reports and the 'ritual quotation of extreme and atypical examples' (Ball 1984: 134) became the common currency of what passed for a political debate on education. By the early 1990s Prime Minister Major sounding like a *Daily Mail* editorial told his audience the deterioration was so acute there was no alternative to putting the clock back:

> 'When it comes to education, my critics say I'm 'old-fashioned'. Old-fashioned? Reading and writing? Spelling and sums? Great literature – standard English grammar? Old-fashioned? Tests and tables? British

> history? A proper grounding in science? Discipline and self-respect? Old-fashioned? Well, if I'm old-fashioned, so be it.'
>
> (Conservative Party Conference 1992)

To ensure this counter revolution was successful, trainee teachers were to be given 'basic subject teaching, not courses in the theory of education. Primary teachers should learn how to teach children to read, not waste their time on the politics of gender, race and class' (ibid.).

Pervasive messages of failure were sustained by negative reporting of events at specific schools. Initially these were high-profile comprehensives, with headteachers committed to modernising the curriculum, eradicating corporal punishment, creating a community presence and involving students to some extent in the decision-making process. Beginning in 1965 with Risinghill described by the *Sunday Times* as London's 'toughest school' and followed by Summerhill Academy (1974), Countesthorpe Community School (1974), Sutton Centre (1977), and Madeley Court (1984) a series of causes célèbres resulted in the departure of the head and a high proportion of the teachers. At Countesthorpe and Sutton, the attacks were orchestrated by a hostile local press, but in all cases the schools were besieged eventually by reporters from the '*Sun*, *Mirror*, *Daily Express* and *Daily Mail*' who left staff feeling they were 'virtually damned and utterly defenceless' (Fletcher, Caron and Williams 1985: 1). One victim implied schools like his own contributed to their downfall by 'going public' and as a consequence enabled 'those that don't make waves to wallow on' (Ellis *et al.* 1976: 141). Fletcher and his colleagues agreed, concluding the willingness of the staff to engage in debates within the local media proved naive and mistaken. The fate of these schools and their headteachers ensured that most adopted a nervous and defensive attitude towards the media. As Reader notes, fear more than anything else came to 'characterise the relationship between schools and the media' (Reader 1992: 127). School-based innovation became viewed as hazardous, something best avoided or undertaken surreptitiously. The memories of such campaigns linger but they have less and less purchase although the London *Evening Standard* still delights in exposing dangerous leftie teachers as the headline 'Threat of the militant teacher' indicates. 'Tony Garwood' the story continues 'clashed constantly with a hard core of Left-wing teachers over his attempts to throw out discredited Sixties teaching methods. His departure from Islington Green school in North London will be seen as a victory for the Trotskyites who dominate Islington Teachers' Association' (quoted in Wolchover 1998).

The current paucity of such vendettas owes less to media indifference than the irresistible pressure to conform post-1979. Radicals and non-conformists have been driven from teaching, discouraged from entering or become frightened to attract attention. Adverse media coverage and government policy have done for them so effectively that now such stories lack credibility and are in short supply.

Inevitably sites of disorder remain but progressives are rarely blamed directly. They are merely held responsible for creating comprehensives and training their teachers. Weak leadership, incompetent local authorities, poor discipline and parenting are now blamed. These provide such front-page banner headlines as 'Thugs who rule our schools' (Roberton 1998) which on examination turned out to be based on a report about expulsions from three schools. No example encapsulates better this interpretation than the Ridings School in Calderdale. It acquired national and international notoriety during autumn 1996. Reputedly on a single day, the Ridings as a world story, was eclipsed only by Yeltsin's heart attack and Clinton's re-election (Clark 1998a: 62). Like most previous cases a local paper, the *Halifax Courier*, initiated interest this time by drawing attention to a doubling of exclusions. However, Lumley's (1998) study shows attention quickly moved from local anxiety over this to Ridings becoming a focus of national concerns about children being 'beyond control' and 'failing schools'. Politicians preparing for a general election shamelessly jockeying to appear tough on juvenile crime and disorder then exploited Ridings as an opportunity to ground the debates in real-world events, to extemporise as they had on the Bulger case (Jeffs and Smith 1994, 1996). The coverage given to Ridings far exceeded anything previously devoted to 'failing schools'. The most publicised episode was the V-sign made by two pupils as they accompanied the Head, Karen Stansfield, into the school. Clark contextualises this:

> After asking the photographers to stay outside the school grounds, as she [Karen] turned her back on the cameras to walk up the now infamous steps a photographer shouted encouragingly to some of the pupils, 'Flick some Vs'. Two girls enthusiastically obliged, and the moment was recorded for posterity . . . I later discovered that, although the picture had been set up by one of the photographers, it was pure bad luck that it had been recorded for television. Most of the cameras had been switched off, but one cameraman had been distracted and left his running. Those pictures made an enormous, and unfair, impact across the nation – and the world. They struck a chord with all those who like to see young people as nasty, violent and anti-authority, and epitomized the Ridings as the 'school from Hell'. What upset Karen most was that she had accompanied the two girls back to meet the press, and they had apologized tearfully and profusely in front of the cameras, but that interview had only been shown once – and at a time when few people were watching.
>
> (1998: 37)

Reporters were bent on collecting unflattering evidence. They followed staff, harassed governors and spied on the school. The *Panorama* team employed a hoist to film into classrooms. Journalists pinned their own 'school closed' notice to the gate before photographing it. The story line ignored by the news media, including the 'in-depth' *Panorama* programme (4 November 1996), was their own role in the events prior to closure and the Head's dismissal. Certainly none investigated or reported the instances recounted to them by the Head of journalists paying pupils to misbehave, let off fireworks in school and recount fictitious misbehaviour (Clark 1998a: 7).

The Ridings may be an extreme example but it is not unique. For it flows from the Government's decision to enforce its writ via league tables and OFSTED reports which, along with frequent, aggressive, sometimes brutish, inspection, are designed to beget biddable teachers and cowed LEAs. This is not simply a return to the Victorian past for central government has resolved to expropriate control from professionals and local authorities. To achieve this, virtually any stratagem seems acceptable. So whereas beforehand the tip-off came from alienated parents, outraged neighbours or disgruntled councillors now it is largely governmental in origin. Post-1990 Ministers have employed a slavish media to name and shame schools. Headlines such as 'Britain's 18 worst schools' have become commonplace alongside stories about 'The worst school in Britain'. None are to be spared: in addition to the 'failing schools', now the 'Complacent schools are to be named' (*Independent*, 12 November 1998). Reports are sent and phone calls made to ensure journalists and TV cameras descend on those near the foot of a league table or given a 'bad report'. By lunchtime the ritual humiliation begins. To frighten the rest this must be total so they receive the minimum time to marshal a defence. One headteacher recalls after 'naming and shaming':

> Angry parents and local politicians held a secret meeting, at which there were calls for the school to be shut. Two politicians announced that they would not send their children to the school. The press had a field day. The *Daily Mail* sent a reporter and a photographer who sat in a car outside the school gates all day waiting for an incident to develop. Mr Varnava recalls: 'It was really terrible, very hurtful. It was destroying morale at a time when the school was beginning to make progress. We were in the middle of our second OFSTED review and we didn't need that.'
>
> (Hoare 1998)

Besides schools Conservative and Labour governments alike exhibit a parallel determination to humble LEAs. Recently reporters were deliberately briefed on a critical report about Manchester LEA before the authority received a copy. This ensured headlines such as 'The city that lets down its pupils' along with details about 'The worst schools' were published with only time for a vague and hurried response from the council leader. This sleight-of-hand allowed the minister Stephen Byers, by contrast, to pose as dynamic and decisive ordering Manchester 'to take urgent action to protect some of its most vulnerable children' and demanding 'a report within a month on how the authority intended to meet its statutory responsibilities' (Judd 1998). One education correspondent (anxious not to be identified) who has attended numerous briefings given by Labour ministers believed this behaviour confirmed his view 'they actually hate local government and the [teacher] unions more than the Tories did. If that was possible', an opinion reflected in Blunkett's description of teachers as 'miserable sneering cynics' (*Teacher*, November 1998). Brenton (1998) gives an account of a Blair briefing to an eminent journalist in which he claimed the government is 'planning to "take on" the NUT (National Union of Teachers) and the NASUWT (National Association of Schoolmasters and Union of Women Teachers), in the same way that Margaret Thatcher took on the NUM (National Union of Mineworkers) . . . their power has to be broken once and for all'.

League tables receive blanket coverage even though few who understand their origins treat them seriously. Their simplicity and lack of rigour, however, make them easily digestible, providing instant copy plus the excitement of a football league table. Papers eagerly print them whilst radio and TV provide highlights. But as John O'Leary, *The Times* education editor, admitted, they show 'only the leading A-level scores and are not intended to mark out the 'best' schools. Selective schools, which enjoy advantages over comprehensives in the academic ability of their intake, inevitably fill most of the leading positions' (quoted Hattersley 1998: 23). Yet the *Sunday Times* published two 56-page supplements entitled *Parent Power* which assured the gullible. These listed the top 500 state and 500 independent and preparatory schools. To fortify this claim they were introduced by an article by Chris Woodhead, Chief Inspector of Schools. This smugly assured parents that such tables 'show schools there is nowhere to hide' (*Sunday Times* 1998: 2). The *Parent-Power* supplements were marketed with the *Sunday Times Equitable Schools Book* (a guide to independent secondary schools) and the *Sunday Times State Schools Book*, with each sold as definitive guides detailing what gives these schools their 'edge' and the names of primary schools which sent most pupils to the 'country's best secondary schools'. Unfortunately squeamishness prevented them, like the rest, from supplying better-off parents with the key information many crave when choosing – the proportion of pupils from working-class and ethnic-minority homes. Currently they must ascertain that themselves (Gerwitz, Ball and Bowe 1995).

What is particularly dishonest has been the reluctance to report research exposing the tests' unreliability. Even when the Chief Inspector finally questioned their validity arguing 'the tests are vague, unreliable and administered creatively by schools' (Judd 1998b) this made one midday news bulletin, but was then dropped.

League tables like OFSTED reports, while supplying 'facts', have helped asphyxiate debate. By telling us 'all we need to know' about the state of schools and colleges in an easily digestible fashion they seem to make discussion superfluous. A mood well formulated in an *Independent* editorial published on the day another set of league tables appeared. This confidently proclaimed:

> At last, education is not a political battleground. Today's publication of examination league tables is no longer the cue for party political arguments. This is the welcome sign of a new consensus on education policy: as the public debate shifts to the mechanics of teaching and the details of raising schools' performance, so the ideology that so marred the Seventies and Eighties has been fading into the background.
>
> (*Independent*, 1 December 1998)

What the editorial failed to acknowledge was that not only are the content and direction of education no longer to be debated – that was settled in 1988 – but also the mechanics. For as Woodhead informed us, successful schools all adopt the same methods of 'challenging direct teaching, often to the whole class' (Woodhead 1998: 2) and the methods teachers should employ in the compulsory literacy and numeracy hours. League tables tell all what they must achieve and inevitably create boundless insecurity by ensuring more fail than succeed. To disagree or try to debate objectives therefore merely identifies one as a member of the awkward squad, someone uncommitted to the enterprise of education as the following introduction to a phone-in illustrates:

> 'Well on the day the new League Tables come out the Government announces plans for performance related pay for teachers. The teachers it seems don't like the idea and as usual are moaning. Why don't you phone in and let us know what you think about league tables for schools and performance related pay for the top teachers.'
>
> (Mike Parr, BBC Radio Newcastle, 1 December 1998)

A *Northern Echo* editorial discussing critical comments about the quality of OFSTED reports suggested that this 'sounds like another whinge from a profession which, sadly, can sometimes appear more concerned about a cushy life for its members than co-operating with any attempt to improve services to the schools' customers – the children' (*Northern Echo*, 13 November 1998).

Disagreements relating to the purpose and direction of education, about what is worthwhile and useful knowledge are, of course, perennial. They occupied Aristotle and Plato and will not dematerialise because governments and managers find them uncomfortable or journalists assume readers find them a 'turn-off'. Currently every attempt is made to restrict such discussions to a clique of tame government appointees. A good example of this was the decision not to make the document *Developing the School Curriculum* available to the public (and that means the teachers who deliver the curriculum) because 'Ministers have no intention of distracting attention from the primary standards drive by launching a major debate on how the curriculum should be shaped' (Pyke 1998).

A growing interest

Heightened media interest in education reflects their hopes of securing lucrative advertising income from the educational sector, but it also mirrors the expansive scale of the enterprise. Thirteen million pupils and students are taught and serviced by over one million full- and part-time staff: nearly a quarter of the population are directly involved in education and this proportion continues to escalate. Successive generations seem to start earlier and remain longer; more voluntarily proceed to further and higher education then return to study. In advocating 'lifelong learning' the government are pushing at an open door. The expansionist case has long held sway with only insufficient resources, sub-standard provision and access difficulties curtailing yet higher take-up. Indeed the view that governments must sell education to a reluctant population is the opposite of the truth. For 82 per cent want more spent on education and are willing to pay the higher taxes required (HMSO 1998: 121). We are it appears a pro-education society ruled by politicians following, not shaping, public opinion in this matter.

As public involvement develops so the media responds. Thirty years ago few national and virtually no local papers employed specialist education correspondents. Now the broadsheets have at least two, the tabloids one apiece, and some local papers have a journalist with some claim to the nomenclature. The former also have weekly education sections or pages containing a mix of specialist news and general articles: one of these, I learnt, was established solely to secure revenue from universities and private schools selling places. The content of these sections falls into two broad categories. First there are articles designed to attract the attention of parents and students. Often problem-centered these tend to dwell on parental fears such as under-achievement, unhappy pupils and dealing with professionals. Those directed at university students endlessly revisit the themes of – surviving your first week or term, avoiding debt, dealing with personal relationships (predictably sex and drugs dominate), plus an array of celebrity tales of success or failure. The *Daily Telegraph* even has an agony column hosted by the Education Editor, John Clare. Second, alongside these general articles is material written either by journalists, researchers or practitioners which, although accessible, is aimed primarily at professionals. Again, material is often issue- and problem-orientated but also covers policy questions. Education also features in unexpected quarters; for example, 'Miriam's Photocasebook' featured the story 'Her son's being bullied' (*Daily Mirror*, May 1998). Whilst agony columns regularly include items such as 'Sex with my teacher has stopped my studies' (*Sun*, 3 July 1998) the day after 'Sex case sir's suicide agony' (*Sun*, 2 July 1998).

Expansion of higher education from 94,000 undergraduates in 1960 to currently over a million has not just impacted on national papers. Newcastle now has more students than England and Wales in 1939. Sunderland, a major shipbuilding and mining town before the 1980s, now finds the university as its largest employer. Consequently, whereas the *Sunderland Echo* once featured launching ceremonies and reports of orders lost or secured, items relating to the comings and goings of academic staff, degree ceremonies, research completed, grants secured and the doings of students, currently proliferate. Physically universities dominate many city centres. Less obviously as major employers and generators of income they have inherited the virtual immunity from local media criticism always enjoyed by big firms. Partially this is because their public relations staff hide damaging stories and manage the local media by offering academics who provide hard pressed journalists with ready copy and quotes, add gravitas to thin items, or fill radio slots at short notice. What is good for the university becomes axiomatically good for the area; therefore only positive impressions are promulgated and serious discussion regarding their impact upon local communities excluded.

Stories about schools, further education and higher education seem almost ready to swamp local papers. The weekly *Chester Chronicle*, for example, regularly devotes three out of thirty pages to school and college news besides the numerous education-linked items scattered elsewhere. Some comprise recycled DfEE material pushed by press offices or local MPs under instructions from Millbank to 'get on message'. One example is the £500,000 Summer Numeracy Scheme involving fifty-one English schools and catering for just 1,500 children which gets blanket national and local television coverage before percolating down to local papers as 'Summer school maths for pupils leads the country' (*Sunderland Echo*, 9 June 1998). Another example is 'Truants to face police crackdown' (*Chester Chronicle*, 5 June 1998), 1,500 words of banal ministerial quotes reprinted without comment and augmented by a critical 300 words from a local headteacher. The bulk of local education coverage comprises these bland puffs based on press releases complemented with smiling-face photographs, thinly disguised adverts to lure students from feeder schools or paybacks to commercial concerns who require flattering publicity for sponsorship. What is largely absent is serious discussion of local education policy.

Coverage is often just a backcloth for advertising. As private schools expand, more parents seek nursery and day care, and funding mechanisms incite competition between educational institutions, so this potential revenue eclipses that traditionally linked to jobs. This bounty ensures the rigour and analysis within local education supplements tends to approximate to that of the motoring section. With education correspondents as fearful of losing the goodwill as the motoring correspondent is of offending the dealers and manufacturers who provide their revenue, good news abounds. Thus only Skoda College with a minuscule advertising budget and low rent clientele fears a poor press.

Not only the marginal are obsessed with publicity. The foyer of an LEA secondary in the *Sunday Times*' top 500 reflects this. It is a cultural desert devoid of works of art, with a trophy cupboard on one wall, with a plaque of remembrance to the war dead on another obscured by equipment, and on a third a substantial noticeboard illuminated by a brass picture light. This displays highlighted photocopies of local newspaper articles showing pupils receiving certificates, taking part in drama productions, sitting in rowing boats, and so on. It speaks volumes regarding the school's priorities and values. Here, like so many others, image is now all, procuring a 'competitive edge' and balanced books having fostered pressures which drive management decision-making 'towards commercial and away from educational or social considerations' (Gerwitz, Ball and Bowe 1995: 92). Such ends and desires may not always be mutually exclusive but they are not the role of education. As O'Connor notes, once the 'tatty and partial reporting' (O'Connor 1989: 218) of many journalists meant schools shunned and feared them. Now they are courted for financial and commercial ends whilst educational aims are diluted.

Growing centralisation of policy making has encouraged more coverage of education in national papers. However, volume is not all. The increasing size of the *Times Educational Supplement* (TES) does indicate heightened interest as well as expanding advertising revenue. Initially one edition covered all sectors; now there is one for schools and further education plus another for higher education. The former grows like Topsy as it spawns sub-sections. The number of journalists has not kept pace with growth. Therefore news is predominately repackaged handouts and briefings, research summaries, human interest stories often just giving an 'educational spin' to a big news story, articles by academics often seeking Brownie points rather than to stimulate debate, features from teachers (overwhelmingly uncritical and often shameless examples of smug self-promotion), and thinly disguised advertising features. All this is padded out with teaching tips, thin reviews and advice columns with scant critique or any evidence of investigative journalism. It says much about the tameness of the *Times Educational Supplement* and broadsheet education sections that possibly the most significant education story of recent years, namely the financial corruption and nepotism within further education and parts of higher education since local authority control and auditing ended, was largely exposed by *Private Eye* whose 'High Principals' column is now almost essential reading.

Despite rhetoric to the contrary the collective result of recent legislation, circulars and central government bullying and bluster has been 'to reduce diversity and stultify risk and experiment' (Gerwitz, Ball and Bowe 1988: 68). As differences between schools become less significant regarding what is taught and how it is delivered so trivial distinctions become ever more significant. Like soap powder and tyres, both indistinguishable to the untutored, schools are obliged and encouraged to market themselves by creating or magnifying trivial differences. Uniforms, logos, web sites, minor sporting accomplishments and pseudo-events (often more accurately termed stunts) acquire spiralling salience. The media, crucial for the success of the enterprise, rather than keeping the schools and colleges at arm's length have been seduced by this flood of easy-to-process froth. Editors and owners are delighted to report the doings and happy to fall into line. As the local media become awash with 'happy school tales', lingering relics of past serious discussions of education as a process are forgotten.

Centralisation

The Assisted Places Scheme introduced in 1980 marked an important departure. This transferred a sizeable sum from central government to independent schools to reduce or waive fees for the academically 'very able'. It was a vote of no confidence in the LEAs' ability to offer 'appropriate' education for such students. This programme required the government to find ways of talking directly to parents. It was a key moment in the onset of 'policy making by press release, by speech or by "informal" leak' (Reynolds 1989: 191).

In a centralised educational system teachers and local communities are no longer trusted to make even minor decisions. Once cooks managed unaided to compose school dinner menus but this is no longer so. Now the government must supply compulsory nutritional standards, covering portions by weight for primary and secondary sectors suggesting fish once a week and sample menus such as 'grilled gladiator beef or veggie burgers with carrot spears'. Ministers arrogantly notify teachers regarding how many minutes of homework to set. As the bureaucracy gathers momentum instructions become more outlandish. First teachers are ordered to have a daily literacy hour, then a numeracy hour. Blunkett then informs teachers, via the media, how to teach maths – no calculators – tried and trusted methods only. Told to balance fiction with non-fiction in the literacy hour, it is assumed teachers are too ignorant to tell these apart so the DfEE defines the former for them as 'a text which is invented by a writer or speaker' (quoted in Cooling 1998).

In replacing local democratic control with management by central government diktat the latter has created a series of problems for itself. How can it ensure that educators find out what they must do and prevent directives going astray or being communicated unsympathetically by union officials and local government officers? How can it also enthuse teachers who possess scant control over their working lives? How can some sense of collective educational purpose be generated when institutions are set against their neighbours and teachers told to fight off the claims of colleagues if they want improved status or pay? Such matters have caused sufficient concern for ministers and officials to initiate 'off the record' discussions with education correspondents regarding how they might communicate directly with the chalkface and get teachers to receive the message.

The result has been a new DfEE Strategy and Communications Directorate to organise media offensives. Each policy is now pre-released via leaks, then officially launched and constantly re-released. It is also dressed up in different ways for different audiences. Government spokespersons tell the *Daily Mail* how they are going to be tough on teachers, whilst making pro-teacher noises to the *Guardian* (Brenton 1998). Education correspondents are kept busy commuting between events and briefings. When their coverage is lack-lustre or hostile, DfEE spin doctors punish them by withholding the next 'scoop', or by belligerently phoning them for an explanation, or after a briefing demanding to know how they will cover it, and by giving education news to other correspondents on the same paper to undermine their standing with the editor who wants to know why they 'missed it'. Then following a national launch each initiative is farmed out to the local press, radio and television to ensure it filters down. Ministers are dispatched to provide added publicity and tame local MPs dragooned into drumming-up additional coverage.

Sometimes it goes horribly wrong, such as when Charles Clarke, a junior minister, briefed education correspondents concerning his wish that baseline assessment of incoming pupils would, given his 'sympathy with more setting in primary schools', encourage streaming. Although assumed by sceptics that this was always intended, such views had not previously been articulated. A hostile front-page piece in the *Daily Express* followed producing angry reactions from teachers' leaders who like others felt deceived by earlier assurances that the tests were solely to help formulate learning strategies and calculate value-added elements within Standard Assessment Tests (SATs), thus enabling schools in 'poor areas' to avoid permanent stigmatisation as league-table failures. Faced with this criticism Clarke retracted and wrote to the national papers saying he 'saw no direct relationship between baseline assessment and setting or streaming and that I did not believe the assessments were the vehicle to achieve more setting' (quoted by Ghouri 1998b).

Another ruse has been the growth in 'personal communications' from ministers. Blunkett, for example, wrote to all teachers in September 1998 to thank them for their help in raising standards and 'to tell them about our forthcoming consultation document on modernising the teaching profession' (Blunkett 1998). The same month also saw each school getting a copy from him of a leaflet with the snappy title *Taking Forward our Plans to Raise Standards for All*. Earlier, one million parents received letters prior to their children undertaking compulsory baseline assessments urging them to refrain from coaching as this might 'hide the real situation'. Perhaps this was a strange message from a department which also distributed advice leaflets to parents, via all 21,000 primary schools, listing seven ways they should support their children's learning. A video was also being prepared explaining forthcoming legislation for dispatch to every school. The communication needless to say does not assume a reply and is designed as an alternative to dialogue not as a stimulant to aid meaningful consultation.

Gimmicks designed to offer individuals an impression they can influence policy have been tried. For example when the White Paper *Excellence in Schools* was launched, copies were distributed in supermarkets and newsagents so ministers might learn by some ill-defined osmosis what people thought. A four-page summary appeared in the *Sun* and a hotline was provided with

Stephen Byers, a junior minister, plus fourteen civil servants spending a day listening to *Sun* readers telling them what they thought about education.

Centralised control of the curriculum and therefore school timetables means those anxious to change content or balance must now secure the ministerial ear. Policy formulation becomes more akin to a Byzantine court than a democracy with groups indulging in special pleading and exaggeration to get pet items onto the timetable. Organisations (voluntary and statutory) use the media to achieve this bypassing teachers or parents. The whole process is transparent. First scare stories emerge – 'without X then crime will increase or performance fall', then questions or early day motions surface in Parliament, and finally a minister promises action. Recent examples include NACRO (1998) advocating an anti-crime strategy imposed on schools to reduce offending, the Institute for Public Policy Research (Ghouri 1998a) pressing for citizenship teaching to be placed on the curriculum to prevent social exclusion, the Youth Sports Trust arguing that less PE will harm literacy (Barnard 1998), the Navy pleading for swimming lessons (Marsh 1998), Lord Menuhin proclaiming that music, dancing and singing civilise young people and more music would cut crime rates (*Daily Telegraph*, 13 November 1998), and the Secondary Heads Association proving that drama teaching builds confidence and team-building and must become a compulsory part of the curriculum (SHA 1998).

Again it can all too easily fall apart. As different groups jockey for position ministers are tempted to take the easy way out. A favourite ploy has been to set up working parties stuffed with safe names and sprinkled with celebrities to aid publicity. Currently the list includes ones on citizenship, sustainable development, personal, social and health education, creative and cultural and moral and spiritual values (established in response to the Bulger Case). All will eventually report during 1999 to a hurriedly convened group set up to oversee their work. Proposals for a new national curriculum will be published in summer 1999. A consultation process will then take place. This will be so thoroughgoing that it will be possible for the new national curriculum to be published by the autumn (DfEE 1998: 11). One assumes this is another example of the government following advice given to its predecessor that 'it will be important to ensure that any . . . consultation [with staff and pupils] does not unduly slow down decision-making, nor reduce management flexibility' (Coopers and Lybrand 1988: 34). What is certain, given the timescale, is that the consultation will be farcical and conducted via media briefings, stunts and celebrity events with neither teachers nor schools allowed a meaningful opportunity to engage in a debate regarding what they should or should not teach.

Conclusion

In 1901 George Cadbury purchased the *Daily News*, then the *Morning Leader* and *The Star* to campaign for education and welfare reform. He also voluntarily taught adult literacy classes every Sunday, opened his gardens and home to local children, anonymously funded higher education and built model schools to shame the government and local council into improving their standards. Cadbury lost a lot of money in running those newspapers but he never regretted it for he had a 'profound conviction that money spent on charities was of infinitely less value than money spent in trying to arouse my fellow countrymen to the necessity of measures to ameliorate the condition of the poor' (quoted Bradley 1987: 136). Since his demise it is unlikely any media proprietor has prioritised a desire to improve educational standards above the urge to secure a profit or personal power.

Such altruism is inconceivable today. Education, like art and culture, has become something to privatise first and then exploit. The media are not solely to blame for this but they have made a major contribution towards reducing current exchanges on education policy and practice to a torpid monotone which sticks close to the safe and predictable. When the main channels offer forty plus cookery programmes a week and only one magazine programme on education and when one surveys the press coverage it is difficult not to share the conclusion of George Walden that despite all the verbiage and heat 'the debate on education is not an educated debate' (1996: 14).

The press and television have done much to police the teaching profession and create a cowed workforce terrified of serious experimentation. It has also unquestioningly accepted the destruction of local democratic control and the centralisation which has followed. As a respected educational journalist has noted serious journalism in this area has not totally disappeared but it is seriously endangered, for:

> Trivialization and superficiality and political bias are not the prerogatives of the tabloid press, although they reach their apogee there. And in an atmosphere where the government is positively hostile to research results which tell them things they do not want to hear, the dislike of the message touches the messenger too, and the editorial response is too often to take the easy way out, and leave the uncomfortable truth unsaid. The market exerts its malign influence too: if it's difficult it must be dull, and if it's dull we daren't print or broadcast it.
>
> (O'Connor 1989: 221–222)

Education is a complex and difficult arena to understand. Issues are not straightforward and there will never be definite answers regarding what comprises useful and worthwhile knowledge, how education should be funded, how control should be distributed between educators, politicians, students, parents and local communities, and whose interests should be prioritised. A healthy system requires us to create ways which enable such topics to be constantly discussed and revisited; for dialogue to develop in which the greatest number might thoughtfully engage. Our present structures make that virtually impossible. Politicians determined to stifle debate and manage events for short-term electoral advantage, combined with a news media which are run on the cheap (and therefore ever more dependent on pre-packaged news) alongside companies seeking to manipulate education for the meanest of ends, contrive to militate against such debates taking place. Yet they will inevitably surface because they are too important to remain stifled for long. Just as we are obliged to constantly revisit the question of how justice can be balanced with freedom however much those in powerful positions may tell us it can all be left to them, so discussion of what our schools should teach and whose ends they should serve will constantly demand our attention. If the existing media will not help those debates to flourish then new alternative ways will undoubtedly be found.

References

Adams, R. (1991) *Protests by Pupils: Empowerment, Schooling and the State*, Lewes: Falmer.

Ball, S.J. (1984) 'Becoming a comprehensive: facing up to falling rolls', in S.J. Ball (ed.) *Comprehensive Schooling: a Reader*, Lewes: Falmer.

Barnard, N. (1998) 'PE lobby warns of threat to literacy', *Times Educational Supplement*, 22 May.

Bradley, I.C. (1987) *Enlightened Entrepreneurs*, London: Weidenfeld and Nicolson.

Blunkett, D. (1998) Letter sent to all Labour Members of Parliament, 16 September.

Brenton, H. (1998) 'Beware: spin-doctors are after the unions', *Times Educational Supplement*, 4 December.

Byers, S. (1998) 'Speech to NAHT Conference, Eastbourne', DFEE Press Release, 29 May.

Clark, P. (1998a) *Back From the Brink: Transforming the Ridings School – and our children's education*, London: Metro.

Clark, P. (1998b) 'To hell and back', *Times Educational Supplement*, 16 October 1998.

Cooling, M. (1998) 'Scripture's place in the literacy hour', *Times Educational Supplement*, 4 December.

Coopers and Lybrand (1988) *The Local Management of Schools: A Report to the DES*, London: Coopers and Lybrand.

Denscombe, M. (1984) 'Control, controversy and the comprehensive school', in S.J. Ball (ed.) *Comprehensive Schooling: a Reader*, Lewes: Falmer.

Department for Education and Employment (1998) *Taking Forward our Plans to Raise Standards for All*, London: DfEE.

Donnachie, I. and Hewitt, G. (1993) *Historic New Lanark*, Edinburgh: Edinburgh University Press.

Ellis, T., McWhirter, J., McColgan, D. and Haddow, B. (1976) *William Tyndale: the Teachers' Story*, London: Writers and Readers.

Fletcher, C., Caron, M. and Williams, W. (1985) *Schools on Trial: The Trials on Democratic Comprehensives*, Milton Keynes: Open University Press.

Gerwitz, S., Ball, S.J. and Bowe, R. (1995) *Markets, Choice and Equity in Education*, Buckingham: Open University Press.

Ghouri, N. (1998a) 'Clarke backpedals on primary setting', *Times Educational Supplement*, 11 September.

Ghouri, N. (1998b) 'Civil rights integral to citizenship, says report', *Times Educational Supplement*, 22 May.

Gribble, D. (1986) 'Dartington closes', *Libertarian Ed* 2(3).

Gribble, D. (1987) *That's All Folks*, Devon: West Aish Press.

Halpin, T. (1998) 'Don't expel drug pupils', *Daily Mail*, 17 November.

Hattersley, R. (1998) 'Silly exam tables actually do harm', *Times Educational Supplement*, 11 September.

HMSO (1998) *Social Trends* 28, London: HMSO.

Hoare, S. (1998) 'Beware editors and predators', *Times Educational Supplement*, 16 October.

Humphries, S. (1981) *Hooligans or Rebels? an Oral History of Working Class Childhood and Youth*, Oxford: Blackwell.

Jeffs, T. and Smith, M. (1994) 'Young people, youth work and a new authoritarianism', *Youth and Policy* (46): 17–32.

Jeffs, T. and Smith, M. (1996) '"Getting the dirtbags off the streets": curfews and other solutions to juvenile crime', *Youth and Policy* (53): 1–14.

Judd, J. (1998a) 'The city that lets down its pupils', *Independent*, 18 June.

Judd, J. (1998b) 'National tests criticised by schools chief', *Independent*, 18 December.

Lumley, K. (1998) 'Teeny thugs in Blair's sights: media portrayals of children in education and their policy implications', *Youth and Policy* (61).

NACRO (1998) *Children, schools and crime*, London: NACRO.

Marsh, A. (1998) 'Schools blamed as Navy reveals 10 per cent of recruits cannot swim', *Daily Telegraph*, 17 September.

O'Connor, M. (1989) 'Reflections from an observer', in A. Hargreaves and D. Reynolds (eds) *Education Policies: Controversies and Critiques*, Brighton: Falmer Press.

Pyke, N. (1998) 'Prescription pruned back', *Times Educational Supplement*, 22 May.

Reader, P. (1992) 'Liasing with the media', in N. Foskett (ed.) *Managing External Relations in Schools*, London: Routledge.

Reynolds, D. (1989) 'Better schools? past and potential policies about the goals, organization, and management of secondary schools', in A. Hargreaves and D. Reynolds (eds) *Education Policies: Controversies and Critiques*, Brighton: Falmer Press.

Roberton, C. (1998) 'Thugs who rule our schools', *Sunderland Echo*, 23 February.

Secondary Heads Association (1998) *Drama Sets You Free*, Leicester: SHA.

Spiller, P. (1998) 'Schools in drugs storm', *Newcastle Evening Chronicle*, 17 November.

Walden, G. (1996) *We Should Know Better: Solving the Education Crisis*, London: Fourth Estate.

Weeks, A. (1986) *Comprehensive Schools: Past, Present and Future*, London: Methuen.

Wolchover, J. (1998) 'Head quits after war with militant staff', *Evening Standard*, 5 June.

Woodhead, C. (1998) 'The forces driving up standards in schools', *Sunday Times*, 25 October.

Chapter 11

Exorcising demons

Media, politics and criminal justice

John Muncie

Media discourse is saturated with crime. Crime consumes an enormous amount of media space as both entertainment and news. Whether it be TV cop shows, crime novels, docudramas, newspaper articles, comics, documentaries or 'real life' reconstructions, crime, criminality and criminal justice appear to have an endless capacity to tap into public fear and fascination. Indeed much of our information about the nature and extent of crime comes to us via the secondary source of the media. We should expect, then, that they play a significant role in our perception and understanding of the boundaries between order and disorder. But despite the powerful 'commonsense' view that news media merely provide the facts of a process in which crime occurs – police apprehend criminals and courts punish them – the relationship between crime and media reportage is far from simple.

This chapter is written in the context of an ongoing debate over the complexities of media content, news sources and media effects. In the 1960s and 1970s a critical media analysis alerted us to the ways in which crime news is not only a cultural product but the result of a particular configuration of institutional definitions and priorities. Media, political and criminal justice discourses, it was argued, share a hidden ideological consensus, reproduce the same crime agenda and deliver the same message. In the process, fears of crime and disorder are exacerbated, legitimating a shift to an authoritarian law 'n' order society (Hall 1973a). By the 1990s, this 'media as hegemonic' stance was substantially revised by detailed empirical studies which revealed a plurality of competing voices battling to gain media access. It was stressed that no direct relation existed between media discourse, public opinion and political action. Each was dependent on a wide variety of subtle, diverse and contingent relations (Ericson 1991; Ericson, *et al.* 1987; 1991). At the same time a postmodern imagination emerged which claimed that in a forever growing 'mediatised' world crime narratives generate an 'insecure security' in which it has become increasingly impossible to draw clear boundaries between media image and social reality (Barak 1994; Osborne 1995).

This chapter sets these debates in the context of the 'youth crime problem' of the 1990s and in particular the political fallout from the murder of James

Bulger in 1993. In the past six years, in Britain at least, theoretical and empirical evidence tends to lend weight to the former view that a generally right-wing press and politicians, whilst not always agreeing, have shared an affinity on issues of law and order. This period has witnessed a sustained media and political attack on crime in general, and on young people in particular, despite contrary statistical evidence that suggests that much of this may be misplaced.

Reading crime news

Since at least the mid 1880s, crime news has been a staple diet of the popular press. Roshier (1973) found that between 1938 and 1967 on average 4 per cent of total news space was devoted to crime. It is a percentage though that has increased significantly in the past decade. Williams and Dickinson's (1993) analysis of ten national dailies in 1989 put the figure at almost 13 per cent and Reiner (1997) reports that data from the *Daily Mirror* and *The Times* between 1945 and 1991 shows a rise from an average 8 per cent to 21 per cent. It is probably no coincidence that law and order has also grown as a significant political issue during this time.

But as the amount of crime news has increased the type of crime reported has stayed remarkably constant. Since Davis' (1952) pioneering research in Colorado, comparisons of crime news and crime statistics have produced consistent results. For example, studies of the provincial press by Ditton and Duffy in Strathclyde and Smith in Birmingham both revealed that newspapers distort the 'official' picture of crimes known to and recorded by the police. In Strathclyde an over-reporting of crimes involving violence and sex was noted to the degree that during March 1981 such crimes constituted 2.4 per cent of reported incidence yet occupied 45.8 per cent of newspaper coverage (Ditton and Duffy 1983: 164). In Birmingham personal offences such as robbery and assault accounted for less than 6 per cent of known crimes but occupied 52.7 per cent of the space devoted to crime stories (Smith 1984: 290). Smith also reported biases in terms of the media's identification of key 'criminal areas' of a city although they did not have the highest reported crime rate, and a tendency to link issues of race with crime. The first research of crime news in all of the national dailies in Britain in the late 1980s similarly found that newspapers regularly devoted over 60 per cent of the space given to crime reporting to stories dealing with cases of personal violence even though they only constituted some 6 per cent of crimes reported by victims (Williams and Dickinson 1993: 40).

Clearly, whilst newspapers do inform the public, they can also help to create a public awareness that is substantially different from any 'reality' contained in victim surveys and the official statistics (Smith 1984: 293). Young (1974), for example, noted how the type of information which the mass media select and disseminate to the public is coloured throughout by the notion of newsworthiness. He argued that, rather than providing a pure reflection of the social world, 'newspapers select events which are *atypical*, present them in a *stereotypical* fashion and contrast them against a backcloth of normality which is *overtypical*' (Young 1974: 241). The criminal is then usually depicted as violent, immoral and a threat to an otherwise peaceful social order. Crime – despite its ubiquity – is presented in a way in which it continually breaches our 'normal' expectations about the world.

The media appear to be involved in a continual search for the 'new', unusual and dramatic. This is what makes the 'news'. Chibnall (1977: 77) notes five sets of informal rules of relevance which govern the professional imperatives of popular journalism: 1) visible and spectacular acts 2) sexual or political connotations 3) graphic presentation 4) individual pathology and 5) deterrence and repression. It is around such themes that news values are structured. According to Chibnall, press reports cannot simply be a reflection of real events because two key processes always intervene: *selection* – which aspects of events to report, which to omit; and *presentation* – choosing what sort of headline, language, imagery, photograph and typography to use. As he argues, the violence most likely to receive coverage in the press is indeed that which involves sudden injury to 'innocent others', especially in public places. Concern with such violence has typified newspaper accounts throughout the past fifty years, bolstered by such media labels as 'cosh boys', 'bullyboy skinheads', 'vandals', 'muggers', 'hooligans', 'joyriders', 'blood-crazed mobs' and 'rampaging thugs'. The concentration on these forms in media and public discourse does, however, reinforce limited concepts of crime and violence. Domestic violence, unsafe working conditions, pollution of the environment and the mental violence involved in repetitive jobs are all cited by Chibnall as phenomena that have caused equal suffering but have received less sustained press attention because they do not conform to the criteria of spectacular newsworthiness (Chibnall 1977: 78). The same applies to white-collar crime, corporate corruption, state violence and the regular and unhindered denial of human rights.

The graphic presentation of events also plays its part in constructing a particular image of crime and criminality. Headlines of catch-all phrases and derogatory labels combine to sensitize us to certain types of crime. Similarly, the choices of photograph are governed by an ideological procedure. By appearing to reproduce the event as it really happened, news photographs suppress their underlying selective, interpretive and ideological function (Hall 1973b: 188). The drama also depends on the easy identification of opposing factions: young people versus adults, hooligans versus police, black people versus white, 'violent' protesters and 'innocent' victims. In this way, crime is depicted in terms of a basic confrontation between the symbolic forces of good and evil. Complex social events are collapsed into simplistic questions of right and wrong. The intricate history and consequences of an event necessary to provide a fuller and more complex picture are rarely provided, or only at a later date when the terms of debate have already been firmly set (Hall *et al.* 1975; Hall 1978).

However, the media do not necessarily adopt a unitary approach to crime news. Important degrees of emphasis appear between the quality, mid-market and tabloid press and between the national dailies and television news. Schlesinger, Tumber and Murdock's (1991) research, for example, found that the tabloids are more likely to feature violent crime, whilst television gives more attention to offences relating to public order, to the justice system and to the state. Roshier's (1973) analysis also found that it is not only the dramatic and exceptional that is considered newsworthy. Rather, incidents of petty theft and those with 'whimsical circumstances' also feature strongly, usually in the inside pages as a reliable form of trivial, light entertainment. However, as he acknowledges, in certain cases, such as drug offences and football hooliganism in the 1960s, there emerges a noticeable tendency to dramatise offence seriousness and publicise 'get tough' responses. Nowhere was such unanimity most clearly seen than in the media reaction to the Bulger murder in 1993.

On 12 February 1993, sixteen video cameras in a shopping centre in Liverpool filmed two 10-year-old boys abducting 2-year-old James Bulger. He was found two days later battered to death by a railway line. This particular murder was to form a significant watershed in media and political responses to youth crime, and not simply because of its apparent brutality. The Bulger case had at least three related consequences. First, it initiated a reconsideration of the social construction of 10-year-olds as 'demons' rather than as 'innocents'. Second, it coalesced with, and helped to mobilise, a moral panic about youth crime in general. Third, it legitimised a series of tough law and order responses to young offenders which came to characterise much of the 1990s.

Franklin and Petley (1996) and Davis and Bourhill (1997) have provided detailed assessments of the newspaper reportage of the trial of the two boys who were eventually convicted for the murder in November 1993. For all but the *Financial Times* and the *Morning Star* it was the front-page headline story. The *Daily Mail* carried twenty-four separate articles, the *Daily Express* an eight-page supplement. One of the *Daily Mail*'s headlines 'The evil and the innocent' (25 November 1993) set the tone for some intensive media agonising over 'How could it happen?' However, it was the video footage from a security camera of James Bulger being led hand-in-hand by one of the 10-year-olds out of the shopping centre that made the case famous. The blurred and shaky image was replayed endlessly on television, as Alison Young (1996: 112) argues, inviting feelings of helplessness and horror as we watch the boys slowly disappear from view with the voyeuristic knowledge that death is to follow. As such, the event 'always existed as much as an image of itself as it did in itself' (Young 1996: 137). A recurring theme in media representations of the case was the juxtaposition of childhood innocence and children as inherently evil. Innocence was easily imputed to James Bulger; he was the symbolic epitome of an ideal child. Normally 10-year-old children would also be media-idealised as innocent victims. But, as Hay (1995) argues, herein lies the crux of the event. We are forced to confront the uncomfortable notion that ten-year-olds may not be innocent at all. As the *Sunday Times* (28 November 1993) put it: 'we will never be able to look at our children in the same way again . . . Parents everywhere are asking themselves and their friends if the Mark of the Beast might not also be imprinted on their offspring'. At the end of the trial, the judge described the two defendants as 'wicked and cunning' having committed acts of 'unparalleled evil and barbarity' (*The Times*, 24 November 1993). And so it was that one of the preferred media explanations of 'why it happened' dwelt on the theme of 'evil'. The *Daily Mirror* (25 November 1993) described the 10-year-olds as 'Freaks of nature' with 'hearts of evil'. Elsewhere, terms such as 'boy brutes', 'monsters', 'animals' and the 'spawn of Satan' abounded. For many the case demanded that all children be regarded as a threat and that childhood should be redefined as a time of innate evil. As James and Jenks (1996) suggest, it was not just two children who were put on trial, but the very nature of childhood itself. Other dominant explanations dwelt on an assumed decline in moral responsibility as a result of '1960s permissiveness'. The disintegration of the nuclear family, single parenting and the influence of media violence (particularly the film *Child's Play 3*, 1991) were all cited as key precipitating factors. William Golding's novel *Lord of the Flies* (1945) was repeatedly referenced as 'evidence' of the horror and evil that is unleashed when children are free from the discipline of adults (*Guardian*, 16 February 1993; *Daily Mail*, 25 November 1993). As a result, any number of alternative 'readings' based on welfare, health, psychology, victimology, psychiatry, behavioural science or economics were subsumed by, or were ruled out in favour of, the law. Once the killing was coded as 'crime', it was the legal process and the assumption of individual responsibility which 'laid down the agenda for what could be reported and commented upon as "news"' (King 1995: 173).

The Bulger case also came to symbolise something much broader; it became a signifier for a generalised 'crisis' in childhood and a breakdown of moral and social order (James and Jenks 1996; Davis and Bourhill 1997). As the *Daily Star* (30 November 1993) put it: 'much of Britain is now facing a truly frightening explosion of kiddie crime . . . too many kids are turning into hardened hoods almost as soon as they've climbed out of their prams'. In a climate of general anxiety about crime, the exceptional murder of an infant by two boys, barely at the age of criminal responsibility themselves, was viewed as symptomatic of a prevailing youth crime wave, even though they bore no obvious relation to each other (Hay 1995).

In the early 1990s, a raft of youth troubles, most notably truancy, drug taking, disturbances on housing estates in Oxford, Cardiff and Tyneside following police clampdowns on joyriding and images of 'youth out of control' and 'one-boy crime waves' had already raised levels of public concern. Notable was the case of 'Ratboy'. Alleged to have committed fifty-five offences by the time he was fourteen, one boy in north-east England first came to the notice of the police, when he was ten, for burglary. After two cautions his parents volunteered him for local authority care, from which he absconded thirty-seven times. In February 1993 he was found hiding in a ventilation duct. A local newspaper could not print his name, so invented the nickname 'Ratboy'. Next day he was front-page national news. With the construction of images of sewers, of a hidden underworld and of secret tunnels running beneath the urban landscape, the boy became a symbol of all juvenile crime against which the police and courts were 'impotent' to act. But in many other respects, the boy did not live up to the prevailing stereotypes of dangerous and outcast youth. He did not come from a broken home . . . he was not violent . . . he did not grow up in some 'urban wasteland' . . . he became a 'symbol surrounded by cliches' (*Independent*, 9 October 1993).

Individual TV images, such as that of an 11-year-old in a balaclava mask being arrested after crashing a stolen car, also galvanised politicians of all parties, the police, judges and magistrates to demand more effective measures to deal with young offenders. As Bill Jordan argues, it is difficult to underestimate the impact the Bulger case has made on subsequent political discourse and policy formulation (see Chapter 12). Just ten days after the Bulger murder, the Home Secretary announced plans to establish a new network of secure training centres for 12–15-year-old offenders. He opined that no excuses could be made for 'a section of the population who are essentially nasty pieces of work' (*The Times*, 22 February 1993). The two 10-year-olds – Jon Venables and Robert Thompson – were eventually sentenced to be detained for a minimum of eight years. This was raised to ten years by the Lord Chief Justice and to fifteen years by the Home Secretary (a decision subsequently declared to be illegal in July 1996). Much of this punitiveness was inspired by the *Sun* urging its readers to plead with the Home Secretary that the boys should be locked up for life. In 1998 The European Commission on Human Rights ruled that there was a prima facie case that both their trial and their sentencing was in violation of the European Convention on Human Rights. In most European countries Venables and Thompson would have been considered much too young to be prosecuted at all. There would have been no trial and no question of guilt or innocence. Most pernicious, perhaps, was the way in which reaction to the death of James Bulger firmly located violence solely with youth. As Scraton (1997: 164) astutely concluded: 'what a terrible irony this represents given the apparently insatiable appetite that much of the adult, patriarchal world has for violence, brutality, war and destruction'. At which point it is also worth reminding ourselves that young people are more likely to encounter crime as victims than as offenders. More than 10 per cent of the 600 homicides in Britain each year are perpetrated by parents against their under-16-year-old children. This too tends to remain absent from media and political discourse.

Producing crime news

The news media have little direct access to crime as such. The majority of crime stories come to them via the police, the courts and the Home Office. Agencies of crime control are the primary sources of crime news. As such they are in a position to provide initial definitions of crime and locate them within the context of a continuing crime problem. The credibility of their definitions is in turn enhanced by their 'official' and 'institutional' standing. Rarely does the criminal's own interpretation figure in this defining process, and thus the possibility of obtaining any counter definitions is diminished. The regular access of control institutions to media reportage is both open and 'acceptable'. They are the institutions in the front line of crime control; they have an everyday knowledge of the 'fight against crime'. It thus appears quite 'natural' that they should be the main source of news about crime.

As Chibnall (1977: 49) argued, crime stories have historically been the bread and butter of popular journalism. The nineteenth century developed the tradition of sensational crime reporting in the Sunday newspapers, the *Police Gazette* and the *Illustrated Police News*. These were dependent largely on court cases, but as popular journalism expanded in the twentieth century, information about the earlier, and potentially more sensational aspects of criminal proceedings became highly sought after. Thus the press came to rely increasingly on one major institutional source – the police. Reporters' increased contact with the police gradually became more informal and their role more secure and autonomous. In 1945 these specialist journalists formed the Crime Reporters' Association in order to improve press–police relations. Today it remains a common – though declining – practice for journalists to be trained on local newspapers by attending court cases. Contemporary news values and commercial interests have tended to give an ever greater weight to the particularly horrific, the exotic or events with a celebrity angle at the expense of the vast majority of crime now considered 'routine' or 'mundane'. In the 1970s the police also had considerable success in elevating themselves as authoritative political advisors, not only on the implementation of crime control but also on matters of criminal justice policy and reform. Under the guidance of Sir Robert Mark, former Commissioner of the Metropolitan Police, a new and more 'open' press relations policy was instituted, in which press conferences and direct communication between editors and senior police officers were commonplace (Mark 1979). And by the 1980s police forces began hiring corporate image specialists to improve their public standing and were actively encouraging audience mobilisation, especially in the more sensational cases, through such television programmes as *Crimewatch UK* and *Crimestoppers* (Schlesinger and Tumber 1994).

Stemming directly from such policies the possibilities for 'news management' by the police have been greatly enhanced, such that the dissemination of crime news is controlled by a 'deviancy defining elite' involving collaboration between police, news media and private organisations (Ericson *et al.* 1991). The media and criminal justice systems are increasingly penetrating each other. This is not to argue that journalists and broadcasters are incapable of presenting views that are controversial or unacceptable to established politicians or the control agencies, but that in the vast majority of cases their accounts are grounded in the interpretations provided by these 'authoritative' primary sources (Schlesinger and Tumber 1994: 20). These interpretations are in turn dependent largely on the rate of reported crime, the focused and organised police response to certain crimes, and the reports of Home Office statisticians reliant on eventual rates of conviction. The partiality of public knowledge about crime is then further exacerbated by the reproduction of judicial and police statements, the shaping power of news values and the practices of news presentation. Indeed, most crime news usually occurs through the subsequent representation of criminal acts in court proceedings, rather than at the moment of the act itself. Many of the most dramatic headlines are taken directly from a judge's summing up or reflection on the state of society as a result of a particular event. For example, much media reaction to the mods and rockers conflicts on Brighton, Clacton and Margate beaches in 1964 famously reproduced the public pronouncements of the Margate magistrate, Dr George Simpson:

> Virtually every court report quoted Dr Simpson's 'Sawdust Caesars' speech in full and his terminology significantly influenced the mass media symbolisation and the process of spurious attribution. His phrases were widely used as headlines: '"Sawdust Caesars hunt in pack" says magistrate', '"A Vicious Virus" says J.P.', 'Town Hits Back on Rat Pack Hooligans'.
>
> (Cohen 1980: 108)

The judge's comment that the killing of James Bulger was an 'act of unparalleled evil' was also widely used to headline stories about the child's murder. In this way it has been argued that the media do not simply reflect social reality but define it in a particular way, subsequently affecting the quality of public opinion. In analysing this effect Hall *et al.* (1975: 2) propose replacing the 'everyday' assumption that crime → apprehension → crime report, with the more complex model of:

> Crime (volume and incidence unknown) → 'crime' (product of institutional definition by crime control agencies) → news values (the selective institutional practices of 'news making') → 'crime as news' (the selective portrayal of crime in the media) → public definition of crime (consequence of information provided by official and media sources).

As such it appears that popular images about crime are 'popular' only in so far as they are consequences of information provided by official sources with a vested interest in expanding crime control, and by media sources with a vested interest in maintaining profitable news values (Muncie 1996: 49).

In some contrast detailed analysis of the production of crime news in the 1980s and 1990s has maintained that the media are not hegemonic but the site of different group interests (Ericson 1991; Schlesinger and Tumber 1994; Sparks 1992). Increasingly, pressure groups, penal reform organisations and civil liberties groups have gained access to the news media and have become ever more sophisticated in designing their own media strategies to which the established law enforcement agencies have been forced to respond. Such oppositional and alternative entries into the policy agenda process may indeed lead us to query conceptions of all-powerful 'primary definers'. Schlesinger, Tumber and Murdock's (1991: 413) analysis, for example, found that whilst the quality newspapers tended to 'source' judges, lawyers and court officials, similar weight was also given to members of lobby and pressure groups. In the tabloids law enforcement agencies were again prioritised but not at the expense of victims, suspects' relatives and criminals. But such diversity may mask continuing inequalities in media access and in particular may not be able to withstand the dramatic and political purchase of certain mediatised events. As Franklin and Petley (1996) found, there was total unanimity amongst the British media following the Bulger murder, characterised by a 'brutal and hysterical press vilification' with an 'unrelenting retributivist and punitive character'. At such moments alternative and oppositional voices are rarely, if ever, heard.

Consuming crime news

It has long been argued that the process of delivering news does not necessarily end with the representation of crime in press reports. For a story about crime, especially when singled out as significant by a senior police officer or by a judge in court, can legitimise the press taking on a more active and editorial role (Young 1974; Hall 1978; Cohen 1980). The press can play a role in orchestrating the concern they have helped to create. Sections of the press frequently use these causes of concern as the basis for stimulating the public into a moral panic, and through a process of 'repetitive retribution' are able to make a significant impact on major policy decisions (Sanders and Lyon 1995).

Of the numerous publicly debated and dramatised social problems from the late 1960s to the present, law and order has been one of the most prominent. High visibility of this particular problem holds certain advantages for some groups in society. Politicians, for example, often align themselves with the forces of the police and the law in order to gain public appreciation and improve their electoral chances. Similarly, crime journalism (following the success of Rupert Murdoch's sensationalist formula in the *Sun* from 1969 onwards) found that increasing the audience for, and profit from, crime news depends upon promoting a generalised belief that law and order are breaking down. Neo-conservative ideologues have collapsed together such diverse phenomena as truancy, sadism, drug taking, vagrancy, violence in the streets, student revolt and illiteracy (Joseph 1974, cited by Chibnall 1977: xii) and identified them all as symptomatic of lawlessness. In the 1970s, Patricia Morgan readily equated violence and destruction with youth, and talked of this 'new barbarism' as the major cause of urban breakdown and moral decline in Britain (Morgan 1978: 12–13). In the 1990s, Digby Anderson echoed such sentiments by claiming that the 'yobs and criminals' had been 'allowed to take over' (*Sunday Times*, 2 June 1996). Government ministers have foreseen the imminent destruction of society epitomised by Margaret Thatcher's denunciation of the football hooligan in 1985 as the 'new enemy within'. The threat of youth violence was equated with trade union militancy and international terrorism. MPs have called for flogging and the use of stocks to punish offenders (*The Times*, 14 March 1981), with one Conservative MP contemplating the ultimate spectacle of flogging criminals live on television before or after the weekly National Lottery draw in order to humiliate and deter (*Independent*, 20 March 1995).

Law and order campaigns have clear commercial and political consequences, as well as sensitising the public to 'moral panic'. Young (1974) has argued that the tendency to sensationalise the news also carries with it a tendency to amplify the phenomenon being reported. For once a social problem has been identified and labelled, the attention of journalists and readers tends to be directed to finding more examples of the same problem. For example, following the release of the 1981 official crime statistics, the *Daily Mirror* devoted 8 of its 32 pages (including front page and centre spread) to an analysis of 'Our Violent Cities'. Each of the reports detailed incidents of gang fights, pub brawls, muggings and violent attacks. But, such reporting is rarely related to an actual increase in such incidents at any particular time. As Lea and Young state, 'whatever this achieves in promoting the sale of newspapers, it certainly creates quite detrimental effects on public consciousness and fear of crime' (Lea and Young 1984: 25). By clustering a number of unrelated events under a single headline, the press can indeed create a trend, a trend which then becomes newsworthy in its own right.

Pearson (1983) has also catalogued how leading politicians, the police and the media appear to collude in their condemnation and explanation of youth disorder. Of note is the often repeated notion that such disorder is progressively becoming more serious. The usual historical reference is 'twenty years ago'. By restating this premise the impression is given that the problem of youth and crime is new. As a new problem, new and urgent measures are called for, particularly a return to unequivocal discipline and retributive measures. Frequently, the so-called 'permissiveness' of the 1960s is used as a catch-all to explain youth's present unruliness. In contrast, the distant past of the 1950s is idealised as a time free of such troubles. But in a sequence of backward glances through English social history, Pearson shows how images of a more peaceful, orderly and harmonious past (against which the present can be unfavourably compared) fail to stand up to close scrutiny: for example twenty years before the moral outrage surrounding the 1981 riots similar fears and responses centred on the lawlessness of the Teddy Boys; in the interwar years, the folk devils were football rowdyism and the demoralising influence of the American cinema. Edwardian and Victorian England meanwhile was 'plagued' by the 'un-English' hooligan in the 1890s, the garotters of the 1860s and the street urchins of the 1840s. Such research alerts us to key continuities in a history of 'respectable fears'. Pearson reveals a remarkable consistency in the identification of youth as the source of social problems and in the nature of the dominant culture's condemnation. Moreover he concludes that preoccupations with youth disorder are not simply about crime but are invariably associated with wider social tensions. Moral panics about youth are characteristically the surface manifestation of deeper concerns which revolve around the place and passivity of the working classes. For example, the original Edwardian hooligan was part of a much wider debate of the boy labour 'problem' and their moral degeneration in dead-end jobs. This in turn signified a growing concern over urban degeneration and national decline at the turn of the century. Analysis of 'moral panics' and 'crime waves' tells us more of the condition and stability of society at particular historical moments than it does of any particular incidents called 'crime'.

This is a view with which many media researchers would now concur. Katz's (1987) study of news stories in the New York and Los Angeles daily press concluded that public fascination for crime news emanates not from a concern for crime per se, or from a naive belief that such news will provide some empirical truth, but from the way in which crime news provides material for a working out of moral dilemmas that are confronted in everyday life. It is this which helps to explain the constant reader fascination even when the substantive distortion of types of crime news is blatantly obvious. So for Katz in order to understand why the reader voluntarily submits to a daily bombardment of disturbing images and emotions we must recognise how crime news serves a similar purpose to that of any other daily ritual: it is an acknowledgement of a 'personal burden for sustaining faith in an ordered social world' (Katz 1987: 72).

As a result it has been argued that whilst media representations do have an effect, they are unlikely to be received passively, but rather interpreted by an 'active audience' as but one element in their lived experience (Livingstone 1996; Ericson 1991; Roshier 1973). But that 'active audience', as Osborne (1995) reminds us, increasingly lives in a media saturated world. Trying to isolate a specific media effect may be particularly problematic when the boundaries between drama and reality are becoming more and more blurred . . . and when the parameters of 'lived experience' are harder to define.

Public fear, political discourse and social control

Whilst there may be an almost unanimous belief that the media affects public opinion in some way which in turn plays a part in the formulation of criminal justice policy, the exact relationship between these three 'voices' is far from clear. Attempts to measure the impact of the mass media in promoting fear have generally found that readers of those newspapers that report crime in the most dramatic and distorted fashion also have the highest levels of fear of crime. Moreover, the majority of people attribute their knowledge of risk to information received from television and press reports (Williams and Dickinson 1993). However a causal link cannot be unequivocally established. Sparks (1992: 13–14), for example, argues that risk may well be evaluated differently at the time of the committing of a crime and once that crime has entered the 'circles of punishment, retribution, reporting, rhetoric and rebuttal, election platforms and the multitude of communicative exchanges which compose the public sphere'. Perceptions of fear are always indelibly tied up with issues of representation, interpretation and meaning of which the media form a significant but only one part.

Nevertheless some strong parallels have been found between media biases and public misperceptions. Using data from the 1996 British Crime Survey, Hough and Roberts (1998) found that, whilst the national recorded crime rate fell by 8 per cent between 1993 and 1996, 96 per cent of the public believed rates to have risen or stayed the same. When asked how much crime involves violence, 78 per cent replied 30 per cent or more, whilst Home Office statistics record it at just 6 per cent. Conversely substantial underestimates were routinely made about the extent to which the courts use custodial disposals for convicted offenders. A view, not that dissimilar to that propagated by most of the media, emerges of a forever spiralling crime rate and an over-lenient criminal justice system. Neither could be further from the truth. Indeed this study directly implicates the media in such public misunderstanding: 'media news values militate against balanced coverage. Erratic court sentences make news and sensible ones do not. As a result large segments of the population are exposed to a steady stream of unrepresentative stories about sentencing incompetence' (Hough and Roberts 1998: x).

Between 1993 and 1996 the prison population in Britain increased by 50 per cent. This occurred without any significant increase in the number of convicted offenders and with a decline in the crime rate. There was however a great deal of political rhetoric about 'prison works' and about being 'tough on crime and tough on the causes of crime'. Howard's 'prison works' slogan first surfaced at the Conservative Party conference in October 1993. This claim was based on the simple premise that incapacitation would ensure that offenders could not reoffend whilst they were inside and thus the crime rate would be reduced. Notwithstanding contrary Home Office research which concluded that even a 25 per cent increase in the prison population would only reduce the crime rate by 1 per cent, the policy was widely hailed as progressive by the tabloids, Tory activists and the police. What followed was a succession of Criminal Justice Acts between 1993 and 1997 designed to overturn the decarcerative principles of previous legislation. In particular the 1997 Crime (Sentences) Act introduced mandatory minimum sentences for certain offences, extended electronic monitoring to 10-year-olds, allowed juveniles to be 'named and shamed' in court, ended automatic parole and curtailed conditions of sentence remission. All such measures may have had a dubious rationale in penological terms but their intuitive appeal remained strong. In a period of public anxiety, of economic stringency and of considerable electoral unpopularity for the Conservatives, such appeals to penal severity spoke powerfully to 'popular sensibilities'. By the time of the 1997 general election there was a marked convergence of Conservative and Labour Party law and order politics – each, it seemed, trying to outdo the other in not being seen to have in any way 'gone soft' on crime. Boot camps, curfews, parental control orders, child jails, fast-track punishment, the abolition of the presumption of childhood innocence for 10- to 14-year-olds, zero tolerance campaigns, the abolition of repeat cautioning, tougher community penalties and so on were all on the agenda. In 1994 the Conservative Home Secretary had denounced 'do-gooders' who in his view simply rewarded offenders for their crimes (*Independent on Sunday*, 21 August 1994), while in 1996 the shadow Labour Home Secretary blamed 'liberal elements' who used poverty and deprivation as an excuse for a do-nothing approach (*Guardian*, 19 September 1996). For both, the faults of the present were laid firmly in the hands of inadequate parents, welfare professionals and penal reformers. And by 1998, just one year into the New Labour administration, the Crime and Disorder Act put most of these proposals onto the statute book. Whilst Labour rhetoric has promoted a communitarian logic to this expansion of penal powers, it retains a firm commitment to populist authoritarianism. It reclaims, rather than disturbs, the remoralisation thesis once firmly associated with Conservative ideology (Muncie 1999). The problem of crime is once again viewed as a breakdown of morality associated with unruly youth, dysfunctional families and a parenting deficit. Its solution lies in locking up more people and in enforcing parental and community responsibilities.

In many respects much of this enduring punitive mentality can be traced back to the barrage of public, political and media outrage following the Bulger murder in 1993. This one event alone has been the catalyst for successive years of authoritarianism heralded by the headlines 'Tory blitz on teenage crime' (*Daily Mail*) and 'Home Secretary pledges: I'll lock up young villains' (*Daily Express*) on 22 February 1993. Images of teenage thugs, public horror, spiralling crime, persistent villains, ineffective court powers, failing teachers and social workers and a widespread loss of moral values have continued to dominate media and political discourse and to inform criminal justice policy. As Osborne (1995: 31) put it: 'Reactions to crime representations are deeply irrational and that is what makes the media's love of crime so dangerous'. Any cursory glance at the prison statistics over the last decade will confirm such a view. From a previous high of some 50,000 in 1987 the prison population fell to a low of 42,000 in January 1993 (the month preceding the Bulger murder). Since then it rose year-on-year to reach an all time high of 67,000 in July 1998. As the *Financial Times* – in a rare self-reflexive moment – commented on 13 March 1993:

> . . . the British media exercise a uniquely decisive influence on national political life . . . in no other country would what has been termed the 'moral panic' over juvenile crime have provided the basis of such a concerted campaign that led to almost instant action on the part of government.

Conclusion

Whilst the relation between media, public, politics and policy is complex and contingent, it is clear that any number of issues – from moral decline, teenage lawlessness and single parenting to the royal family – would not have acquired such a central importance without their promotion by the press and broadcasting. In the past decade the media and political reaction to the Bulger murder has been pivotal. We have shifted from a position of discrete 'panics' about particular events and people, such as the mods and rockers of the 1960s or the 'black mugger' of the 1970s, to a seemingly endless and perpetual period of moral 'crises', criminal spectacles and media-generated justice. In a media-saturated and self-referential world the distinction between fictional and factual narratives is eroding. Some crimes (particularly car crime) are selected because of their presentational value (and low cost) to be broadcast around the world literally as they happen. The police arrange arrests for times when cameras can be present. The actions of the media are cited as legal grounds in numerous trials. Law enforcement agencies and pressure groups have adopted public relations departments precisely to construct and manage the news in particular ways. Facts are fused with institutional values, beliefs and myths. Crime-as-news blends into crime-as-entertainment. Mass media and law-enforcement agencies have become inextricably related in the defining and constituting of the realities of crime, justice and social order. And successive governments in the 1990s, keen to secure short-term political gain by capitalising on public misgivings and misperceptions, have brought their power to bear by continually extending the reach and intensity of criminal justice interventions.

References

Barak, G. (ed.) (1994) *Media, Process and the Social Construction of Crime*, New York: Garland.

Chibnall, S. (1977) *Law and Order News*, London: Tavistock.

Cohen, S. (1980) *Folk Devils and Moral Panics*, second edition, Oxford: Martin Robertson.

Davis, J. (1952) 'Crime news in Colorado newspapers', *American Journal of Sociology* 57: 325–330.

Davis, M. and Bourhill, M. (1997) 'Crisis: the demonisation of children and young people', in P. Scraton (ed.) *Childhood in Crisis*, London: University College London Press, 28–57.

Ditton, J. and Duffy, J. (1983) 'Bias in the newspaper reporting of crime news', *British Journal of Criminology* 23(2): 159–165.

Ericson, R. (1991) 'Mass media, crime, law and justice', *British Journal of Criminology* 31(3): 219–249.

Ericson, R., Baranek, P. and Chan, J. (1987) *Visualising Deviance*, Buckingham: Open University Press.

Ericson, R., Baranek, P. and Chan, J. (1991) *Representing Order*, Buckingham: Open University Press.

Franklin, B. and Petley, J. (1996) 'Killing the age of innocence: newspaper reporting of the death of James Bulger', in J. Pilcher and S. Wagg (eds) *Thatcher's Children*, London: Frances Pinter, 134–155.

Hall, S. (1973a) 'A world at one with itself', in S. Cohen and J. Young (eds) *Manufacturing the News*, London: Constable.

Hall, S. (1973b) 'The determinations of news photographs', in S. Cohen and J. Young (eds) *Manufacturing the News*, London: Constable.

Hall, S. (1978) 'The treatment of football hooliganism in the press', in Ingham *et al.* *Football Hooliganism*, London: Inter Action Imprint.

Hall, S. *et al.* (1975) *Newsmaking and Crime*, Birmingham: Centre for Contemporary Cultural Studies.

Hay, C. (1995) 'James Bulger, juvenile crime and the construction of a moral panic', *Social and Legal Studies* 4(2): 197–223.

Hough, M. and Roberts, J. (1998) *Attitudes to Punishment*, Home Office Research Study No. 179, London: HMSO.

James, A. and Jenks, C. (1996) 'Public perceptions of childhood criminality', *British Journal of Sociology* 47(2): 315–331.

Katz, J. (1987) 'What makes crime news?', *Media, Culture and Society* 9(1): 47–75.

King, M. (1995) 'The James Bulger murder trial: moral dilemmas and social solutions', *International Journal of Children's Rights* 3(2): 167–187.

Lea, J. and Young, J. (1984) *What is to be done about Law and Order?*, Harmondsworth: Penguin.

Livingstone, S. (1996) 'On the continuing problem of media effects', in J. Curran and M. Gurevitch (eds) *Mass Media and Society*, London: Arnold.

Mark, R. (1979) *In the Office of Constable*, London: Fontana.

Morgan, P. (1978) *Delinquent Fantasies*, Aldershot: Temple-Smith.

Muncie, J. (1996) 'The construction and deconstruction of crime', in J. Muncie and E. McLaughlin (eds) *The Problem of Crime*, London: Sage/Open University.

Muncie, J. (1999) 'Institutionalised intolerance: youth justice and the 1998 Crime and Disorder Act', *Critical Social Policy* 59 (forthcoming).

Osborne, R. (1995) 'Crime and the media: from media studies to postmodernism', in D. Kidd-Hewitt and R. Osborne (eds) *Crime and the Media*, London: Pluto.

Pearson, G. (1993) *Hooligan: a History of Respectable Fears*, London: Macmillan.

Reiner, R. (1997) 'Media made criminality: the representation of crime in the mass media', in M. Maguire, R. Morgan and R. Reiner (eds) *The Oxford Handbook of Criminology*, second edition, Oxford: Clarendon Press.

Roshier, B. (1973) 'The selection of crime news by the press', in S. Cohen and J. Young (eds) *Manufacturing the News*, London: Constable.

Sanders, C.R. and Lyon, E. (1995) 'Repetitive retribution: media images and the cultural construction of criminal justice', in J. Ferrell and C. Sanders (eds) *Cultural Criminology*, Boston, Mass.: NE University Press.

Schlesinger, P. and Tumber, H. (1994) *Reporting Crime*, Oxford, Oxford University Press.

Schlesinger, P., Tumber, H. and Murdock, G. (1991) 'The media politics of crime and criminal justice', *British Journal of Sociology* 42(3): 397–420.

Scraton, P. (1997) 'Whose "childhood"? What "crisis?"', in P. Scraton (ed.) *Childhood in Crisis?* London: UCL Press.

Smith, S. (1984) 'Crime in the news', *British Journal of Criminology* 24(3): 289–295.

Sparks, R. (1992) *Television and the Drama of Crime*, Buckingham: Open University Press.

Williams, P. and Dickinson, J. (1993) 'Fear of crime, read all about it', *British Journal of Criminology* 33(1): 33–56.

Young, A. (1996) *Imagining Crime*, London: Sage.

Young, J. (1974) 'Mass media, drugs and deviance', in P. Rock and M. Mackintosh (eds) *Deviance and Social Control*, London: Tavistock.

Part 3

The Media Reporting of Social Policy

Case Studies

Chapter 12

Bulger, 'back to basics' and the rediscovery of community

Bill Jordan

The need for strong, responsible communities is one of the main themes of New Labour's programme for reforming the British welfare state, and remodelling British society. Commentators seeking to define the essence of Tony Blair's political philosophy are agreed that communitarianism is one of its central features (Driver and Martell 1997; Smith 1997; Marquand 1998). After all, in a key essay, published in 1996, he had written of the need to promote a society 'where the community works for the good of every individual, and every individual works for the good of the community' (Blair 1996a: preface).

This chapter traces the origins of New Labour's conversion to the notions of responsibility, obligation and community to the media response to the murder of James Bulger, a Merseyside toddler, in February 1993. The circumstances of the murder itself – a small child 'abducted' by two boys aged ten from a shopping arcade, sustaining a number of injuries during a long and frequently-observed walk to waste ground, and then killed and dumped on a railway track – provoked an outcry about the moral condition of Britain. In the media soul-searching of those weeks, *The Times* editorialised about a shift in political discourse: 'even Labour now wants people to talk about right and wrong' (*The Times*, 22 February 1993). It was the first step in the redefinition of the social agenda that was propelled forward by Tony Blair, and that now underpins the government's reform of the welfare state.

I shall show how the media coverage of the murder, the arrest of the two boys, and their subsequent trial, all shaped the specific form of communitarianism – backward-looking, nostalgic, authoritarian and focused on social control – that now drives New Labour's programme (Jordan 1998a, b, c). The rediscovery of community began cautiously under John Smith, but accelerated as Tony Blair recognised a winning theme in his election campaign, and a central rationale for his government's programme for social justice and social inclusion (Lister 1998).

But this in turn was largely provoked by the ill-fated 'back to basics' initiative, launched by John Major at the Conservative Party Conference of October, 1993. At the time, his government stood low in the opinion polls, and his party was deeply divided over Europe. Desperate for a unifying slogan, his Cabinet think-tank came up with an ill-digested compound of crime control, traditional moral values and personal responsibility. Despite its homespun, cobbled-together provenance, the 'back to basics' message was surprisingly successful, and allowed Major a brief respite that even promised to be something of a revival.

But as I shall show, this quickly foundered early in 1994 on the series of sex scandals surrounding a number of his ministers and backbench MPs. The media linked 'back to basics' with these indiscretions, and ridiculed the whole enterprise of remoralising society. Under fire from the Eurosceptic 'bastards', Major could not sustain his new focus, or carry the fight to Labour. 'Back to basics' was largely abandoned, and no other theme emerged around which to forge party unity or mobilise electoral support.

Instead, after the death of John Smith, Labour made a bold bid for the moral high ground under Tony Blair, dwelling increasingly on the unintended consequences of excessive individualism, the sequilia of selfishness, and the spillovers from Tory sleaze. Community was the positive antidote to all these evils, and New Labour adopted it as its banner, pre-empting Major's attempt to capture the sentiments associated with mutuality and social discipline.

But – as I shall demonstrate – the Bulger trial and the consequent communitarian agenda had already influenced policy in criminal justice, and created a climate in which many of the authoritarian measures now integral to Labour's programme became feasible. The Major government could never have sponsored such an unequivocal attack on 'claimant passivity', 'benefit fraud' and 'free riding' as was launched by the Green Paper *A New Contract for Welfare* (Department of Social Security 1998). Nor would it have dared to introduce curfews for children, or to abolish benefits for all asylum seekers. New Labour can put a positive spin on all these measures only because it can appeal to a sense of responsibility and obligation to the common good, a notion that – even under conditions of globalisation and postmodernity – there are recognisable duties that all citizens owe each other, that work contributions through formal employment are at the heart of these reciprocal duties, and that membership of the polity can be precisely defined, and its obligations rigorously enforced by the state (Jordan 1998a).

I shall question and criticise all these assumptions, and trace their origins to a series of muddles and mistakes about the nature of community under present-day conditions. All these can in turn be found in the media response to the Bulger case, in which New Labour's communitarianism was born.

Bulger and the debate about morality

It is not my purpose in this chapter to review the whole media response to the death of Jamie Bulger, the arrest of the two boys who killed him, or their trial in November 1993. Rather it is to show how the rediscovery of community occurred in a media-generated frenzy of breast beating about society, morality and the socialisation of children. This ensured that the particular form of communitarianism adopted by New Labour was one that was primarily addressed to the phenomena of crime, truancy and violence, with some tangential concerns about the corrupting influence of videotapes and magazines. This is still the main focus of the debate about morality and community; it displaces deeper concerns about solidarity, inequality and redistribution as elements of social justice (Jordan 1998a).

Other scholars have more thoroughly charted the media's coverage of the Bulger case (Franklin and Petley 1996; Davis and Bourhill 1997). The case attracted enormous media attention, both during the police investigation into the murder (late February 1993) and again during the trial of Robert Thompson and Jon Venables (November). As soon as the charges were made against the two 10-year-old boys, feature articles and editorials at once addressed the case in terms of moral and social disintegration, the threat of juvenile delinquency to the whole social fabric, the hidden evil within children, the vulnerability and corruptibility of childhood, and the need for a new sense of responsible community. In addition to this reportage, editorialising and the contributions from selected 'experts', there were also articles from interviews with ministers, other politicians and religious leaders, all on much the same themes.

The fact that the tabloid press devoted enormous attention to the story is hardly surprising, since it contained such obvious elements of newsworthiness in terms of its themes of the past two decades. The *Daily Mirror* ran fourteen pages of coverage the day after the boys' sentence, and the *Sun* fifteen pages; the *Daily Star* followed a banner headline of 'How do you feel now you little bastards?' with nine pages of stories (Franklin and Petley 1996: 47). The broadsheets and 'quality' press, with the exception of the *Financial Times*, gave almost equal prominence to the investigation and to the trial, and took a similar line, devoting many pages to analyses of social fragmentation and irresponsible parenthood. The *Sunday Times*, for example, on 21 February 1993 ran a leader on 'The brutality of Britain', which intoned:

> For those living in some council estates, [their lives] have got so much worse, to the point where law and order have, in effect, broken down . . . Institutions such as family, school and community, which once gave children, regardless of background, a sense of discipline and moral compass have declined in their ability to impart these values.

It describes '"sink" estates, inhabited by a largely white underclass which has come to resemble . . . the black ghettos of urban America', and – in a feature article titled 'Are our children out of control?' – interviewed Charles Murray on the disastrous effects of absent fathers, and Frank Field on responsibility. *The Times* on 26 February 1993, in a report entitled 'Public fear grows of a breakdown in law and order', quoted a MORI opinion poll which recorded a doubling of concern about this issue since the end of the previous month.

The trial itself, with its evidence by many witnesses who saw the two boys leading James Bulger to his death, stirred more fears about the loss of community, with a strong link again to the theme of crime control. *The Times* reported 'The story Britain could not bear to hear', as the child was brutalised 'in full view of dozens, perhaps hundreds, of honest citizens' (7 November). The tabloid papers were more focused on the 'evil' in the two boys, and the need for savage retribution. They subscribed to biological determinism rather than social causation, the standard reference being William Golding's novel *Lord of the Flies* – cited in three newspapers in the week of 25 November (Franklin and Petley 1996: 47).

From the first reports of the murder, government ministers made links between juvenile crime, permissiveness (including violent and pornographic films and videos) and the need for greater individual and social responsibility. On 21 February 1993, Prime Minister John Major told the *Mail on Sunday* 'I would like the public to have a crusade against crime and change from being forgiving of crime to being considerate to the victim. Society needs to condemn a little more and understand a little less'. Home Secretary Kenneth Clarke wrote in the *Daily Mail* that:

> the courts should have the power to send really persistent nasty little juveniles away to somewhere where they will be looked after better . . . John Major and I believe it is no good that some sections of society are permanently finding excuses for the behaviour of the section of the population who are essentially nasty pieces of work.
>
> (22 February 1993)

Education Secretary John Patten warned of a 'battle ahead to bring youngsters under control' and added that 'we face a very long haul of five to ten years before we undo some of the changes of the sixties and seventies' (*Daily Express*, 23 February 1993). The Secretary of State for Wales linked the killings with violent films and videos (one notorious film involving a child, *Child's Play 3*, having been found in Robert Thompson's family's house), writing of:

> a generation bombarded by TV images of gratuitous violence, loveless sex and amoral behaviour – or hooked on computer games. The average teenager today has seen something like 30,000 killings on the cinema and TV screen . . . If that doesn't lead to delinquency, what does?
>
> (*Mail on Sunday*, 28 February 1993)

Thus the case provided the government with cultural and rhetorical resources for launching a combination of policies on crime and community, linking the need for greater control over youth with the virtues of traditional families and neighbourhoods. The Labour Party's position on this was still unclear, but it failed to criticise or modify the government's initiatives during 1993.

'Back to basics' and the Bulger trial

At the Conservative Party conference in October 1993, the Prime Minister was beset by the low poll ratings of his government and by internal divisions (especially over Europe) in his party. Searching for a theme for his conference address, he came up (at the last minute) with an appeal for a return to past moral values. On 9 October, *The Times* reported a favourable reception of his speech, which announced a crackdown on child pornography, and supported a return to traditional standards in the areas of crime, education and the family. He said:

> 'It is time to get back to basics: to self-discipline and respect for law, to consideration for others, to accepting responsibility for yourself and your family, and not shuffling it off on to the state.'

He lined this up with tough new measures by Michael Howard, the new Home Secretary, for tackling rising crime, which would be the centrepiece of his government's legislation for the next year. He said that understanding and persuasion had been tried – it was time for a 'harsher approach'.

At first, it looked as if the Prime Minister's initiative had been rather successful in its two aims, to catch Labour off guard on an issue over which it was still unclear, and to unite the Conservative Party around a strong theme, popular among its supporters. A private Tory poll on 'back to basics' indicated that the response was 'very encouraging, and could halt the decline in moral standards during 14 years of Tory rule' (*Sunday Times*, 9 January 1994). In November, the Policy Unit at 10 Downing Street issued a memo to all Cabinet ministers on back to basics, which included the fateful words 'going back to basics means expecting and respecting personal responsibility' (ibid.).

During the media feeding frenzy in the aftermath of the trial of Robert Thompson and Jon Venables, the Home Office minister David MacLean attacked the Church of England for failing to provide moral leadership for a nation in crisis over standards of behaviour and control of youth (*The Times*, 26 November 1993). The link between the trial and this foray was clear from its timing. On 17 December, Michael Howard introduced the Criminal Justice and Public Order Bill to the House of Commons. He said the new law was intended '. . . to make it easier to catch, convict and punish criminals', and *The Times* linked this (and especially the harsher sentences for young offenders introduced) to the James Bulger case in its leader of the following day (*The Times*, 18 December 1993).

Unfortunately for the government, in less than a month the 'back to basics' initiative was in tatters. A junior minister, Tim Yeo, had been revealed in the tabloid press as having fathered a child outside his marriage. There was an embarrassing delay, during which further revelations occurred, before he resigned. *The Times* noted that it was the 'back to basics' line that forced his resignation, since his actions discredited the policy. In the next few weeks, further scandals surrounding the sex lives of Tory MPs were revealed in the tabloid press. Each new revelation further undermined John Major's claim to the moral high ground, and the whole initiative was quietly abandoned by the government.

Meanwhile, these scandals had made it easy for the opposition to leave the government to suffer the consequences of its own folly. Labour was not forced to clarify its stand on any of these issues, nor did it do so under John Smith. After his death, and with the election to the leadership of Tony Blair, the inauguration of New Labour's consultations and focus groups quickly gave rise to a fresh version of 'back to basics', the same mixture of homespun communitarianism, traditional values and anti-crime, retributivist invective as John Major tried to mobilise for his party. The difference was that Tony Blair was able to unite his troops for the 1997 election, and to combine the appeal to moral values with more Labourist appeals for social inclusion and social justice, and hence to sustain a very similar campaign, appealing to very much the same sector of the electorate (readers of the *Daily Mail* and even *The Times*) as John Major had tried to address.

New Labour, New Community?

Communitarianism has been an important element in Tony Blair's winning combination of free-market economics and moral rearmament. It is his distinctive response to the economic individualism of the Thatcher era, and to Old Labour's statism, providing a cement for society and a discipline for his party. Social inclusion replaces redistribution as Labour's key aim, and a responsible community counters lawlessness. Blair takes up Bill Clinton's theme of rights and responsibilities – 'you can take, but you give too' (Blair 1996b: 2) – in a vision of a society in which 'the community works for the good of every individual, and every individual works for the good of the community' (Blair 1996a: preface).

New Labour's welfare reforms seek to translate these principles into policies, and through these a 'change of culture among benefit claimants, employers and public servants, which will break the mould of the old [welfare state]' (Department of Social Security 1998: 3). Above all, they seek to put work back at the centre of a welfare state as both the surest way out of poverty, and the best way of distinguishing between those who can and should provide for themselves, and those in 'genuine need' (DSS 1998: 23). But these same values of self-responsibility for active citizens in a flexible labour market, and authoritarian measures against 'free riders' and deviants, influence a whole range of policies on crime, homelessness, education and immigration – for example, in measures to compel rough sleepers to enter hostels, to impose curfews on young people, or to deny benefits to asylum seekers.

Blair's communitarianism, like Clinton's, is strongly influenced by the conservative version of this tradition, epitomised in the work of Amitai Etzioni. In asserting that above all there must be no new rights without corresponding responsibilities, and that the state should be the fifth in line as a source of care, after self, family, kin and neighbours (Etzioni 1993: 145–146), he provided the ideas to legitimate a backward-looking appeal to the social controls of the traditional, monocultural, disciplinary, working-class community that is characteristic of New Labour (Driver and Martell 1997; Marquand 1998; Smith 1997; Hughes and Little 1998). In this, Blair follows directly the path set by John Major at the height of the Bulger moral panic.

The Blair–Clinton line emphasises that social inclusion through community requires contributions to the common good, and this is the basis for social justice. It insists that citizens' claims against the state should stem primarily from their merits and performances as economic participants and only by default from their needs. In prioritising equality of opportunity over equality of outcome (i.e. redistribution), and retributional or deterrent forms of criminal justice, it appeals to moral intuitions from the sphere of family and neighbourhood relations; but it emphasises that formal employment contributions must take precedence over informal work (such as childcare by lone parents).

In one sense, this view of community is indisputable. In any mutual-benefit club, obligations are always prior to rights, in the sense that the club only has something to distribute if members contribute (material resources or labour power). But this truism about small voluntary associations is very difficult to translate into principles for large, complex polities with market economies. Nation states rely on the power of government to compel contributions in the form of taxes or military service, but the primary distinction between regimes is between those which minimise such coercive potential (liberal states), and those which rely on central power for enforcement in all spheres of interaction between citizens (totalitarian states). New Labour often seems to have forgotten this (Jordan 1998a: Chapters 1–3).

Conversely, markets cut right across human associations of all kinds, from households to nation states, by maximising the potential for advantageous exchange without obligation. The principle of markets is that they enable transactions between individuals who are unencumbered by traditional bonds, family loyalties or archaic authority, as Adam Smith pointed out (Smith 1776: part IV, section vii, chapter 80). Capitalism, after all, saved us from what Marx and Engels aptly described as 'the idiocy of rural life' (Marx and Engels 1848: 11). In an age of globalisation, capitalists owe only weak contractual duties to workers, and can relocate production to anywhere in the world at any time. Mobile, skilled workers can likewise choose to work almost anywhere, and consequently to make their social contributions where they will. Welfare states can no longer tie down either companies or their most skilled workers, or force them to make high contributions for social redistribution; indeed this is the main reason why New Labour has abandoned Old Labour's tax and spend policies (Jordan 1998a: Chapter 2).

What national governments can still do is compel those who are least mobile, most adversely affected by global competition (with lower-paid workers abroad), and most vulnerable to insecurity and exploitation. They can be made to do forced labour, for the state, for factory owners, or for rich households (the protest slogan of lone parents against the Secretary of State's announcements of cuts to their benefits – 'We won't clean Harriet's toilet' – was especially apt). Tony Blair's ideal society has three different levels. At the top are the international capitalists – Bernie Ecclestone, Richard Branson – whom he so admires, and who live in a kind of global anarchy, where they can make their own rules, and enforce these on national governments. In the middle are the employed and self-employed, driven by a new work ethic, rather in the manner of postwar Germany (the Germans now work at a far more leisurely pace) for the sake of 'national renewal'. And at the bottom are the poor, cajoled, persuaded, counselled or coerced, in an ironic imitation of the state socialism of the Soviet era. In this sector, the old slogan of the central Europeans under Stalinism ('we pretend to work, you pretend to pay') is once more appropriate (Jordan 1998a: Chapters 2 and 3).

Tough luvvies

New Labour's communitarianism draws its moral arguments from the sphere of family and small voluntary associations, and transposes them into the economy and the polity, as work obligations and civic duties. This violates the liberal tradition of politics, and the conditions for free markets. It relies on notions of reciprocity and responsibility, backed by authority and power, where liberalism relies on free choice and markets for material advantages and incentives. In this sense it is not so much a return to Victorian values as a return to pre-liberal, pre-capitalist authoritarianism.

The codes that govern communal relationships are reciprocal bonds of love and care; ideally these give rise to sharing and redistribution according to need of what is produced according to ability. Such relationships are functional (indeed optimal) when transactions concern goods and services that cannot be divided up and priced (Jordan 1996: Chapters 1 and 2). Labour services are exchanged according to a rule of give and take, whether in households or in small associations (e.g. taking your turn to mark the pitch or make the tea at the hockey club). But such idealised community relations seldom occur in real life, and the politics of small-scale interactions are often transacted through patriarchal, racist, religious or other power-laden norms, or through absurd archaisms like folk dancing and duck racing (Jordan 1998c).

Under present-day labour market and social conditions, the notion of reimposing a reciprocal regime of work obligations is ridiculously inefficient.

Where sufficient incentives exist, people are easily moved to 'contribute to society' – but they are primarily motivated by self-interest, not duty. As free individuals, they can choose what work to do, and they attract no criticism if they prefer to work in less-productive occupations, or for shorter hours, or to quit their national economy to work abroad. Their duties are fulfilled the minute they comply with the terms of their employment contracts; for the rest of their lives they can choose whether simply to consume, or to give time and energy to their community.

In the deregulated labour market established during the Thatcher-Major years, however, a large proportion of employment cannot provide subsistence-level wages, especially for families. Hence the phenomenon, often mentioned in New Labour texts, of the 3.4 million households of working age without a member in work; hence also the large number of individuals classified as lone parents or disabled claimants. For these, there are no incentives to take the various bits and pieces of low-paid work that are offered on the labour market. For them, a more rational strategy is to establish a claim to a long-term benefit (and any additional services), and to work 'on the side' for cash, to pay for 'extras' – irregular or large expenditures. Poor people not only practise this strategy routinely; they also justify it, in terms of the irregularity of available work, and the slowness and unreliability of means-tested supplements such as family credit and housing benefit (Jordan *et al.* 1992; Evason and Woods 1995; Dean and Melrose 1997; Rowlingson *et al.* 1997).

New Labour's answer to this is to tighten up still further on enforcing work conditions and prosecuting fraud (DSS 1998: chapters 3 and 8). In addition to legislating (eventually) for a minimum wage – easily circumvented by employers who will make their workforce 'self-employed' – the government will rely on an army of 'personal advisers' to give all claimants individualised, 'tailor-made packages of help'. In other words, it will substitute various kinds of pressure, backed by threats of disqualification and exclusion, for the incentives and choices that a free labour market is supposed to provide. The obligation to work 'for the good of the community' is in fact an enforced duty to work for the state. The form that this will take is various kinds of subsidised employment and training by private firms and agencies, or in public services, or 'community work' in voluntary organisations. (The experience of the 1980s 'Community Programme' shows that much of the latter turns out to be low-skilled, low-productivity drudgery, indistinguishable from the kind of work done by offenders under court community service orders.) As the DSS Green Paper says, there will be no 'fifth option' of claiming and organising one's own work, not even if this is valuable local voluntary effort, such as the social support groups through which lone parents sustained many communities during the Thatcher-Major years (Jordan 1997). Instead, claimants must take bureaucratic orders to avail themselves of opportunities to stack supermarket shelves, serve hamburgers, or do dreary computer courses.

American and European experiences show that welfare-to-work measures at best cream off the top 50 per cent of claimants (who would sooner or later have found work anyway), and involve far higher costs for the rest in training, surveillance and enforcement activities (Wiseman 1991; Schuyt 1998). The result is that workfare expenditures are higher than old-fashioned welfare spending; and this calculation does not include the costs of providing hostel, hospital and prison places for the high proportion of claimants who are excluded from benefits, or withdraw claims, and try to subsist outside the labour market and the social protection system (the greater reason for the fall in claims of unemployment-related benefits between 1992 and 1996 took the form of 'disappearance' from either the labour market or the benefit statistics, but there was also a rapid growth in the prison population during this period). The proposed Working Families Tax Credits will marginally improve incentives for the few who get long-term jobs, but again US experience shows that such systems have built-in complexities that limit take-up, and are by no means strategy-proof.

Above all, New Labour's policies, while appealing to the spirit of an idealised past working-class community, in practice substitute state officials for the informal controls that such communities supplied. Because community was rediscovered in a moral context of panic about the collapse of order and the growing lawlessness of the young, it cannot supply a justification for trust, empowerment, or the bottom-up regeneration of local economies and social support systems. New Labour's communitarianism needs a new brand of buromotivator to stimulate the active, participative yet dutiful claimant, service user or pupil for the common good.

It was no coincidence that, during the debate about the Bulger case, the journalist Melanie Philips – herself a neo-communitarian in the Etzioni mould – formulated the concept of 'tough love' (*Observer*, 13 June 1993). Very much in the same spirit as Bill Clinton's New Covenant and Personal Responsibility Act, this notion captures the mixture of charisma and authority that is required of the new breed of public servants who must implement Tony Blair's programme. Tough love is most convincing when embodied in the kind of judges who run the new drugs courts in many American cities – authority figures with exceptional powers of empathy and communication, capable of putting high demands for personal change on groups of resistant and disadvantaged people; or in the equally demanding and challenging regimes run by reformed alcoholics and drug users in self-help groups and therapeutic communities. Tough love combines high levels of support (in the personality of the authority figure, and from the user group) with refusal to accept excuses or evasions. It either produces personal change, or personal collapse; it is a high-risk approach to social policy.

New Labour desperately needs tough luvvies in all its new programmes – in the various New Deals, in the transformed probation service (now to be called something like 'community corrections'), in services for homeless people, in the new psychiatric units, and so on. It also needs them in the classrooms of sink schools, on the beats of deprived neighbourhoods after dark, in prisons and in its revamped children's homes. But where are they to be found? It is likely that they are not among traditional recruits to the social work and teaching professions, over-educated and over-professionalised, with all the spontaneity and charisma they may ever have possessed squeezed out of them by years of academic study and soft living. They are unlikely to be present, too, among the traditional recruits to the police and prison services, or the armed forces, whose version of authority cuts no ice at all among the dispossessed, and who lack the flexibility to learn new ways.

There is a contradiction at the heart of New Labour's communitarianism. Because it was forged in an atmosphere of moral condemnation and mistrust, it cannot harness the indigenous energies of deprived communities, or channel their informal economic activity (including crime), or mobilise their informal support systems, to improve their quality of life. It must rely on top-down, authoritarian methods to achieve its ends, but it lacks the moral authority to do this – as anyone who heard Tony Blair's rushed and stumbling delivery when he introduced the Social Exclusion Unit in a speech on a housing estate in Peckham could easily recognise. Community cannot be artificially constructed by bureaucrats or professionals; it relies on shared experiences (including sufferings), shared facilities and co-operative relationships (sometimes forged through conflicts). The best social workers and teachers, youth leaders and therapists, can create these conditions, by skill and force of personality, even in the most adverse circumstances. But run-of-the-mill officials cannot; they lack the courage and commitment to engage with really disadvantaged and deviant people in a moral dialogue, and to put themselves on the line for the sake of real change. A million words about social inclusion and social justice are worth less than the open heart and steely will of one of that rare breed. Labour is taking an absurd gamble to rely on a massive supply of such spirits.

Conclusions

The rediscovery of community has worked very much to the advantage of the British Labour Party. The Bulger case epitomised, in the most powerful symbolism, the crisis of the economic individualism ushered in by Margaret Thatcher. Captured on security videotape, a small and vulnerable child, standing alone outside a supermarket, was taken away, battered and killed on waste ground by children already beyond the reach of parental, educational, communal or professional controls by the age of 10 years. In the very temple of consumerism, the anarchy of markets and the anomie of individualism combined to produce a 'killing of innocence' (Franklin and Petley 1997); this was what happened when there was no such thing as society. Community had to be reinvented, by common consent – the media demanded it. But the government of John Major was in no position to do this; his 'back to basics' initiative foundered in scandal and sleaze. It was left for Tony Blair to mount the moral crusade the media wanted, and were prepared to support.

I have argued that New Labour's communitarianism rests on a shallow understanding of community, and a complete muddle about how it can be sustained in a complex, multi-cultural society with a free-market economy. Notions of responsibility, reciprocity and obligation cannot simply be enforced by public services, or inculcated by political speeches. They rely crucially on informal relationships of trust and co-operation, built up through voluntary exchanges of respect, value and mutual support, sustained by bonds of affection (and sometimes fear, at least fear of public shaming), and negotiated through a myriad of changing circumstances. Such relationships can only flourish in conditions of shared commitment to a good quality of life, and shared resources. Community has survived in the unlikeliest of places during the Thatcher-Major years, but its rediscovery depends on patient and humble grass-roots investigation and support, not top-down imposition, arrogant assumption or authoritarian enforcement.

Law-and-order issues do provide opportunities for the development of radical community approaches (Hughes and Little 1998), but the Blair government has got off on the wrong foot with these also. If it really believes in the merits of tough love, it should aim to recruit from the survivors of the Thatcher economic debacle, not to oppress them.

Social policy in Britain is clearly at a crossroads, and already anticipates future developments in Europe, still lagging miles behind. Professors who write to the *Financial Times*, and ordinary people who voted Labour, should not really be shocked by the government's meanness and authoritarianism. The writing was clearly on the wall, from Tony Blair's earliest speeches on social issues, and from his undisguised admiration for Bill Clinton.

What has been lacking is a strong critique, from within the Labour Party and outside it, and an alternative social policy programme. For far too long the mainstream social policy community (academia and administrators) relied on a mixture of moral outrage over the excesses of Thatcherism, and nostalgia for the good days of Beveridge, Swedish Social Democracy and George Brown-style corporatism. When these hopes faded, the best they could do was turn to Germany and Japan, or even Singapore, rather than think through the full implications of the global economy and the 'flexible' labour market.

In the new situation, where Tony Blair has realistically indicated that there will be no return to these discredited and exhausted models, the social policy community is largely bereft of new ideas. Yet Blair's project for welfare reform is in deep trouble, as the sacking of Harriet Harman and the resignation of Frank Field betray. There is still an opportunity to influence the government's thinking, as long as administrators are not seduced onto the gravy train of new project money (see the *Guardian* job advertisements every Wednesday), and intellectuals do not collapse into mouthing platitudes from New Labour brochures, like 'what we need now are joined-up solutions to joined-up problems' (Mulgan 1998).

My preferred option is the combination of a citizen's income for all (a modest sum guaranteed before individuals enter labour markets or households, and paid unconditionally, as the basis for personal autonomy and social justice), underpinned by all kinds of backing for local, grass-roots initiatives for economic regeneration and social support (Jordan 1998a, c). Others would have different answers: let them proclaim them loudly, soon.

References

Blair, T. (1996a) *New Britain: My Vision for a Young Country*, London: Fourth Estate.

—— (1996b) 'Speech in South Africa', *Guardian*, 15 October.

Davis, H. and Bourhill, M. (1997) 'Crisis: the demonisation of children and young people', in P. Scraton (ed.) *Childhood in Crisis*, London: University College London Press.

Dean, H. and Melrose, M. (1997) 'Unravelling citizenship, the Significance of benefit fraud', *Critical Social Policy* 16(48).

Department of Social Security (1998) *A New Contract for Welfare*, London: HMSO.

Driver, S. and Martell, L. (1997) 'New Labour's communitarianisms', *Critical Social Policy* 17(52): 27–46.

Etzioni, A. (1993) *The Spirit of Community: the Reinvention of American Society*, New York: Touchstone.

Evason, E. and Woods, R. (1995) 'Poverty, deregulation of labour markets and benefit fraud', *Social Policy and Administration* 29(1): 40–54.

Franklin, B. and Petley, J. (1996) 'Killing the age of innocence: newspaper reporting of the death of James Bulger', in S. Wagg and J. Pilcher (eds) *Thatcher's Children: Politics, Childhood and Society in the 1990s*, London: Frances Pinter, 134–155.

Hughes, G. and Little, A. (1998) 'New labour, communitarianism and the public sphere in the UK', paper given at seventh BIEN Congress, University of Amsterdam, 10 September.

Jordan, B. (1996) *A Theory of Poverty and Social Exclusion*, Oxford: Polity Press.

Jordan, B. (1997) 'Service users involvement in child protection and family support', in N. Parton (ed.) *Child Protection and Family Support*, London: Routledge, 212–222.

Jordan, B. (1998a) *The New Politics of Welfare: Social Justice in a Global Context*, London: Sage.

Jordan, B. (1998b) 'Justice and reciprocity', *Critical Review of International Social and Political Philosophy* 1(1): 63–85.

Jordan, B. (1998c) 'New Labour, New Community?', *Imprints: Journal of Analytical Socialism*, forthcoming.

Jordan, B., James, S., Kay, H. and Redley, M. (1992) *Trapped in Poverty? Labour Market Decisions in Low-Income Households*, London: Routledge.

Lister, R. (1998) 'From equality to social inclusion: New Labour and the welfare state', *Critical Social Policy* 18(55): 217–229.

Marquand, D. (1998) 'The Blair paradox', *Prospect*, May: 16–24.

Marx, K. and Engels, F. (1848) *The Manifesto of the Communist Party*, authorised English translation 1888, London: Reeves.

Mulgan, G. (1998) 'Speech to conference on social exclusion', Exeter: University of Exeter, 22 September.

Rowlingson, K., Wiley, C. and Newburn, T. (1997) *Social Security Fraud*, London: PSI.
Schuyt, K. (1998) 'The basis for basic income', paper given at seventh BIEN Congress, University of Amsterdam, 9 September.
Smith, A. (1776) *An Inquiry into the Nature and Causes of the Wealth of Nations*, ed. R.H. Campbell and A.S. Skinner (eds) Oxford: Clarendon Press (1976).
Smith, J. (1997) 'The ideology of "family and community", New Labour abandons the welfare state', in L. Panitch (ed.) *The Socialist Register 1997*, Ipswich: Merlin Press, 176–196.
Wiseman, M. (1991) 'What did the American work-welfare demonstrations do? Why should the Germans care?', Zentrum für Socialpolitik, University of Bremen, Arbeitspapier, September 1991.

Chapter 13

The ultimate neighbour from hell?

Stranger danger and the media framing of paedophiles

Jenny Kitzinger

> 'I talked to other senior managers who were in the same hot seat I was in. The general feeling was: this is difficult, this is *new*. I don't know why that is. I'm quite sure abusers were being released from prison ten years ago and going and living places. But no one was taking any notice. This was something that happened new, different, over the last two years'.
>
> (Deputy Director of Housing in a London Authority, interviewed in 1998)

What happens once convicted sex abusers are released from prison? Where do they live? How are they monitored? Do neighbours have a right to know who is living in their street? These questions gained a dramatic media prominence and public profile during the second half of the 1990s. In 1996 the government unveiled plans to establish an official register of sex offenders which triggered media and public demands for community notification. People began to agitate for 'the right to know' when convicted sex abusers were housed in their communities: the government and 'the professionals' rapidly lost control of the news agenda and information distribution. The names and photographs of offenders were publicised in the press and passed on to neighbours. In some cases direct action was taken to drive these men out of their homes. Monitoring, supervision, 'treatment' and housing of offenders was disrupted and policy makers had to reconsider legislation, policy and practice.

This chapter examines the role of the media in shaping and responding to this crisis. It illustrates how particular events, combined with coverage in the local and national media, fuel debate and examines how media coverage tapped into existing community fears and frustrations. The chapter concludes by exploring how the 'paedophile crisis' built on pre-existing discourses about 'the paedophile' as a particular type of threat. The concept of 'the paedophile', I argue, locates dangerousness in a few aberrant individuals who can be metaphorically (if not literally) excluded from society and it focuses attention on stranger danger in ways which ignore the scale and nature of sexual violence throughout society and, especially, within families.

In addition to providing a substantive case study of the media's role in relation to social policy I also point to different strands which might usefully be examined in any such enquiry. This chapter argues against casual and inappropriate use of terms such as 'moral panic' or 'media hysteria' and suggests ways of moving beyond a media-centric analysis towards an understanding of the motives of media sources such as, in this case, neighbourhood pressure groups. I also argue for the importance of historical context. Analysis confined to the peak of media concern with a particular problem, is inadequate since it is important to interrogate the historical frameworks and 'common sense' assumptions which inform public discourse.

The rise of the paedophile problem

Child sexual abuse was 'discovered' by the modern media in the mid-1980s. In the UK, this 'discovery' began in 1986 when Esther Rantzen devoted an entire programme called *Childwatch* to the issue and launched the children's helpline 'Childline'. This was quickly followed by a dramatic increase in attention to the issue of child abuse in the rest of the media. Analysis of *The Times*, for example, shows a four-fold increase in coverage of sexual abuse between 1985 and 1987 (Kitzinger 1996) and it became a regular topic for documentaries such as *Everyman* (BBC1, 8 May 1988), *Horizon* (BBC2, 19 June 1989), *World in Action* (ITV, 20 May 1991), and *Panorama* (BBC1, 7 December 1992). By the early 1990s, the issue began to appear in chat shows and drama programmes too. Sexual abuse storylines were incorporated into regular series such as *The Bill* (ITV, 29 January 1993) and *Casualty* (BBC1, 6 February 1993) as well as soap operas such as *EastEnders* and *Brookside* (see Henderson 1998).

Throughout this media attention a constant (but often shadowy) figure lurked in the background: the figure of 'the paedophile'. He appeared in silhouette in Ester Rantzen's original *Childwatch* exposé. He was 'unmasked' in press reports as the Jekyll and Hyde character who posed as a caring priest or committed director of a children's home (Aldridge 1994). He was introduced as 'psycho Trevor' in *Brookside* (Henderson 1998). More recently he even put in a controversial appearance on the chat show *Kilroy* boasting about his offences against children (*The Times*, 23 July 1997).[1]

It was not until the second half of the 1990s, however, that public debate began to focus on the dilemmas posed by convicted sex offenders released back into the community. Although sporadic concern, especially around particular individuals, was evident earlier (see Soothill and Walby 1991), it was only in 1996 that media and public outrage focused on these men (and some women) who might invisibly slip back into society free to abuse again.

The origins of this particular focus can be located in 1996. Initial media attention to the 'paedophiles-in-the-community' problem was generated by central government policy initiatives. In March 1996 Michael Howard (then

Home Secretary) proposed legislation to monitor sex offenders, details of which were published in June. This led to headlines such as: 'National paedophile register to be set up' (*The Times*, 23 March 1996), 'Paedophiles to be "marked men" on national register' (*The Times*, 18 May 1996) and 'Howard plans paedophile curbs' (*Guardian*, 13 June 1996). The legislation was introduced in December of that year prompting further headlines including: 'Paedophile lists for police' (*The Times*, 19 December 1996) and 'Crackdown on sex offenders unveiled' (*Guardian*, 19 December 1996).

Such reporting followed routine media practice whereby media agendas are traditionally set by high-status official sources (such as government bodies) (Tuchman 1978). But media coverage and public debate shifted rapidly as particular communities and sections of the media began to agitate for public access to the register and demand that communities be notified when dangerous individuals moved into their neighbourhood. Journalists and pressure groups picked up on similar community notification legislation in the USA know as 'Megan's Law'. Introduced in 1996 this legislation was named after a seven-year-old New Jersey girl, Megan Kanka, who was raped and murdered by a twice-convicted sex offender who lived across the street. Towards the end of 1996, and early 1997, the 'big story' for the media, but the major headache for policy makers, became not government initiatives, but public fear and anger. Headlines in the national press included: 'Parents in dark as paedophiles stalk schools' (*Guardian*, 24 November 1996), 'Paedophile out of prison "fearful for life and limb"' (*Observer*, 15 December 1996), 'Jeering mothers drive paedophile off council estate' (*The Times*, 11 January 1997), 'Stop hiding perverts say protest mums' (*Daily Mail*, 3 February 1997) and 'Town not told of paedophiles' stay' (*The Times*, 12 October 1997).

Protest rapidly spread from one area to another, and concern quickly escalated: the role of the local press in voicing these concerns was crucial. Although often ignored when thinking about the media, the local press can play a key role. Indeed, the local media influence many national and international policy-making processes from road building to the disposal of nuclear waste (Franklin and Murphy 1998). The theme of 'paedophiles within-the-community' received extensive regional media coverage across the UK from Aberdeen to Brighton, from Leicester to Belfast, from Teesside to Lancashire. Indeed, many of the national stories about paedophiles began life on the front page of local papers and some neighbourhood protests were sparked by local press reports rather than vice versa. Headlines from local papers announced: 'Angus mums on alert over local sex offender' (*Press and Journal* (Aberdeen), 17 June 1998), 'Parents besiege abuser's house' (*Press and Journal*, 17 July 1997), 'Residents pledge to continue campaign' (*Leicester Mercury*, 4 July 1998), 'Give us the right to know' (*Torquay Herald Express*, 2 September 1997), 'Parents' paedophile poster campaign' (*Evening Gazette*, (Teesside), 26 January 1998), 'Panic hits town over perverts' (*Belfast Telegraph News*, 22 March 1997) and 'Sex offender's home torched' (*Belfast Telegraph News*, 6 October 1997).

Such articles often included quotes from the host of local residents' groups which formed in response to the 'paedophile' threat: organisations such as 'Freedom for Children', 'People's Power', 'Parents Opposed to Paedophiles' and 'The Unofficial Child Protection Unit'. Reports were also often accompanied by photographs of local people marching with banners declaring 'Perverts out', (*Press and Journal*, 9 June 1997) or children carrying placards reading: 'Make me safe' (*Torquay Herald Express*, 2 September 1997). The *Manchester Evening News* published a front-page spread about a local sex offender alongside a photograph of him in his car behind a smashed windscreen after 'a vigilante mob had vented their anger' (cited in Thomas 1997: 68). The tone of some of this reporting was overtly provocative and clearly 'fed the flames' of protest.[2]

Many newspapers adopted a more proactive role rather than merely reporting local unrest with whatever degree of approval or urgings of restraint. Some papers assumed the role of guardians of public safety, especially in relation to particular dangerous individuals. Robert Oliver, involved in the brutal sexual assault and killing of Jason Swift, was repeatedly pursued by journalists. The *Sun* asked readers to phone an emergency number if Oliver was spotted (*Guardian*, 18 October 1997) and, when he moved to Brighton the local paper, the *Evening Argus*, published his picture on their front page with the headline 'Beware this evil pervert' (*Evening Argus*, 14 October 1997).

In other cases, newspapers alerted people to the presence of 'paedophiles', either through knocking on the doors of neighbours and asking how they felt about living near a sex offender or through 'outing' them on the front page. The *Sunday Express* printed photographs and details of offenders with their last-known address under the headline 'Could these evil men be living next door to you?' (cited in Thomas 1997). The Scottish *Daily Record* produced a similar campaign, devoting the bulk of one issue to asserting a 'Charter for our children' and demanding 'The legal right for communities to be told when a pervert moves into the area' (*Daily Record*, 25 February 1997). Alongside articles headed 'End the suffering', 'Pervert's playground' and 'Monster freed to kill', they published a double-page 'Gallery of shame' with thirty-eight photographs and names of convicted offenders and details of their offences.[3] Four of these were described as 'people power' success stories. One man was 'hounded out of Drumchapel housing scheme because of his sick background' and another 'forced into hiding' while 'people power drove sick child molester, Christie, 50 out of Stirling' (*Daily Record*, 25 February 1997).

'Moral panics' and 'lynch mobs'?

Such media coverage and the public reactions it reflected, triggered and amplified, presented a major problem for those involved in monitoring and housing convicted sex offenders. The media were accused of whipping up 'hysteria', creating a 'moral panic' and encouraging a 'lynch mob mentality'. Routine community notification and the automatic right of public access to the sex offenders' register is opposed by chief constables, chief probation officers and the NSPCC (*Guardian*, 19 February 1997). The main reason for their opposition is the belief that it will not protect children. Instead it may result in vigilante action and drive offenders underground making it less possible to monitor or 'treat' them. Indeed the Association of Chief Officers of Probation (ACOP) documented ten cases where the press had given editorial authority to campaigns to identify and expel offenders, leading to disruption of supervision and, even, to acts of violence (ACOP 1998). Convicted abusers were beaten up and driven from their homes, leaving behind arrangements put in place to monitor them (such as electronic tagging and video surveillance) and often absenting themselves from any treatment programmes. The notorious Robert Oliver was obliged to move from London to Swindon to Dublin to Brighton. Refused hostel accommodation, his location was repeatedly exposed by the media and he finally took refuge in a police station. Ironically, the police and probation services were obliged to protect sex offenders from the public rather than vice versa. The cost of protecting Oliver is estimated at around £25,000 (Adams 1998).

In addition, other people are often caught up in the violence and harassment aimed at 'paedophiles'. Hostels have been attacked (whether or not convicted sex offenders are in residence). The wife and child of one offender were named and driven from their home after it was set on fire. In an earlier case a young girl died after a house in which she had been staying was burnt down (*Guardian*, 10 June 1997). In Birmingham, the 81-year-old mother of a convicted sex offender was forced to move and her home was wrecked when the *Birmingham Evening Mail* twice publicised the address where she lived with her son. In Manchester, a man was badly beaten by a gang who mistook him for a paedophile named by the *Manchester Evening News*.

The panic about paedophiles has also been used to victimise individuals with no known official record of sex offences (and with no connection to convicted offenders). Sometimes it seemed little more than a convenient way of harassing unpopular or minority members of the community (reading between the lines, it appears that gay men and those with mental disabilities are particularly likely to be victimised). The *Sunday Times* documented '30 cases where men wrongly suspected of abusing children have been beaten and humiliated by gangs bent on driving them out of their homes' (*Sunday Times*, 2 November 1997). While writing this chapter, the sensitivity and ongoing nature of some of the controversies was illustrated by reactions to requests I made for information. One newspaper said they would only send out a copy of their exposé on sex offenders if my request was made in writing because of 'the sensitive nature of the material'. A children's charity refused to disclose their policy on this issue over the phone; they would only supply it in print form because 'you have to be so careful'. A media complaints body said they could, at present, release no information beyond saying that they were 'in discussion' and 'looking at' the questions raised by the media 'outing' of offenders.

Clearly the media contributed to the spiral of unrest across the country and some coverage was at the very least counterproductive if not blatantly irresponsible. The media, however, did not create community protests out of thin air and it is fundamentally unhelpful to dismiss media and community reactions as a 'moral panic'. This concept implies that the panic is totally unjustified and that it is state-sanctified; neither could be asserted in this case without qualification. More fundamentally the theory fails to pay attention to the processes through which a 'moral panic' is engendered and therefore offers a way of glossing over rather than truly investigating public reactions (Miller *et al.* 1998). To accuse the media of whipping up 'hysteria' and creating 'lynch mob' violence is equally inadequate and ignores key sites through which community reactions evolve. (The very term 'lynch mob' is used to signal irrationality in ways which, in addition, obscure the history of lynching and its position in relation to institutional racism.)

Instead of dismissing public and media reactions as proof of their failure to match the rationality and objectivity of the policy makers, it is crucial to give detailed attention to the questions raised by 'the public' and to examine the processes which led to the policy makers and 'the professionals' losing control of the agenda. This is essential if we are to understand the many complex levels on which the media can play a role in social policy issues.

Theorising community and media protest

The 'paedophile-in-the-community' coverage was driven by factors operating on three levels: the first concerns policy and practice initiatives; the second relates to local community responses and the role of local media; the third involves the underlying construction of 'the paedophile' which underpinned the whole debate.

Policy and practice: initiatives, developments and unanswered questions

The initial decision to establish a register placed the issue of 'paedophiles-in-the-community' on the public agenda: it begged more questions than it answered. How should these offenders be monitored and who should have access to this information? Policy and practice on this issue were clearly underdeveloped and often inconsistent. Legal rulings and professional disputes received extensive media coverage. There were, for example, several cases exposing uncertainty about sex offenders' housing rights: 'Town considers banning sex offenders from council houses' (*Guardian*, 9 January 1997) and 'Eviction of paedophile justified, court rules' (*Guardian*, 20 February 1997). Confusion also surrounded probation officers' responsibilities to pass on information about their clients to prospective employers. The Home Office originally advised probation officers not to notify employers of sex crime convictions in case employees were sacked leading to court actions for damages. This advice was quickly withdrawn leading to headlines such as: 'Home Office confusion on paedophiles' (*Guardian*, 5 December 1996).

Policy on notification to the general public seemed to develop in a similar ad hoc fashion. Particularly high-profile cases raised the following questions. If a housing officer takes it upon himself to inform tenants about a released sex offender on their estate should he be disciplined? Should schools be told, but not pass on the information to parents, or did this place headteachers in an untenable position? Should the police inform the public, but only under very special circumstances? One couple in North Wales, for example, was granted legal aid to sue police for publicising details about their sexual offences (*Manchester Evening News*, 9 June 1997). In some cases public warnings were released: 'Police warn of threat to young males: town on paedophile alert' (*Guardian*, 15 October 1997). In other cases communities were not informed, or only provided with information after media exposure. In a graphic illustration of direct interaction between the media and policy decisions one London Council decided to warn parents about a 'very dangerous' convicted abuser who had moved into their area, but only after learning that a television documentary was to name the man (*Guardian*, 27 March 1997). It was not until September 1997 that guidelines came into force clarifying procedures. Police were given the power to warn headteachers, youth group and play-group leaders and local child protection agencies that a convicted sex offender had moved into their area. But these guidelines did not empower the police to broadcast the names of paedophiles generally unless a professional risk assessment said this was necessary. ('Paedophile guidelines expected to end "outing"' *Guardian*, 12 August 1997).

Public fears and critical media interest were also enhanced by the loopholes in the Sex Offenders Act. These loopholes were readily illustrated by high-profile cases such as that of Graham Seddon – a convicted sex abuser, detained by officers in June 1997 carrying a bag containing toys. He was, he said, looking for a child. Seddon was (briefly) detained in a Liverpool hospital but could not be kept against his will. The notorious Robert Oliver (convicted in 1985) also slipped through a loophole. Judged to be neither repentant nor rehabilitated this man was released without any compulsion to comply with supervision; legislation compelling such compliance only applied to those released after a certain date.

Consequently, in the second half of the 1990s there was a confluence of events (such as the release of particular notorious individuals) and the development of policy and procedures which heightened public awareness of this threat. The original highly newsworthy government initiatives set the news agenda, but that agenda was rapidly revised by the questions it posed about obvious areas of uncertainty.

To suggest that events drove the news agenda would be mere tautology. Some events became 'newsworthy' because of existing news hooks (the court case concerning the eviction of a 'paedophile', for example, would not have received so much media coverage outside this time). Minor events quickly become newsworthy because they are 'topical'. Thus 'satellite' reporting included escorted visits of convicted sex offenders to play-parks and fun-fairs and plans for a commercial UK 'paedophile directory'.

In addition, some of the events which generated peak news coverage around this time were also, of course, not official events (such as court cases, government announcements or inquiries); much of the coverage focused on the surrounding community action. In order to understand the extent of local neighbourhood and media protest it is also necessary to look more closely at these responses.

Neighbourhood reactions: democracy, trust and local information exchange and representation

The local media clearly fed into neighbourhood responses and helped to identify targets for popular anger. Concern about children's safety, however, was certainly not a new phenomenon. 'The paedophile' had already been established as 'public enemy number one' and, long before 1996, fear of the predatory paedophile was etched into the bedrock of parents' anxieties. In focus groups I conducted in the early 1990s, it was clear that fears of child abduction were woven into the fabric of parental experience. Parents talked about the heart-stopping moment when they looked round and realised their young child had disappeared from their side or described the daily pattern of worry every time a son or daughter was late home. One woman summed up her fears and sense of lack of control by stating 'When Andrew goes round the corner he could be off the end of the earth'.

In these focus groups it was also clear that some communities already felt under siege. People spoke about predatory men coming on to the housing estates and, in almost every group, parents described incidents where 'shady' individuals had been seen behaving suspiciously around playgrounds or children had been approached by strangers. Such events inevitably become the topic of conversation (e.g. outside the school gate) and parents felt they had a duty to seek out and share such information. By contrast assaults on children by men within the family were rarely shared with the community (Kitzinger 1998).

Given this background it is hardly surprising that the idea that known sex offenders were to be secretly housed in their neighbourhoods triggered grave concern. The very names of some of the community protest groups express their anger at the restrictions placed upon their lives (e.g. 'Freedom for Children') and their desire to assert their rights (e.g. 'People's Power'). Some protest groups also chose names which encapsulated their disillusionment with official protection and monitoring procedures (e.g. 'The Unofficial Child Protection Unit'). This disillusionment (and some hope and expectations) was vividly articulated by the founder of the (anti-vigilante) 'Scottish People Against Child Abuse'. Speaking to the *Scotsman*, she commented:

> 'People must be able to sit back and be responsible. If they saw something constructive being done, maybe they would start having trust again in the authorities. The Government is there because we trusted them to look after us and protect our children, but they are not doing that yet'.
>
> (*Scotsman*, 16 October 1997)

Official incompetence was a recurring theme both in local discussion and in national coverage. Internationally high-profile cases of multiple sex abusers (from Dutroux in Belgium to Fred and Rosemary West in Cromwell Street) suggested that 'the professionals' could not be trusted to monitor and investigate properly. Dutroux was able to continue his activities even though police were notified that he was building dungeons to imprison abducted children (Kelly 1997). The police were regular visitors to Cromwell Street but the Wests were able to continue to rape and murder their victims. Both these cases served as a backdrop to public concern. In 1997 this concern was underlined, with the murder of Scott Simpson in Aberdeen by a known 'paedophile'. The boy's murderer was under social-work supervision but this did not prevent him committing this crime. The bungling of the Scott Simpson case received extensive coverage (particularly in Scotland). The case was blamed on a failure of social services to follow guidelines and to convey relevant information to the police. The police were also criticised for 'serious corporate failure' in investigating the nine-year-old's disappearance ('Inquiry into blunder as paedophile gets life' *Scotsman*, 11 November 1997). The name of Scott Simpson case was evoked by those campaigning for community notification in future cases. His murder suggested the 'experts' and 'professionals' could not provide sufficient protection on their own.

If such cases inspired little faith in 'the authorities', then housing inequalities further exacerbated the crisis. Released prisoners, including convicted sex offenders, tend to be placed in hostels or offered housing in working-class areas and often on council estates. Where offenders were offered social housing, rather than returning to private accommodation, this also raised particular questions about policy. Many protesters expressed anger and frustration at the fact that their fate was to be decided by faceless bureaucrats who rarely lived in such areas themselves. The question often asked in public meetings called to reassure people was: 'How would *you* feel if he was living next door to you and your kids?' Residents often seemed to feel that council tenants were expected to put up with living next to an incinerator, playgrounds built on polluted sites, damp housing or a failing local school. Now they were also expected to tolerate the country's most dangerous predators dumped on their doorsteps. People living on council estates are also, of course, less likely to have access to private transport, or even decent public transport, safe play areas and consistent childcare, all of which may mute concerns about children's safety.

For some protesters it was clear that direct action (ranging from seeking media publicity to vigilante activities) represented the only way of having their voices heard. The local media, for their part, were usually happy to co-operate and have a special remit to respond to local pressure groups and address community reactions. Local newspaper editorials demanding (or in effect providing) community notification presented the papers as standing up for their constituents, asserting a strong neighbourhood identity and fulfilling their functions as representative of 'the people'. While local media have problems representing some local concerns (such as pollution from a factory which is key to providing local jobs), the sex offender presented an apparently clear-cut 'enemy' and 'outsider'. As the *Daily Record* declared: 'the Record believes action must be taken now to confront the plague of abuse that wrecks young lives and disgusts all right-minded Scots' (*Daily Record*, 25 February 1997).

In understanding media and public reactions, therefore, it is important not to be dismissive when 'the public' come into conflict with 'the experts' or when local 'NIMBYISM' seems to come into conflict with the 'wider public good'. Community concern and the conditions under which people are forced to live should not be underestimated. As feminist journalist and author Beatrix Campbell points out, community notification may not be the best way of protecting children, however:

> 'There is a piety around the notion of "the mob" which doesn't take responsibility for what some communities endure. A liberal disposition can't cope with what these communities are facing. There are communities, there are children, who live in a permanent panic about when he's going to get out of prison. That fear, and the dreadful consequences for individuals and communities, don't always infuse the debate.'
>
> (Beatrix Campbell, conversation with author)

The issue of former neighbours returning from prison to live near their victims has certainly enjoyed considerable media prominence. A housing worker faced with press coverage of such a situation expresses some ambivalence about the media's role. The press focus was unhelpful and resulted in a defensive reaction from parts of the housing authority and generated unnecessary fear on the estate. But media coverage did trigger an official acknowledgement of the problem. Indeed:

> 'The media were useful in that the tenants had tried telling their housing officer and had not succeeded in persuading her to listen. It is a shame that the council obviously felt inaccessible so that they had to go to the press. There are lessons to be learned from that. But the press made sure that the council reacted.'
>
> (Housing Officer, interview with author)

In this particular case, local and national media attention also led to further enquiries from tenants about other individuals on this estate. This, in turn, led to the exposure of a further case in which children might be at risk and where there had been a failure in inter-departmental communication. According to the housing officer, this led to 'significant policy shifts about the sharing of professional information and adoption of protocols and guidelines to support that.'

The media then should not be seen as merely 'interfering' in an area best left to 'the experts'. Public debate and involvement in social policy issues is a democratic and practical imperative. Questions from the media and 'the public' (as neighbours, tenants, and citizens) can disrupt important policy initiatives, but they can also be effective in pushing issues onto the policy agenda and refining procedures.

There were far more fundamental problems, however, with the way in which the debate about paedophiles was framed in public discourse, including media coverage and policy making. These problems have far deeper roots than the immediate concerns raised in the second half of the 1990s and this chapter concludes by problematising the way in which 'the paedophile' was constructed as an object of social policy and by identifying some of the problems which were obscured by the media focus on convicted offenders.

Framing paedophiles: public, media and policy gaps in addressing child sexual abuse

Throughout this chapter the word 'paedophile' has appeared in inverted commas: the intention has been to signal the constructed nature of the term. 'The paedophile' has become the dominant way through which sexual threats to children are conceptualised and articulated, but the concept is laden with ideas and assumptions which confine thinking about this issue to a very narrow focus.

'The paedophile' is a concept enmeshed in a series of crass stereotypes which place the child sexual abuser 'outside' society. In the tabloid press abusers are 'animals', 'monsters' 'sex maniacs', 'beasts' and 'perverts' who are routinely described as 'loners' and 'weirdos'. Right across the media it is also implied that paedophiles, far from being 'ordinary family men', are more likely to be gay (for systematic analysis of this see Kitzinger and Skidmore 1995). Such conceptualisations were amply illustrated in the press reporting about 'paedophiles-in-the-community'. The *Daily Record*'s 'Gallery of shame', for example, perpetuated all the old stereotypes, highlighting particular words in bold block capitals. Struggling for variety of negative epithets to describe their gallery of thirty-eight sex offenders the paper ran through the usual list warning readers of: 'TWISTED Dickons [who] got eight years for raping two young sisters'; 'WEIRDO Sean Regan 'who 'was dubbed "The Beast"', and 'DEPRAVED paedophile Harley' who 'preyed on terrified children as young as six.' Other convicted offenders were variously described as: 'EVIL Herriot', 'PERVERT teacher', 'SEXUAL predator', and 'SEX BEAST'. In among these highlighted adjectives one man was simply described as 'BACHELOR Paritt' (with its gay implications) and three of the descriptions highlighted a disability (e.g. 'DEAF Duff posed as a priest as he prowled the street' and 'DEAF MUTE Eaglesham, 66, carried out a series of sex attacks on a 10-year-old girl') (*Daily Record*, 25 February 1997).

Portraits of 'paedophiles' do more than simply stereotype and reinforce prejudice against particular minority groups. They also imply that paedophiles are a separate species, subhuman or 'a breed apart' (Hebenton and Thomas 1996). The term also singles out the sexual abuse of children, as if there were no connection between the acts of sexual abuse and exploitation perpetrated against children and those perpetrated against adult women. One interesting piece of information released by the Home Office during the height of the paedophile crisis was the fact that, by the time they are forty, one man in 90 has been convicted of a serious sex offence, such as rape, incest or gross indecency with a child (Marshall 1997). This fact, combined with evidence that most perpetrators of sexual assault are never convicted, suggests that every community is likely to have its share of sex offenders. The release of the Home Office statistic received some media attention, but was quickly forgotten and rarely integrated into the narrative of stories about 'paedophiles-in-the-community'. The fact that most 'paedophiles-in-the-community' were undetected and probably well integrated into their neighbourhood was rarely raised. The fact that most people would already know a sex offender was ignored.

To acknowledge that sexual violence was quite so endemic would have undermined the narrative thrust of most 'paedophile-in-the-community' stories. By confining their attention to a minority of convicted multiple abusers and defining those who sexually abuse children as a certain type of person, 'a paedophile', the media were able to focus not on society but on a few dangerous individuals within it. The problem of sexual violence was represented by the newspaper image of the man with staring eyes or the evil smirk, the 'beast' and 'fiend' who could be singled out, electronically tagged, exposed and expelled. If paedophiles are literally 'evil personified', then such evil can be exorcised by exclusion of these individuals from society. This individualised approach fits in with certain strands in criminological discourse (see Hebenton and Thomas 1996); it also fits in with the whole media shift towards 'dumbed down' personalised stories whereby, for example, journalists focus on the noisy and antisocial 'neighbour from hell' rather than examining the problem of 'sink estates' through analysis of employment, recreation facilities and housing condition (Franklin 1997). Paedophiles are, of course, in this sense the ultimate neighbour from hell.

The concept of 'the paedophile' is flawed. It locates the threat of abuse within the individual (rather than in social, cultural or bureaucratic institutions). In the context of abuse in children's homes, for example, attention can be focused on the cunning infiltrator while ignoring the nature of care system, funding and resourcing. In the case of other sites of abuse attention is confined to 'the outsider' and 'the loner' leaving the role of fathers, and the institution of the family unquestioned. The paedophile is presented as a danger which 'prowls our streets' and is used to reinforce the media's and policy makers' disproportionate focus on 'stranger danger' (Kitzinger and Skidmore 1995). Indeed, 'the paedophile' is a creature that embodies stranger danger. He reflects and sustains a focus on abusers as outcast from society rather than part of it. As feminist activist and academic, Liz Kelly, argues the concept of 'the paedophile' helps to shift attention away:

> . . . from the centrality of power and control to notions of sexual deviance, obsession and 'addiction'. Paedophilia returns us to . . . medical and individualised explanations [. . .]. Rather than sexual abuse demanding that we look critically at the social construction of masculinity, male sexuality and the family, the safer terrain of 'abnormalities' beckons.
>
> (Kelly 1996: 45)

If we adopt the word 'paedophile' and see it as synonymous with 'child sexual abuse' then we narrow the policy agenda. The fact that most children are assaulted by someone that they know virtually disappears from the debate and policies which would be deemed unacceptable if applied to 'ordinary men' become allowable. Commenting on government initiatives in relation to 'paedophiles' Kelly draws attention to the fact that 'paedophiles' may be denied the right to work with children or even to approach playgrounds, yet such proposals would cause outrage if applied to fathers (Kelly 1996: 46). Indeed, women are often forced by the courts to allow violent and abusive partners access to their children, even where those children have also been sexually abused by him.

The fundamental critique here is that the notion of the paedophile restricts definitions of 'the problem' and thus limits how we can envisage solutions. The term helps to obscure important aspects of sexual violence and shifts attention 'away from political solutions addressing male power and the construction of masculinity toward a range of "problem-management" solutions'. [Such as] . . . 'long term incarceration' (*Mail*), 'risk assessment tribunals for dangerous men' (*Guardian* and *The Times*) and 'individual therapy (*Guardian*)' (McCollum 1998: 37).

Conclusion

This chapter has explored the role of the media, particularly the local media, in the 'paedophile crisis'. It has attempted to highlight the positive as well as the negative impact of coverage and to identify those factors which shaped and maintained the momentum of media attention. In presenting this case study

I have tried to demonstrate the intertwined levels of analysis which can contribute towards theorising the relationship between the media and social policy. It is not sufficient simply to focus on media coverage. It is important to consider the motives of source organisations who seek out media publicity. It is also unhelpful to dismiss the media as 'interfering' or 'sensationalist' or to blame the press for 'media hype'. Instead, it is necessary to recognise their role as a forum for public debate. At the same time, however, it is vital never to accept the terms of that debate as cast in stone and always to question what is left out of the policy agenda as well as what is addressed. In this way one can combine detailed analysis of crisis coverage with critical reflection on the underlying assumptions which frame public discourse and limit visions for social policy.

Notes

1 For discussion of the emergence of the child abduction threat (in the USA) see Best (1990); for discussion of the media creation of the popular image of the 'paedophile priest' see Jenkins (1996).

2 Other reports urged caution and restraint. The (Aberdeen) *Press and Journal*, for example, reported efforts to reassure the public and condemn vigilante action: 'Crowd (self) control' (*Press and Journal*, 6 August 1997) 'Police and community condemn vigilantes' *Press and Journal*, 10 June 1997) and similar reports and editorials appeared in other papers e.g. 'Sex crime vigilantes not answer' (*Yorkshire Evening Post*, 6 February 1997); 'Have faith in the police to shield our children' (*Express on Sunday*, 10 August 1997).

3 The *Bournemouth Evening Echo*'s 'Protect our children' campaign involved setting up a register of convicted sex offenders, compiled from newspaper reports. This was, however, available only to workers with children. Other papers, such as the *Guardian*, adopted a policy of only 'outing' offenders if there was evidence that supervision had broken down and children were at risk.

References

Adams, D. (1998) 'The "at risk" business', *Police Review*, 30 January, 16–17.

Aldridge, M. (1994) *Making Social Work News*, London: Routledge.

Association of Chief Officers of Probation (1998) *Recent cases of public disorder around sex offenders which have impeded surveillance and supervision*. London: ACOP.

Best, J. (1990) *Threatened Children*, Chicago: Chicago University Press.

Franklin, B. (1997) *Newzak and News Media*, London: Arnold.

Franklin, B. and Murphy, D. (1998) *Making the Local News: Local Journalism in Context*, London: Routledge.

Hebenton, B. and Thomas, T. (1996) 'Sexual offenders in the community: reflections on problems of law, community and risk management in the USA, England and Wales', *International Journal of the Sociology of Law* 24: 427–443.

Henderson, L. (1998) 'Making serious soaps: public issue storylines in TV drama serials', in Philo, G. (ed.) *Message Received*, London: Longman.

Jenkins, P. (1996) *Pedophiles and Priests: Anatomy of a Contemporary Crisis*, Oxford: Oxford University Press.

Kelly, L. (1996) 'Weasel words: paedophiles and the cycle of abuse', *Trouble and Strife* 33: 44–49.
—— (1997) 'Confronting an atrocity', *Trouble and Strife* 36: 16–22.
Kitzinger, J. (1996) 'Media representations of sexual abuse risks', *Child Abuse Review* 5: 319–333.
—— (1998) The gender politics of news production: silenced voices and false memories', in Carter *et al.* (eds) *News, Gender and Power*, London: Routledge.
—— (forthcoming) 'A sociology of media power: key issues in audience reception research', in Philo, G. (ed.) *Message Received*, Harlow: Longman.
Kitzinger, J. and Skidmore, P. (1995) 'Playing safe: media coverage of child sexual abuse prevention strategies', *Child Abuse Review* 4(1): 47–56.
Marshall, P. (1997) *The prevalence of convictions for sexual offending Research findings* 55, London: Home Office Research and Statistics Directorate.
McCollum, H. (1998) 'What the papers say', *Trouble and Strife* 37: 31–37.
Miller, D., Kitzinger, J., Williams, K. and Beharrell, P. (1998) *The Circuit of Mass Communication: Media Strategies, Representation and Audience Reception in the AIDS Crisis*, London: Sage.
Soothill, K. and Walby, S. (1991) *Sex Crimes in the News*, London: Routledge.
Thomas, T. (1997) 'How could this man go free: privacy, the press and the paedophile', in Lawson, E. (ed.) *Child Exploitation and the Media Forum: Report and Recommendations*, Dover: Smallwood Publishing Group, 67–69.
Tuchman, G. (1978) *Making News: a Study of the Construction of Reality*, New York: Free Press.

Chapter 14

Out of the closet

New images of disability in the civil rights campaign

Ann Pointon

Introduction

The events leading to the introduction of the Disability Discrimination Act 1995 (DDA) dramatically raised the growing profile of disabled people in Britain and prompted media and public recognition that there was a 'disability movement', even though that movement had been in existence for some time. The movement had been seeking comprehensive civil rights for disabled people through a series of Private Members' Bills proposed by the then opposition Labour Party. These attempts were consistently opposed by the Conservative government but such was the heavy cross-party and public support in favour of legislation, that it was forced to make a reluctant U-turn. The limited and piecemeal DDA which was eventually introduced fell far short in its provisions from the Civil Rights (Disabled Persons) Bill preferred by the disability movement. But the fact that it was enacted at all signalled a profound change in the political agenda on disability. 'A very able pressure group' was the headline of an article by Victoria Macdonald in the *Sunday Telegraph* which referred to the 'wind of change' that the government had somehow 'missed'. 'The most remarkable point' Macdonald continued 'was the Government's belief that the civil rights bill could be shelved without such a fuss; for the growth of the disability pressure group – indeed the growth in the numbers of "disabled" – is one of the features of British life in the past 20 years' (15 May 1996).

Over the last decade new images of disabled people have entered the media catalogue, as a result of disabled people taking protest to the streets to publicise a variety of issues – including benefits, lack of access to transport and buildings, patronising television Telethons and demands for civil rights. These images showed disabled people chained to inaccessible buses or trains, blocking traffic in the streets, crawling along the pavement outside the Houses of Parliament, and more recently in 1997 protesting at proposed benefit cuts, smearing symbolically angry red paint on themselves and the pavements of Downing Street.

Although these new images contradicted traditional media stereotypes of dependency, physical limitation, or individual 'courageous' achievement, they were media attractive because of their shock and surprise value. Disabled people are accustomed to 'objectification'; but these were self-generated images that reflected both the reality of effective political action and the growth of assertive self-confidence. Nevertheless, such activities were only partly understood by the general public, and were rejected by some disabled and non-disabled people as counter-productive, but as Jane Campbell, a leading disability activist, argues concerning earlier, less confrontational policies, 'the absence of visible direct action in the streets was to our detriment, because it is only since we have taken to the streets that we have been visible in the media' (Campbell and Oliver 1996: 192).

The 'disability pressure group' referred to earlier in the Macdonald article, however, is not synonymous with the 'disability movement', which might best be characterised as comprising organisations 'of' disabled people rather than organisations not controlled by disabled people but operating 'for' them.

The 'ofs' and 'fors'

The distinction between organisations 'of' and organisations 'for' disabled people is regarded as fundamentally important to the disability movement, with 'of' organisations being recognised as having democratic structures that give control to disabled people. In brief the distinction is relevant to understanding the balance between the mix of disability organisations lobbying for civil rights legislation.

Scope (previously the Spastics Society), Mencap, the RNIB and the RNID are examples of traditional charities controlled by non-disabled people. Some, like Scope and Mencap, were established as parents' self-help organisations to support one specific kind of impairment. Their history is one of speaking for disabled people and, along with medical professionals, being regarded by governments and journalists as the disability experts. The imagery of disability used in their advertising to win donations, represented disabled people as pathetic and dependent individuals. These images were dominant at a time when disabled people were less visible in the media than they are today, and they have improved following trenchant criticisms from disabled people. The charity RADAR (Royal Association for Disability and Rehabilitation) is, despite its protests, also regarded as an organisation 'for' disabled people but it is government supported and does not advertise for funds.

An effective alliance was formed between organisations 'of' and 'for' disabled people to push for civil rights legislation, although there was a discernible note of irony for some disabled people to be working with the disability charity organisations that had been the principal target of their criticisms since the 1970s.

The civil rights agenda had been initiated by disabled people's organisations, in an unequal and under-funded struggle against initial opposition from traditional charities. Although the alliance has been useful in many respects, it could be argued that is has helped obscure perceptions about the disability movement and what and who it represents. Further confusion arises from new corporate images created by many of the big charities in response to the increasingly competitive market, which have included changes in advertising strategies in response to criticisms by the disabled people that they ostensibly represent.

The disability movement

Political activity by disabled people in Britain has a long history (Campbell and Oliver 1996; Pagel 1988). The British Deaf Association was formed in 1890, for example, while in 1899 the National League of the Blind became a trade union. Its 250 members marched to London in 1920 and again in 1933 to protest against low pay. Immediately after the war the Disabled Persons (Employment) Act of 1944 was passed but, between 1945 and 1964, no party manifesto included any further measures to help disabled people. More shocking, however, is the absence between 1959 and 1964 of even a single debate on disability in the House of Commons (Meacher 1985).

Concerns about poverty led to the founding of DIG (Disability Income Group) in 1965. The group expanded rapidly to become a mass organisation and the most significant of a number of groups of disabled people focusing on issues that 'were not freely chosen but arose out of the problems that [people] experienced as they tried to cope with the range of barriers in a community designed for able-bodied lifestyles' (Finkelstein 1997: 6).

The British disability movement has its origins in a letter published in the *Guardian* by Paul Hunt in 1972, calling for a united struggle against all forms of discrimination (20 September 1972). Two years of subsequent correspondence led to the founding of the Union of the Physically Impaired Against Segregation (UPIAS) in 1974 followed by the establishment in 1979 of the British Council of Organisations of Disabled People (BCODP) which was renamed the British Council of Disabled People in 1998. BCODP was formed as an umbrella organisation for affiliate groups controlled by disabled people.

A key development was the redefinition of disability, which challenged the individual or 'medical approach', in favour of what is now called the social model, pioneered by Vic Finkelstein (1980) and Mike Oliver (1990) and adopted by UPIAS and BCODP. The disability movement in Britain was theoretically strong from the outset and proved influential internationally in redefining disability away from the medical model (Oliver 1996: 33 and Dreidger 1989: 53). Conversely, the American civil rights approach to disability, particularly the black civil rights movement and the tactics employed by disabled lobbyists in the campaign for the Americans with Disabilities Act, was influential in Britain (Pagel 1988). The American emphasis on individual self-empowerment rather than collective strength and support, however, has been criticised in the UK (Campbell and Oliver 1996).

Expressed very briefly, the social model argued that 'disability' reflected the way society was organised rather than the person's impairment or condition. Disability could be changed or reduced by changing society, including changes to the environment, to institutional structures and in the provision of technical aids and personal support.

'Tragic' impairment

The social model is in opposition to the traditional, and still prevailing, 'individual' or 'medical' model of disability in which the impairment itself is seen as the 'tragic' and central problem. The responses of 'cure' or 'care' came from medical professionals and charities, with the latter emphasising the tragic aspect in the images and language it used in order to get income. Disabled people's responsibility was, and still is, popularly thought to be somehow to 'overcome' their impairment rather than 'overcoming' or pushing for changes to a hostile environment and institutional barriers.

There are ongoing debates about weaknesses in the model, particularly around the place of 'impairment' within it, but Shakespeare and Watson maintain that 'there is a broad and vigorous consensus [and] the views that have to be debunked are not those of disabled people, but those of non-disabled academics and commentators who continue to view disability as a personal medical tragedy' (Shakespeare and Watson 1997: 293–294). Oliver argues that criticisms raise questions about how the model is used rather than the model itself (Oliver in Barnes and Mercer 1996: 50).

It is impossible in a short essay of this length to explore the forms, sources and cultural outcomes of the imagery around disability and impairment, or to engage with criticisms by Shakespeare (1994) that cultural imagery is neglected within the social model, reflecting the neglect of impairment. But 'the link between impairment and all that is socially unacceptable was first established in classical Greek Theatre. Today there are a number of cultural stereotypes which perpetuate this linkage' (Barnes 1992 citing Hevey 1991). Barnes refers to the twelve common media stereotypes identified by Biklen and Bogdana (1977), which include the disabled person as: 'pitiable and pathetic', 'an object of violence', 'sinister and evil', 'atmosphere or curio', 'super cripple', 'an object of ridicule', 'their worst and only enemy', 'a burden', 'sexually abnormal', 'incapable of participating fully in community life' and 'normal' (Barnes 1992).

It is the first of these mainly negative stereotypes – the disabled persons as 'pitiable and pathetic' – which has received the most prominence in the daily press and magazines, while the stereotype of the disabled person as a 'burden' is an often unspoken theme of benefit and 'carer' stories. The explanation of the popularity of these two prominent images is not simply that stories of tragedy are overwhelmingly attractive to journalists and readers. It reflects the fact that the greater part of advertising which features disabled people has been sponsored and produced by charity organisations and designed to attract donations for such 'needy people': or to induce fear and scare non-disabled people into contributing towards research to eliminate particular conditions.

In the late 1990s, however, active protest work on issues of representation and media portrayal lost ground to work around civil rights. An article in the *Guardian* entitled 'The last civil rights battle' seemed to herald a new period, in which there was greater street activity and disabled demonstrators were prepared to block traffic flows by chaining themselves to buses (20 July 1988). Police forces were at first bemused and uncertain about how to respond. Many members of Campaign Against Patronage (CAP) and Campaign for Accessible Transport (CAT) eventually joined the newly formed Disabled People's Direct Action Network (DAN) and widened the scope and amount of protest activity.

Getting together

BCODP launched its campaign for anti-discrimination legislation in September 1991, although there had been a number of attempts to get legislation onto the statute book during the 1980s. BCODP published a substantial book which represented the first comprehensive account of disability discrimination in Britain (Barnes 1991).

Nineteen ninety-two witnessed the publication of Labour MP, Alf Morris's Private Member's Civil Rights Bill which was reintroduced as the Civil Rights (Disabled Persons) Bill in 1993, 1994 and 1995, sponsored on each occasion by a different Labour MP but opposed every time by the then Conservative government. On 31 January 1992 Social Security Secretary Nicholas Scott (then Minister for Disabled People) famously described his position as 'benevolently neutral', and also said that there was 'by no means unanimity among the disabled community, let alone among others in society, that legislation is necessarily the right way at this particular time' (*Guardian*, 1 February 1992).

This Bill was filibustered out but revived in 1993 and sponsored by Baroness Lockwood. At this time BCODP was part of Voluntary Organisations for Anti-Discrimination Legislation (VOADL), a disability organisations' lobbying consortium of twenty-four organisations that included 'ofs' and 'fors', with a Chair from the Spinal Injuries Association, an 'of' organisation. This was not, however, the first mixed alliance. The Disability Manifesto group, for example, which launched its *Agenda for the 1990s* in June 1991, comprised thirteen of 'the country's leading disability organisations', four of which were controlled by disabled people. This agenda included anti-discrimination legislation in its ten recommendations.

The press climate was relatively sympathetic. The *Sun* (17 February 1993) offered strong support in an article that was unsentimentally headlined 'We don't want sympathy – just equal rights'. The paper quoted George Bush's 1990 comment on the Americans with Disabilities Act that it will 'let the shameful wall of exclusion finally come tumbling down.' But this excellent 'equality' approach to disability was undermined by references to the individual 'tragedy model' which was evident in the newspaper's three 'heartstring-tugging' examples of disabled people: 'a brave young policewoman, crippled as she tackled a gunman, is turned away from a charity event because she is in a wheelchair; a woman who has devoted her life to helping fellow blind people is banned from taking her guide dog to Buckingham Palace . . . [to] receive the MBE; a soldier who lost his legs in the Falklands cannot get into his local cinema because . . . there is no lift for his wheelchair' (17 February 1995).

Rights Now!

The thirteenth and most extensively reported attempt at legislation, sponsored by Roger Berry MP, followed in 1994. The subsequent lobbying and political activism witnessed the maturing of the anti-discrimination pressure group into one which had more media appeal and a clearer image. The clumsily titled VOADL became the more media-friendly Rights Now! campaign, operating as an umbrella and pressure group for eighty-four disability groups. Rights Now! was based at the headquarters of RADAR, and was well organised. It produced the now almost obligatory coloured ribbon (blue for 'unity' and yellow for 'freedom'), which was also being adopted internationally, and which helped increase the sense of solidarity across a broad range of disability organisations.

There were greater hopes for this attempt. Cross-party support was strong, led by the All Party Disablement Group and Alan Howarth, then a Conservative MP with a disabled son, argued the case persuasively in the *Guardian*, drawing comparisons with the USA and attempting to deal with ministerial reservations about costs (26 March 1994). Stephen Hawking's media-credible voice was lent to the campaign, alleging that 'If there were such discrimination against blacks or women, there would be a public outcry' (*Morning Star*, 9 March 1994).

Once again, the *Sun* seemed to be the only newspaper taking a campaigning position, by inviting its readers to fill in a form to send to their MPs urging support at the second reading and the final stage of the Bill (5 March 1994 and 26 April 1994). Regrettably, the paper again referred to 'police officers crippled on duty, the blind, the deaf, war heroes and those hit by illness', the same 'appealing' disabled people that they had listed in 1993.

On 11 March 1994 the Bill had its second reading, with MPs voting 231 to 0 to move the Bill into committee. But when the Bill was sabotaged in May the mood changed from modest hope to a new bitterness. At a demonstration against the Bill's failure some two months later, one disabled activist claimed that 'Writing letters and lobbying parliament wasn't doing much. It was time to cause some real inconvenience'. Disabled people had lost all confidence in the Minister for Disabled People Nicholas Scott, especially when it became clear that despite early denials it had been his own department which had drawn up the eighty wrecking amendments to the Bill.

The publicity immediately following the actual fall of the Bill, however, was not predominantly about the disappointment of disabled people, but the family connection between Nicholas Scott, the Minister, and his daughter Victoria who, as parliamentary officer at RADAR, headquarters for the Rights Now! campaign, was firmly on the other side of the disability fence to her father. Victoria's criticism of her father attracted extensive media coverage including an interview on Radio 4's *Today* programme. Many disabled people had mixed feelings, welcoming the publicity but noting the irony that it was respected but non-disabled Victoria who was getting the headlines and having to put the disability lobby case. Carmichael (1997) noted that disabled commentators were entirely absent from the *News at Ten* report. But Catherine Bennett, writing in the *Guardian*, commented that 'No matter how cynical the interest that flung her on to the front pages, it has made the disabled cause more visible than it had been for years' (14 May 1994: 29). Perhaps more telling were remarks in an article in the *Independent on Sunday*'s supplement a year later (9 April 1995). Journalist Ian Parker wrote:

> 'I'd been trying to get some coverage,' says one campaigner, 'I was ringing the TV – the *Big Breakfast*, whatever – they weren't interested. When the Vicky Scott story broke, they were ringing *us*.' The penny seemed to drop. 'People saw it,' says Rachel Hurst, [a leading activist] 'as a civil rights movement. Not just those poor sods can't get on a bus.' Thanks to the failure of a bill about civil rights, the idea of disabled civil rights seemed to take hold. You could feel an earlier model of pity and passivity slipping away . . . Demonstrations swelled in numbers; individual (rather than institutional) membership of Rights Now! increased eight-fold in one year. And it was a mark of what had happened that articles scornful of 'the disabled lobby' started to appear in national newspapers and magazines: as most campaigners would want it, sympathy – pity – had been removed from the equation.

Another theme in media coverage was the government's alleged estimate of £17 billion to implement the civil rights bill, a figure that was to be pulled apart by government critics in the days following. But as Alan Howarth pointed out, the government had not placed these costings into the library until after the committee stage of the Bill and just one day before its second reading (*Today* Radio 4, 14 May 1994). This ensured its damaging effect.

The Bill was not, however, finally dead, but an attempt by peers to revive it in June, was met by yet another successful blocking manoeuvre. Members of DAN expressed their anger on 23 May by instigating a 'crawl' up the steps to Parliament. This tactic had been famously successful in gaining publicity and expressing anger in Washington during lobbying for the Americans with

Disabilities Act. DAN members had an appointment with Dennis Skinner but, having been refused admission via the fourteen steps of St Stephen's entrance, they crawled 100 metres down the street to the main Carriage Gate entrance where, after a further three-hour wait, the Speaker insisted that they be given access to lobby their MPs. The pictures received the expected good press publicity, and television news coverage.

Almost inevitably the government defeated the Bill, but despite the 'victory', the affair turned out to be a PR disaster for the government. To cite the *Sunday Telegraph* again 'The most remarkable point was the Government's belief that the bill could be shelved without such a fuss' (15 May 1994).

The critics

The press and public support for civil rights legislation was largely sustained, but some political and journalistic voices were critical. Journalists like Melanie Phillips who wished to appear sympathetic ran the 'in their own best interests' line and worried about disabled activists potentially alienating other groups (*Observer*, 7 May 1995).

Other critics, despite their personal 'experience of disability' were more confrontational and dismissive. Norman Tebbit, for example, referring to his disabled wife during a speech at a lunch for hoteliers and caterers, asked them to consider the needs of disabled people but nevertheless said the civil rights bill proposals were 'quite absurd' because of imposing unjustifiable costs (*Financial Times*, 14 July 1994). Wheelchair writing critic and traveller Quentin Crewe, who died in November 1998, confessed that 'Whenever the disabled lobbies get under way, my heart sinks. I know we are in for another bout of preposterous claims, idiot suggestions and gobsful of political correctness' (*Daily Mail*, 7 September 1994: 8).

Richard Ingrams, a regular disparager of disabled activists, warned that the same kind of 'tyranny wielded by American campaigners for the disabled' was starting to happen here (*Observer*, 21 February 1993). Later that year, however, he was possibly quite alone in deploring the fact that a protest had been registered concerning a blind woman who had been refused permission to take her guide dog into Buckingham Palace for an investiture (*Observer*, 29 November 1992). Unusually, in this case, he made no reference to the cost element that was a frequent theme of his and other critics' columns. 'It is surely obvious' he claimed 'however much one sympathises, that disabled people (by which is generally meant people in wheelchairs) cannot enjoy the same freedom of movement and opportunity as the rest of us – unless, that is, billions of pounds are to be spent on altering the environment' (*Observer*, 21 August 1993).

A syndicated piece from Washington by Henry Fairlie a decade before the USA's ADA (Americans with Disabilities Act) was passed put it rather more entertainingly in a long article headlined 'Are handicapped spoiled? Far too much sloppy good feeling about bringing them out of the closet' (*Winnipeg Free Press*, 20 June 1980). His conclusion, of course, was yes! But in the following decade disabled people were not passively 'brought out of the closet', but pushed the door open themselves.

Such criticisms received little coverage relative to the story overall, and indeed the objections seemed 'dated' and old-fashioned rather than fresh, iconoclastic and stimulating. These views nevertheless revealed genuine, if usually hidden and unspoken, fears that are sometimes present if disabled people dare to step out of their supposed dependent place in society and bring their 'odd' appearance into unashamed view.

Stronger expressions of this fear came from A.N. Wilson, although journalists such as Keith Waterhouse hinted at repugnance of disabled people's '*unseemly* scenes outside the Palace of Westminster' [my italics], while making points about costs linked to examples in San Francisco 'where all this wheelchair tomfoolery began' (*Daily Mail*, 8 September 1994).

It was not until the much later 'red paint' demonstration in Downing Street over benefit cuts in December 1997, however, that the most blatant expression of deep prejudice led one to speculate about the ethics of some editorial judgements. It was the broadsheet *Sunday Telegraph* rather than a tabloid that gave editorial space to the crude views of writer A.N. Wilson, whose expression of deep fear of disabled people (or perhaps 'ugly' people) was highly emotive and visual.

> Helpless figures writhe on the pavement . . . it's the disabled, waddling and wheeling their way towards the most popular leader in the democratic world, to protest at the proposed cuts in their 'benefits'. Appearances are all. There was supposed to be something pathetic about the furious Quasimodos who assembled to throw paint over themselves last Monday. But as a demonstration it misfired completely. They seemed not merely visually revolting, but completely horrible, embittered people.
>
> (28 December 1997)

An unsatisfactory act

The Conservative government's decision to introduce its own more limited legislation in the form of the DDA proved to be more dangerous to the disability movement than such reactionary views, although there was undoubtedly a certain satisfaction in seeing a government forced to do something it did not want to do – 'Stung by the outcry' (*Daily Mail*, 7 September 1994: 2) – and trying to redeem its 'pledge' to find practical and affordable ways to fight discrimination (*Sun*, 4 March 1994).

The Bill focused on employment and the provision of goods and services. The disability pressure groups' criticisms included the lack of a general right to reasonable access, the exclusion of education and transport, the lack of an enforcement commission, the exemption of small employers and the limited definition of disability. Subsequent amendments did not redeem the Bill in activists' perceptions.

The campaign had achieved an unsatisfactory success, in the enacting of weak and piecemeal legislation that it did not want. One result was to increase tensions within the Rights Now! alliance, because some organisations were less happy with this compromise than others. This outcome had been predicted in 1995 when Barnes and Oliver argued that the Bill then going through Parliament would not only eliminate discrimination against disabled people, but also present Britain's disabled people's movement with one of its most difficult challenges to date. Having correctly guessed that there would be some form of anti-discrimination legislation before the 1997 general election, they suggested that the 'rhetoric of rights currently echoing through the corridors of power would not be matched by reality. Indeed it is possible that when and if the Government proposals do become law that disabled people in Britain will be worse off than they are today' (Barnes and Oliver 1995: 111).

Barnes and Oliver also argued that 'even fully comprehensive and enforceable civil rights legislation will not, by itself, solve the problem of discrimination against disabled people' (Barnes and Oliver 1995: 114). Like racism, sexism and other forms of institutional prejudice, such discrimination is institutionalised in the fabric of British society, with only a very limited effectiveness for the Sex Discrimination Act and the Race Relations Act. The Disability Discrimination Act 1995 is even weaker, although it can be argued that it has at least changed the climate in which disability is approached.

The government bill ran in the same session as a final attempt was being made to bring back the Labour opposition's civil rights bill, this time sponsored by Labour MP, Harry Barnes. Consequently, the Rights Now! campaigners had three tasks: to promote the Barnes Bill, to oppose the government bill but also to involve themselves in the amendment process in case the government bill became law, as seemed likely. It is not surprising that the newer government bill attracted more media attention and there was relatively little effective comparison between the two proposed sets of measures.

Media coverage in the summer of 1994 when the government's plans were unveiled, reflected the hostility of campaigners to the government's own Bill. By January 1995 after the consultation process, the fears of industry were beginning to be highlighted in media reports with headlines such as: 'Business leaders count the high cost of caring' and 'Plans for disabled "will cost £1.5bn"' (*Daily Telegraph*, 13 January 1995). Cruder critics like Martyn Harris questioned 'the figures and the thinking behind this "bloated sacred cow"' and tried to estimate precisely how many wheelchair users there were to justify the exercise (*Daily Telegraph*, 9 February 1995), while an article in *The Times* bemoaned the dangers of wheelchairs for historic monuments with the barely credible headline 'Disability law "puts historic sites at risk"' (*The Times*, 13 July 1995). When the Bill finally became law in December 1996, the *Daily Mail*, *The Times* and the *Sunday Times*, along with others, ran stories with headlines like 'Firms face flood of claims from disabled people' and 'Flood of employment law threatens small firms'.

What helped in part to undermine these scare stories about business and stop them really running away was the input of the Employers' Forum on Disability, whose members included big-league businesses such as the Midland Bank. The Forum (not an 'of' organisation) was a well-informed and credible voice, able to put the 'business case' for anti-discrimination legislation. Like other disability organisations it pointed to many of the positive experiences of the Americans with Disabilities Act, and counteracted some of the fear and guess-work coming from organisations like the very oppositional Institute of Directors (IoD) and the more supportive but also worried Confederation of British Industries (CBI). RADAR had similar information, but the Employers' Forum on Disability had more credibility with the business community.

The press was playing to a largely sympathetic but relatively uninformed readership. As this fast-moving story unfolded, it was left to broadsheet newspaper features to give context, but it was rarely a headline story. One exception, however, was the emotive issue of AIDS, which triggered the *Daily Mail* into making the Bill front-page headline news, when an amendment proposed recognising people of HIV status as 'disabled'. 'New law puts HIV in the same category as cancer' was the underlined heading above the main headline 'Storm over AIDS victims'. The opening sentence of the story which claimed that 'plans to recognise Aids sufferers as disabled have triggered outrage', made it clear that people with cancer were the 'deserving' disabled as opposed to those who were HIV-positive (28 August 1995).

It was left to the specialist disability press and broadcast programmes to reflect some of disabled people's own 'outrage' at the Bill itself. Ordinary radio and television news coverage was limited to relatively brief items, with 'visual' demonstrations such as blockage of street traffic more likely to extend coverage than long lobby queues outside Parliament. It was not an issue that was regularly attractive to *Newsnight* or *Channel 4 News* and a 15-minute item commissioned for *Channel 4 News* on 11 May 1994 was unusual.

In the 'specialist' disability programmes the events and antipathy towards the government bill could be more fully expressed, but only two radio programmes (the mid-evening Radio 4 *Does He Take Sugar* and *In Touch* on Radio 4) and two television programmes (the Sunday-morning *Link* on ITV and *See Hear* for deaf viewers on BBC2) were running weekly. *Link* regularly interviewed disabled lobbyists and politicians throughout the campaign and its aftermath, but Channel 4's specialist disability programmes and coverage provided by the BBC's Disability Programme Unit were in intermittent short series. A Channel 4 documentary on the May events (*People First: Dirty Tricks,*

Angry Voices) was not transmitted until 5 December 1994. Although there was some notable coverage, it was difficult for these television programmes to give journalistic coverage at a time appropriate to the schedule of events.

Appeasement

Amendments to the Bill were not judged by disabled activists to compensate for a fundamentally unsatisfactory piece of legislation, but optimistic newspaper reporting typified by *The Times* political reporter might well have persuaded the average reader to believe that all was now well. Under the headlines 'Promise of better access to buses, coaches and trains' and 'Ministers make U-turn on help for the disabled', the then Minister for Disabled People, William Hague, announced inclusions in the Bill on transport, education and a widened coverage of people with a history of disability coverage (29 March 1995). That these measures would 'go some way to appeasing six million disabled people and the pressure groups that have lobbied Downing Street in protest' was well wide of the mark.

A *Guardian* leader claimed 'A foot in the door is better than a firmly shut door' and that 'the main pressure groups are right to concentrate on what they have got, rather than reach for the unattainable' (28 March 1995). Given this misleading and self-congratulatory coverage, it is perhaps not surprising that when the Bill finally became law, most ordinary non-disabled people felt that they could warmly congratulate their disabled friends and colleagues on legislation which they assumed to be the equivalent of the Race Relations Act or Sex Discrimination Act.

The election of the Labour government in 1997 undoubtedly brought hope and disappointment to the disability movement, the latter triggered by the government's soon-revealed lack of willingness to tackle the DDA, despite a continuing stated commitment to bring in comprehensive civil rights legislation. The new government offered a task force to consider the establishment of a Disability Rights Commission (DRC) to look at ways to improve the DDA. It was envisaged that a Disability Rights Commission would be an enforcing body with resources and powers similar to those of the Equal Opportunities Commission (EOC) and the Commission for Racial Equality (CRE) which would replace the National Disability Council. Representation on the Task Force included disabled people active in the movement and representing organisations controlled by disabled people. Alan Howarth MP, who had defected to Labour, was appointed as the junior minister responsible, and under his effective leadership a consultation document on a DRC was produced in the summer of 1998.

Howarth's move in a government reshuffle was greeted with dismay, and his replacement Margaret Hodge made an unpromising start by announcing only a minor reduction in the numbers of small employers covered by the Act which still left 92.5 per cent of businesses outside the influence of the legislation. It had been expected that the government would introduce more substantive reforms.

Shared and divergent interests

Although the overall coherence of the Rights Now! drive for civil rights legislation was maintained, the Conservative government's action in promoting the Disability Discrimination Act was, as predicted, highly divisive. There were tensions between organisations willing to work with the government's own legislation (mostly organisations 'for' disabled people) and those who were fundamentally opposed (overwhelmingly organisations 'of' disabled people).

A serious split in 1995 reported in the disability press was caused by the 'big six' charities, Mencap, MIND, RADAR, Scope, RNIB, RNID, making a decision to work closely with the government on implementing the DDA, and furthermore issuing a statement to that effect before consulting other Rights Now! partners. Rachel Hurst, Director of Disability Awareness in Action, and later to become Chair of Rights Now!, said that the move enabled the government to say that disabled people are working with us, but these groups did not express the democratic voice of disabled people.

The split was patched up, but the very existence of the legislation tempted people into further compromises. In November 1996, for example, *Disability Now* reported that a consortium of five major disability charities were negotiating to compete with agencies bidding to provide advice and information when the DDA came into effect. While one of these, the RNIB, said that nothing would compromise its support for full civil rights, Hurst pointed out the difficulties of organisations becoming involved in government-funded service provision and at the same time being powerful lobbyists. In the event the bid was unsuccessful.

A number of organisations, however, including BCODP shunned representation on the National Disability Council, a body that was dismissed as 'toothless', although the existence of the Act had to be acknowledged. In 1995 BCODP's director, Richard Wood, was open about the tensions saying 'There is a degree of antagonism. There is bound to be, isn't there? Because traditional power bases are now being threatened by disabled people' (*Independent on Sunday*, 9 April 1995).

BCODP has continued to grow with 127 affiliates registered in 1998, the year it changed its name from The British Council of Organisations of Disabled People, to The British Council of Disabled People. Nevertheless it was a year in which it had to fight to retain its £30,000 core funding from government, and there is no real comparison to be made between the resources of BCODP and the established charities. BCODP employs only twelve people of whom 100 per cent are disabled. This compares with RADAR's thirty-eight employees (60 per cent disabled), RNIB 2,700 (7 per cent disabled) and Scope 4,000 (3 per cent disabled) (*Disability Now* survey October 1998).

A sign of disabled people's power, and the influence of BCODP and the movement generally, is to be detected more in the makeovers that the big charities have been undergoing in recent years and their efforts to prove their legitimacy by changes in policy and practice. Some like the RNIB protest that their structure makes it an organisation 'of' disabled people, and others point to disabled people in management positions. Indeed the disabled director of RADAR dismissed the 'of' and 'for' issue as 'flummery'. Scope and the RNID have announced plans to seek a wider membership base but Scope's membership will include family members and carers as well as disabled people.

Major charities offer many useful services – the RNIB's technical and information support expertise, for instance, is invaluable and, like a number of other charities, they can afford to employ legal, parliamentary and public relations staff. But they also continue to provide many specialist services which serve to exclude disabled people. Special schools, residential care, special transport and a host of other segregated services are provided under contract to councils and government departments by charities. An important part of their income, however, is derived from donations and legacies. Unlike RADAR, which is the main government-supported disability group, they must maintain a high public profile to maintain their non-government income which they achieve by publishing reports on particular issues and directly by advertising.

The tone of these charities' advertising and organisational image has changed in response to criticisms. Mencap's tearful 'Little Stephen' logo has been replaced by a happier image and in 1995 the RNIB also changed its logo and corporate strategy. The Spastics Society changed the organisation's name to Scope as well as reviewing the content of its advertising campaigns. The latest to relaunch is the Leonard Cheshire Foundation which in 1998 renamed itself Leonard Cheshire and aimed to shift the emphasis away from its residential homes towards its other services. An extensive national advertising campaign around the word 'Enabled' with a wheelchair logo was criticised by disabled people who saw it displayed at bus stops and on inaccessible underground platforms. Press coverage of its corporate makeover was enhanced by the issuing of a headline-catching report based on a MORI poll called 'Access denied: disabled people's experience of social exclusion'. A sign of the times was that it was deemed important to say in the Press Release that the Head of Policy was a disabled person. Nevertheless, a leader in the *Independent* on 17 May 1998 came to the oft-repeated but doubtful conclusion that 'Prejudice is the worst handicap.'

Blind journalist Peter White asks whether charities are supposed to be providers, advisors or campaigners. They have been driven to becoming more of a campaigning force, but with local authority contracts now forming a large part of many charities' income (33 per cent for Scope and 40 per cent for the RNIB) who is their client – the people who award their contract or the people they claim to represent? But the question that White raises which in itself seems indicative of a massive power shift (although struggling local groups of disabled people would not see it that way) is 'Can they adapt to the idea that the people they have regarded as their charges are in fact their masters?' (*Observer*/Charities Aid Foundation 1995).

In the long run the question might prove irrelevant. The rapidly expanding academic field of 'disability studies', developed by disabled people, offers a rigorous and grounded replacement for the previously dominant medical-sociological approach. Politically the movement has come of age, although Oliver (1996) warns of the fine line between marginalisation and incorporation into the establishment.

Cultural expressions of the movement through disability arts have enabled the exploration of identity and the development of disabled people's self worth and body pride. Also, the rejection of concepts of stigma, shame or 'tragic defect' has begun to be recognised by some disability charities. More challenging is the need to convey those ideas that incorporate an assertion of delight or acceptance in 'difference' and a rejection of able-bodied 'normality' which either denies ('look for the ability not the disability') or judges straightforward 'able-bodied' activities undertaken by disabled people as particularly praiseworthy.

Clearly not all disabled people are in this game yet but the opportunity over the last decade to express the aims and philosophy of the movement in an active way while campaigning for civil rights may prove more swiftly persuasive in changing the imagery and expectations that non-disabled people have of disabled people's place in society and of disabled people's expectations of themselves.

References

Barnes, C. (1991) *Disabled People in Britain and Discrimination: a Case for Anti-Discrimination Legislation*, London: Hurst & Co. with BCODP.

Barnes, C. (1992) *Disabling Imagery and the Media: an Exploration of the Principles for Media Representations of Disabled People*, Halifax: BCODP with Ryburn.

Barnes, C. and Oliver, M. (1996) 'Disability rights: rhetoric and reality in the UK', *Disability and Society*, vol. 10: 1.

Biklen, D. and Bogdana, R. (1977) 'Media portrayal of disabled people: a Study of Stereotypes', *Inter-Racial Childrens Book Bulletin*, 8, 6 and 7: 4–9.

Campbell, J. and Oliver, M. (1996) *Disability Politics: Understanding our Past and Changing our Future*, London: Routledge.

Carmichael, A. (1997) 'A family at war', in A. Pointon and C. Davies (eds) *Framed: Interrogating Disability in the Media*, London: British Film Institute, 96.

Driedger, D. (1989) *The Last Civil Rights Movement: Disabled People's International*, London: Hurst and Company.

Finkelstein, V. (1980) *Monograph No. 5 Attitudes and Disabled People,* New York: World Rehabilitation Fund.

Finkelstein, V. (1997) 'From enabling to disabling: an open university?' unpublished valedictory lecture, Milton Keynes: The Open University.

Hevey, D. (1991) 'From self-love to the picket line: strategies for change in picket line presentation', in *Disability and Society*, vol. 8(4).

Meacher, M. (1985) *As of Right*, London: House of Commons.

Oliver, M. (1990) *The Politics of Disablement*, Basingstoke: Macmillan.

Oliver, M. (1996) 'Defining disability and impairment: issues at stake', in C. Barnes, and G. Mercer *Exploring the Divide: Illness and Disability*, Leeds: The Disability Press, 39–54.

Pagel, M. (1988) *On Our Own Behalf – an Introduction to the Self-Organisation of Disabled People*, Manchester: Greater Manchester Council of Disabled People.

Shakespeare, T. (1994) 'Cultural representation of disabled people: dustbins for disavowal?', *Disability and Society* 9(3).

Shakespeare, T. and Watson, N. (1997) 'Defending the social model', *Disability and Society* 12(2): 293–294.

Chapter 15

Social threat or social problem?

Media representations of lone mothers and policy implications

Simon Duncan, Rosalind Edwards and Miri Song

Introduction

In Britain, lone motherhood[1] is not a neutral nor an apolitical status; it evokes strong moral evaluations and therefore easily becomes a political symbol. Although the historical status and treatment of British lone mothers has varied over time (Lewis 1995; Song 1996), they have almost continually been at the centre of public debates about the state of society in general, but more particularly of 'the family' and the role of women. Most recently, political and media attention has focused on the doubling of the number of lone parent families in Britain over the past two decades (reaching around 20 per cent of all families with dependent children, over 90 per cent of whom are headed by a lone mother), on the growth of unmarried mothers as a proportion of all lone mothers, and on their increasing reliance on Income Support (the social assistance benefit) rather than on paid work (Burghes 1993).

Debate has centred around whether lone mothers prefer to live off the state, and may even be created by such policy 'cushioning', or whether they want to be 'self-sufficient' but cannot because welfare policies are unsupportive. Arguably both views are wide of the mark; research reveals that lone mothers' moral views about 'good' mothering, and how this does or does not combine with paid work, is the crucial issue (Duncan and Edwards 1999).

Lone mothers received particularly damning attention at the hands of new right politicians and the popular media in 1993, in the context of the then Conservative government's 'back to basics' campaign. Indeed, 1993 has been dubbed 'The year of the lone mother' (Roseneil and Mann 1996: 192). Lone mothers were depicted as a threat to the fabric of society, supposedly rearing delinquent children without the guidance of a proper father, and scrounging benefits and housing off the welfare state. Social policies were called for that would deal with this menace. Lone mothers received further attention in the media as a legitimate cause for social concern during 1996, again functioning as a sort of symbol as part of a national debate about 'moral values', as policies concerning divorce law reform and working mothers were debated. And towards the end of 1997, lone mothers were once again in the political and media spotlight as a result of the New Labour government's social reforms. Here lone mothers functioned as a symbol in the attempt to restructure social benefits towards welfare-to-work strategies (Lister 1998).

Academics have played an important supporting role in media preoccupations with lone mothers. In particular, new right and revisionist/communitarian academics have gained space in the national media, and have propounded what Judith Stacey calls 'virtual social science' (Stacey 1996: 83–104). Here categorical assertion, anecdote and selective readings of 'facts' are posed as unbiased and fault-free authoritative research, in this case purportedly showing that lone mothers are formative members of a British 'underclass'. The US academic Charles Murray gained particular space in the press in the early-mid 1990s, with Cassandra-like statistical and rhetorical predictions that Britain was heading down the same slippery slope as the US, to extensive urban crime, drug use and disorder – where all this was the result of increasing 'illegitimate' births supported by the benefits system. The answer, in this view, is to stop 'supporting' lone motherhood through social policies and instead support the traditional married family.

Such negative portrayals of lone mothers have not gone unchallenged. Attempts have been made by voluntary pressure groups, such as the National Council for One Parent Families, and liberal left professionals and academics, as well as leading figures in the 'liberal' establishment, such as Church authorities, to (re) insert a public image of lone mothers as 'normal' women who are doing their best in externally constrained and unfavourable circumstances. In this view, social policies should be enlarged to properly support such women in bringing up their children.

Consequently, mainstream political and media debates about lone mothers in Britain – and corresponding policy proposals – have become polarised between seeing lone mothers as a threat to society or as victims of social problems. Each of these positions, their propagation in the media, the role of academics within this, and the social policies that accompany them, is reviewed in more detail below: particular attention is focused on the ways in which the media have depicted black lone mothers. But these polarised positions are not the only ways of understanding lone mothers' situation, or of framing the parameters for social policies in response. Indeed, other views may more accurately reflect how lone mothers themselves understand and experience their lives. These alternative views of lone motherhood are also discussed on pp. 246–247, albeit more briefly, because they have not gained wider legitimacy or currency in national media and political debates, nor influenced policy frameworks to any great extent. (Duncan and Edwards 1999).

The propagation of particular media images of lone mothers and their accompaniment by recommendations for particular social policies, is posed rather simply above. Clearly, the media increasingly inform public understanding and comprehension of the social world, and play a role in placing issues on the political policy agenda – as this volume attests. Nevertheless, the relationship between mainstream media presentations of lone motherhood and the actual or possible social policies that address their situation is not a relationship of simple stimulus-response. As in other policy areas (see Liddiard and Hutson 1998, on youth homelessness for example), this relationship is more complex, not least because government and political agendas influence and inform media coverage (see Chapters 1–4 for the influence of sources on the construction of news agendas). It is perhaps more useful to see ideological issues lying at the root of both, which relate to shared social understandings about the relationship between individuals, states, markets and families, and to how 'explanations' are constructed in dominant western and academic categorical modes of thought.

Representations of lone mothers as a social threat

One perception of lone mothers expounded in mainstream political and media representations sees them as a social threat: both morally and financially. They are formative members of an underclass that has no interest in providing for itself in legitimate ways. This position links into the underclass theory that has developed in the USA in particular, but has been imported into, and gained influence in, Britain – although it also has its roots in a longstanding British 'social pathology' view of the poor (Macnicol 1987; Morris 1994). This theory posits that, in spatially segregated areas, there is a developing class that has no stake in, and is hostile to, the social order. Lone mothers are seen as active agents in the creation of this underclass. In Britain, young single (that is, never-married) mothers have been focused on as the central culprits. (In the USA this theory has long been racialised, with black lone mothers posited as the chief culprits.) Lone mothers allegedly choose to have children outside wedlock to gain welfare and housing benefits, and then, supported by the state, they choose not to get a job. Their sons, assumed to be without male authority or roles, are said to drift into delinquency, crime and the drug culture, while their daughters learn and repeat the cycle of promiscuity and dependency. (See, for example, Segalman and Marsland 1989; Murray 1990; Morgan 1995.)

Popular media depictions of lone mothers as a social threat use emotional symbolism more fully than more 'respectable' academic tracts. Media reports, however, both draw on, and are sometimes written by, academics. The American new right/republican academic Charles Murray has enjoyed particular prominence in the *Sunday Times*, to purvey his virtual social science. Andrew Neil, when editor of this paper, claimed that he had introduced Murray to the British public and politicians, and sponsored his 'research' in Britain (Roseneil and Mann 1996: 195). During the early 1990s and especially in 1993, the *Sunday Times* and other right-wing broadsheets, along with the tabloid press, devoted considerable and regular editorial attention to stories about single mothers and the underclass. They also displayed some raw prejudice in doing so. An editorial in the *Sunday Times* for example argued that:

> It is becoming increasingly clear to all but the most blinkered of social scientists that the disintegration of the nuclear family is the principal source of so much unrest and misery. The creation of an urban underclass, on the margins of society, but doing great damage to itself and the rest of us, is directly linked to the rapid rise in illegitimacy . . . It is not just a question of a few families without fathers; it is a matter of whole communities with barely a single worthwhile role model.
>
> (*Sunday Times*, 28 February 1993)

A headline in the same newspaper queried, 'Wedded to welfare – do they want to marry a man or the state?' (*Sunday Times*, 11 July 1993). The *Daily Mail*, with its ideological and political address to 'middle England', offered a similar viewpoint:

> The Willenhall estate, on the outskirts of Coventry, houses a large number of single mothers. There are also a lot of young, single men, many living on the proceeds of either crime or benefit fraud and more or less attached to the young women . . . It is kept afloat by the niggardly (if costly) charity of the state and the local authority, that is to say the taxes paid by traditional two parent families.
>
> (*Daily Mail*, 17 October 1995)

The targeting of a particular public housing estate with a supposedly high proportion of young 'underclass' single mothers seems to be a virtual social science technique for delivering messages, and for concretising particular views, as used by Murray and journalists in the popular media. The flagship BBC television current affairs programme, *Panorama*, entitled 'Babies on benefit', broadcast on 20 September 1993, used a similar technique. In this case it was the St Mellon's council estate in Wales that was portrayed as an underclass breeding ground. This estate had previously received critical attention from the then Conservative Secretary of State for Wales, John Redwood, in a speech arguing for policies that deterred young women from having babies outside marriage and supported by the tax payer. Indeed, the programme makers claimed that they were investigating his contentions (*Guardian*, 13 September 1994). Both Redwood and the *Panorama* programme implied that St Mellon's was typical and could be extrapolated as representative of all lone mothers – despite more considered accounts revealing inaccuracies about the estate and lone mothers generally (see Phoenix 1996: 185).

Popular media presentations of lone mothers as a social threat link into a conservative new right political view of the state in society, where the welfare provision of housing, benefits and other social provision is castigated as encouraging state dependency, an underclass, and especially single (never-married) motherhood. Peter Lilley's now infamous 'little list' speech at the 1993 Conservative Party conference, for example, alleged that single mothers were having children to secure welfare benefits and housing, while Stephen Green, Chair of the Conservative Family Campaign, argued that 'Putting girls into council flats and providing taxpayer funded child care is a policy from hell' (*Observer*, 14 November 1993). But strands of an underclass discourse are also discernible in the communitarianism underlying the New Labour government's ideas about a 'stakeholder society' (Driver and Martell 1997). The long-term unemployed, which includes lone mothers, are placed as 'socially excluded'; 'family values' are stressed as the key to a 'decent' and crime-free society, and an element of coercion is required to reintegrate the excluded back into society through paid work. New Labour's view that life in a married two-parent family is better for children and for social cohesion, most notably expounded by Tony Blair and Jack Straw, has been widely reported in the media since 1997.

Media, politicians and academics who promulgate this view of lone motherhood as a threat to society also campaign for social policies that do not reward or encourage such 'self-damaging conduct'. Consequently, the New Labour government has implemented the previous new right Conservative government's proposal to remove the extra allowances available to (new) lone parents on both the universal child benefit payment and on targeted income-related benefits – with Harriet Harman (then Minister for Social Security and for Women) stating, 'Life is about work, not just about claiming benefit' (*Guardian*, 11 December 1997). Other policy disincentives to lone motherhood advocated by those who hold a social threat view include restrictions on payments to lone mothers who have more children while receiving benefit (as is the practice in some American states). There are also suggestions that young single mothers on benefit should be placed in hostels where their sexual relations and children's upbringing can be supervised. This policy idea has been floated by the New Labour government, in linking hostels with job training – again revisiting proposals of the Conservative government (Zulauf 1997). Encouragement and reward for traditional male breadwinner/female homemaker couples is also stressed by social threat advocates, with policy proposals to redress the supposed benefit bias towards lone, as opposed to married, parents (another reason given by New Labour for its lone parent benefit cuts). Other policy proposals include a tightening of the divorce law so that fewer lone mother families are created in the first place, as well as advocating 'moral' family and parenting education – the latter being the remit of the government's new National Family and Parenting Institute to be launched in April 1999.

Black lone mothers as a social threat

Until recently, 'race' and ethnicity were muted features of British social threat representations of lone motherhood (in contrast to the situation in the USA). In the wake of the heightened media attention to lone mothers from 1993 onward, however, articles about black (Afro-Caribbean) lone mothers began increasingly to be reported in the white-dominated media. Under the headline 'The ethnic timebomb', for example, the tabloid *Sunday Express* noted that more than 50 per cent of black families are headed by a lone mother and argued that, 'Almost six in ten black mothers are bringing up children on their own, urged on by the benefit system' (13 August 1995), implying a direct causal relationship between the incidence of black lone motherhood and the growing social security bill. Such claims ignore the fact that black lone mothers are more likely to be economically active and in full-time employment than their white counterparts (Duncan and Edwards 1999); research suggests they also provide healthier lifestyles for their children – Dowler and Calvert 1995). The *Sunday Express* article also raises the spectre of 'babyfathers' (allegedly personified by athlete Linford Christie) who – in newspaper accounts – father worryingly large numbers of children with multiple female partners.

Stories about 'babymothers' (young black women who are presumed to have children by multiple male partners) also received considerable attention in the broadsheet press (see for example the *Guardian*, 13 June 1994 and 21 March 1995, the *Sunday Times*, 19 February 1995 and the *Independent*, 2 June 1993 and 30 January 1995). Mainstream radio magazine programmes, such as BBC Radio 4's *The Locker Room* and *Women's Hour*, have also featured discussions about black lone motherhood and its social implications. Much of this coverage has echoed the ongoing debates in black media, especially the tabloid daily, *The Voice* – self-styled 'Britain's best black newspaper' (Song and Edwards 1997) – but there are significant differences between these stories as they are reported in the black press compared with their coverage in the white-dominated media. First, there are no scare stories about social security bills. Second and importantly, there is a sense of debate in the black press, with the black readership responding to 'personal opinion' columns through the letters page. By contrast, coverage of black lone motherhood in the mainstream press tends to be devoid of vigorous questioning or alternatives, with a flat presentation suggesting that 'this is how it is' in the British black population.

It is argued elsewhere that the emergence of a focus on black lone mothers in the British mainstream press is linked to the broader social threat concerns discussed above. It is suggested, moreover, that it is through such 'exotic' media explorations of black family life that white people vicariously play out their fears about social breakdown and relationships between men and women (Song and Edwards 1997).

Representations of lone mothers as a social problem

In contrast to the view of lone motherhood as a self-created threat to the social order, a second perception of lone mothers widely reported in mainstream media, presents them as victims of externally created problems and in need of help. Stress is laid on the 'facts': in Britain, the majority of lone mothers (just over 50 per cent) are 'mature' divorced, separated or widowed women, rather than young single mothers (with less than 9 per cent being teenagers) (Burghes and Brown 1995). Similarly, there is no underclass in the sense of a self-reproducing distinct part of society which stands outside cultural, political and economic norms. Rather, there is a growing number of people in poverty, including lone mothers, who have essentially the same ambitions as the rest of society, but who are stigmatised and marginalised. The economic and social causes of this marginalisation are beyond the control of those they affect, while the shrinking welfare state only exacerbates difficulties. According to this perception, lone mothers are seen as social problems. They want paid work to provide for themselves and their children, but are hindered by the structure and nature of the welfare state. From this social problem position, the appropriate policy prescription signals that lone mothers should receive more, not less, state assistance to help them escape poverty and state dependency (see, for example, Burghes 1993; Morris 1994; Bradshaw *et al.* 1996).

By contrast with the social threat perspective discussed above, the social problem framing of lone motherhood is far less common in the tabloid press. It is mostly limited to broadsheet newspapers with more left wing or 'middle ground' sympathies, such as the *Guardian*, the *Observer* and the *Independent*, which have given a platform to various commentators stressing the poverty and limited options of lone mothers. An article in the *Guardian*, for example, argued that:

> Reducing the number of single parent families is not an issue about the morality of feckless unmarried women who won't use contraceptives. Two-thirds of single parent families are caused by divorce. What is needed is a genuine political commitment to supporting the family. Better childcare provision for starters . . .
>
> (*Guardian*, 13 October 1993)

Despite these broadly sympathetic views, the broadsheets have also published reports by new right/revisionist commentators and, as we noted earlier, they have also been complicit in vicariously playing out social threat views through examinations of black lone motherhood.

Again, academics such as A.H. Halsey and Norman Dennis, taking a revisionist social-problem position, have been given a platform in the mainstream media to advocate a return of the political left to what they call 'ethical socialism', with its 'historic mission to spread the value of the family throughout all the relationships of society' (Halsey quoted in the *Observer*, 14 November 1993). Indeed, Halsey was one of the commentators featured in the *Panorama* 'Babies-on-benefit' programme. New Labour's commitment to 'the family' as the source of social morality and obligation echoes this ethical socialism (Driver and Martell 1997).

The social problem view of lone motherhood, based on a concern with poverty rather than the fate of 'the family', is dominant among academic social scientists (especially in social policy), however, as well as among welfare practitioners and the British liberal establishment, such as church leaders. This often reflects a Fabian political inheritance of enlightened state intervention. Jonathan Bradshaw, for example, an academic advisor to the Church of England's commission on the family, supported the Archbishop of Canterbury in arguing that 'lone mothers should be seen primarily as victims and get more help' (*Guardian*, 13 October 1993). Furthermore, the major lobby group for lone mothers in Britain, the National Council for One Parent Families, has also adopted this view of lone mothers (discussed further below). In contrast with the marginalisation of these arguments during the eighteen years of new right Conservative government, there has been renewed lobbying for intervention with the advent of the New Labour government – some of which was disappointed early on with the continuation of some Conservative policies such as the cutting of lone parent benefit.

In Britain, advocates of the social-problem view argue that day-care costs should be taken into account when calculating in work benefits for lone (and other) mothers. In 1994, under the Conservative government, an earnings disregard for formal day-care costs was indeed made available, although at a niggardly level. This suggests that, despite the prevalence of social threat representations of lone mothers in the media at the time, the social problem approach retained influence in British policy-making circles. This disregard has since been increased by the New Labour government. Other policy suggestions within the social problem mould which have also been taken up by the New Labour government include measures to encourage lone mothers to pursue training and higher education under the New Deal welfare-to-work strategy. Since autumn 1998, lone parents on income support with a youngest child over school age have been invited to an interview with a personal advisor in their local job centre to discuss 'upgrading' their job skills and/or finding paid work. An expansion of 'after school' care services for children is also part of this New Labour strategy (although this goes no way to matching the levels of public day-care in most other west European countries).

In championing the two-parent family, New Labour politicians are usually careful to say that they do not intend to demonise lone mothers. Jack Straw, for example, in a speech stating that strengthening the institution of marriage as a basis for bringing up children was a cornerstone of 'modern family policy', added, 'We are not in the business of making the job of lone parents more difficult by blaming them as some have done in the past' (*Guardian*, 24 July 1998). However, while it might be thought that the social-problem view of lone mothers' position had gained political ascendancy since New Labour's election victory in 1997, another suggestion under this perspective has not had such success in reaching the policy agenda. Rather than increase lone parent 'top up' benefits these have been cut altogether, as we noted above. Indeed, New Labour is effectively combining the social problem view of lone mothers with the social threat view as part of its communitarian approach (a manifestation of its 'third way' between old left and new right). Certainly, lone motherhood continues to be a potent political and media symbol.

Alternative viewpoints on lone motherhood

There are two alternative views of lone mothers represented in mainstream British media. First, lone motherhood can be seen as part of a general change in family forms and lifestyle patterns, resulting from people's choices about how they live their lives and construct relationships, within a context of overarching economic, social and cultural change. Policies would thus be predicated upon creating better conditions, and reconciling paid work and family life, for all families rather than focusing on lone mothers alone. This view is strong at the national level in much of continental Europe, where lone motherhood is less commented on and is much less important as a moral or political symbol than it is in Britain and the USA. While such a lifestyle perspective on lone motherhood may be muted within national media discussions in Britain, appeals to such a view can be seen in the launch of the niche monthly glossy magazine *Singled Out* in 1995. This was aimed at the British 'lone parent' market and covered all aspects of lifestyle, from holidays and cookery, through conducting relationships and child rearing, to financial and legal matters. However, the magazine did not survive its first year – signalling either the lack of a large enough audience who saw themselves as living a 'lone parent' lifestyle, or lone mothers' inability to afford the cover price.

Second, lone mothers can be seen as women who are no longer willing to accept control over their lives by individual men and are thus escaping patriarchy, with access to paid work, contraception, divorce and so on giving them the practical means to be independent. Policies should thus support and encourage this autonomy (including, for some, state support through wages for housework). Such a radical feminist perspective is rarely represented in the national press in its own terms (other than in more marginal publications such as the now defunct *Spare Rib*). Rather, it gets caricatured and castigated as part of the social threat view, where feminists (and socialists) are blamed for supporting lone motherhood and thus social breakdown (Roseneil and Mann 1996). Other media can portray lone mothers, particularly black lone mothers, as deriving strength from their embeddedness in supportive female networks. The low budget black-British film *Babymother*, released in September 1998, thus tells the 'ragga to riches story of single mother Anita, bringing up her children on Harlesden's tough Stonebridge estate, and her struggles to make it as a deejay' (*Guardian*, 6 August 1998). But journalists who are committed to a social threat view can take an entirely different perspective on the same story: '[*Babymother*'s] aim seems to be to encourage immature black women to behave like aggressive, self-pitying trollops, bring up more and more illegitimate children very badly, with no visible means of finance except the taxpayer' (*Daily Mail*, 11 September 1998). Bigotry of this calibre seems unmoved by facts such as black lone mothers' high rates of employment.

While alternative views may not have had much influence on mainstream media representations of lone mothers or on policy development, they do hold sway amongst lone mothers themselves. Research conducted by two of us (Duncan and Edwards 1999) draws on interviews with lone mothers in 1994, just after the furore in the media about the moral and financial threat lone mothers posed to British society. The research revealed that most lone mothers from all social groups held opinions about their position that were congruent with the (nationally muted) escaping patriarchy position, while aspects of the lifestyle perspective were also much in evidence. They often valued freedom to do what they wanted without having to take account of a male partner and were proud of managing on their own. Some also understood themselves to be just a normal part of the diversity of family forms in contemporary British society, especially younger African-Caribbean and white 'alternative' lone mothers who held a more feminist view of families and society more generally (see Duncan and Edwards 1999, for details).

Voluntary organisations' responses to media images of lone mothers

Given the plethora of bad press that lone mothers have received, voluntary groups representing lone mothers in Britain – most notably the National Council for One Parent Families (NCOPF) and Gingerbread – have made concerted efforts to counter such negative portrayals. Various forms of media coverage, including both newspapers and television programmes, have been influential in shaping the strategies of such organisations. In fact, the NCOPF has emphasised the importance of negotiating the 'right' image of lone mothers. While they maintain that they need to make a case for lone mothers' special needs, they stress that they must be careful to avoid potentially incendiary images that emphasise differences rather than commonalities with other families (Song 1996). Thus both lone mother organisations have been prominent in rebutting dominant social threat political and media images.

In particular, the NCOPF evidenced their concern about harmful media portrayals of lone mothers by challenging the content of the *Panorama* 'Babies-on-benefit' programme. This documentary purported to show the reality of lone motherhood, and alleged that feckless, young, single women were having a string of babies, and living off benefits and in council housing. These never-married mothers supposedly saw no point in gaining employment or in having long-term stable relationships with men as providers and active fathers to their children. The programme also examined the 'effective' policy option of benefit capping (as practised in the US state of New Jersey) to deal with this phenomenon. The NCOPF complained to the Broadcasting Complaints Commission and went to court over this documentary. As is evident from the press release the organisation put out at the time, they did this because of fears that negative media representations might fuel moves towards punitive social policies: 'At the time when Government is investigating ways to reduce the benefit bill, this *Panorama* has been a disastrous intervention into the debate.' (*Guardian*, 13 September 1994).

The NCOPF accused the programme makers and the BBC of presenting an 'unfair, misleading and irresponsible' image of lone mothers. Rather, they asserted, for the majority lone parenthood is an unexpected event in people's lives, and the typical lone parent is a responsible, caring, divorced mother struggling to provide for her children. Interestingly, neither the NCOPF nor Gingerbread responded to the treatment of black 'babymothers' in the mainstream press, for fear of promoting racialised debate about lone mothers that would cut across the 'safe' social problem image of their constituency that they wish to portray (Song and Edwards 1997).

Conclusion

The dominant social threat and social problem views of lone motherhood in Britain, including discussion about black lone mothers, have been articulated strongly in the national media over the past few years. These perspectives, by defining issues and setting agendas around lone motherhood, are significant components in the policy process. They assign meaning and causes to lone motherhood and construct the parameters within which social policies towards lone mothers should be constituted or changed. But this is not to imply any direct stimulus-response relationship between media representations and policy formulation; the two interact in complex ways. For their part, the media are highly diverse and, as we have seen, there are alternative ways to frame lone motherhood to those which are predominant in mainstream media: and these do find voice in some niche media (as well as amongst lone mothers themselves).

Relations between media and politicians are reciprocal. It is politicians, along with academics who share their political mission, who have provided copy for the media while, in turn, the media have fuelled public opinion and encouraged particular responses from politicians.

At one level, media and policy representations of lone motherhood as interlinked and mutually reinforcing can be seen simply as the result of a small but influential 'chattering class' of media workers and policy makers (and a few academics) who inhabit a restricted social and geographical world, and who define what is important and what is marginal. What happens in the 'real world' becomes little more than symbolic foils for various political groupings and regroupings. However, even if largely correct, this appealing caricature does little to explain why it is that the social threat and social problem views of lone motherhood are promulgated in the media and by politicians, and not alternative perspectives. The reasons for this dominance are to be found at deeper social levels; first, at the level of shared social understandings about the relationship between individuals, states, markets and families, and second, at the level of how explanations themselves are normally constructed in dominant and 'educated' modes of thought.

On the first level, different welfare state regimes develop different sets of social policy in expressing their particular conceptions of the proper, and gendered, relationship between individuals, families, states and markets (Sainsbury 1994; Duncan 1995), not least with different implications for the position of lone mothers. In Britain, politicians and media workers increasingly seem to share a world view defined in terms of a liberal welfare state regime.

In the liberal welfare state regime (such as the USA) social policy is used to uphold the market and traditional work-ethic norms. Modest and means-tested benefits are aimed at a residualised and stigmatised group of welfare recipients such as lone mothers, and depiction of lone mothers as a social threat more easily attain dominance. Under the conservative welfare regime (with Germany as a type case) states intervene to preserve status difference – including those of traditional gender roles and family forms. Here lone mothers become peripheralised as mothers without male partners, and the social problem view of lone motherhood more easily gains purchase. In social democratic welfare state regimes (where Sweden is a type case), social policy reforms de-emphasise the market and emphasise equality rather than the meeting of minimal needs. Both men and women – including lone mothers – are seen as independent worker-citizens who support themselves through participation in the labour market, and social problem and lifestyle views of lone motherhood merge.

Within this, Britain presents a complex, hybrid case, where some elements of the social democratic regime (classically in the NHS) have been inserted into a liberal welfare tradition. Thatcherism, however, marked a rapid return towards the liberal model and, whatever its political differences, 'Blairism' seems to share the same liberal assumptions about the proper relationship between states, markets, families and individuals. It is the USA that is explicitly taken as a policy role model by both media commentators and politicians rather than the increasingly derided 'European model' (other than by marginalised 'Old Labour' politicians or maverick journalists such as Will Hutton, author of the best-selling book *The State of the Nation*).

On the second level, though, why is it that the dominant view of lone mothers is as a trope for welfare dependency, social marginalisation and even hopelessness? After all, people know from both personal experience and research that most lone mothers do not fit this caricature (Duncan and Edwards 1999). Partly, this type of image building depends upon a particular method of explanation commonly used in western thought. When they use the term 'lone mother' (or 'single parent'), politicians, the media and even voluntary organisations representing lone mothers themselves (such as the NCOPF) are attempting to invoke a particular categorical representation of a type of person – a ready-made classificatory package that serves as a short cut to reading off a particular social situation. 'Lone motherhood' is seen to stand for an a priori, unitary, fixed, coherent, inherent and essentialised set of attributes and characteristics – in other words, the category articulates a particular stereotype – which in Britain easily becomes a negative stereotype to fit in with the preconceptions of the liberal welfare state regime.

This short cut in image building, and in explanation more widely, is often completely misleading because it assumes that the taxonomic group accurately delineates a social group. Taxonomic groups, such as lone mothers distinguished as a particular parental family form, are often different from the real substantive social groups that actually carry through social relationships and actions. It is not just that lone mothers are not a homogeneous or unified population, so that different social groups of lone mothers may behave differently. (The extreme example of the lone mothers among the British royal family makes the point here.) Rather, it may not be lone motherhood in itself that is substantively or causally most important for their social behaviour. It may, for example, be membership of a particular ethnic or class group, or location in a particular area, that explains why some lone mothers take up paid work and others do not (Duncan and Edwards 1999). Underlying social divisions and differences, however, remain unspoken in taxonomic representations. Nevertheless, lone mothers are not the homogenous group, in terms of social characteristics, that media and politicians invoke when they use the term, and it is therefore extremely unlikely that, as a putative categorical group, they will hold similar views and respond to policy development in similar ways, as maintained by media commentators, politicians, and even many academics.

Such categorical thinking, and taxonomic modes of explanation, have their roots in Cartesian thought as a means to produce independent descriptions of social life that are generalisable. This type of conceptualising has received critical attention in a number of ways from philosophers of science such as Wittgenstein to the critical realist, postmodern and feminist theorists of today (Sayer 1992; Stanley and Wise 1993). Nonetheless, as a model of understanding and portraying social life (and thus also as a mode of control) it retains enormous purchase and power, underlain as it is by the idea that experts, through their categorisations, have a correct and authoritative access to reality. This is why academics like Murray and Halsey are given media space to confirm stereotypes of lone mothers.

The media and politicians clearly also have greater access to image production and dissemination than most lone mothers. In this way they have the power to impose their categorical version of the reality of lone motherhood – and thus to assert a particular identity of lone mothers, their motivations and behaviour, and the causes of all this – as superordinate and exclusive. A particular image, such as that of lone mothers as a social threat, may be contested by less powerful lobby groups such as the NCOPF. But such attempts to insert an alternative identity for lone mothers into the categorical space still rely on the same unitary and essentialist mode of thought as that dominant in media and political portrayals. They do not admit, or recognise, diversity within the category, or that the category itself may be cross-cut or even unimportant where other differences (like those of class, ethnicity or location) may be the more influential in explaining motivations, behaviour and causes. This means, moreover, that the 'categorical identity' that ascribes a particular set of characteristics to the taxonomic group 'lone mothers' is not the same as the various 'ontological identities' of lone mothers themselves – how they think about themselves in relation to others and their situation (Duncan and Edwards 1999; Taylor 1998). These ontological considerations have little authority or power, however, and largely remain invisible unless they are used by the media to support pre-existing categories of lone motherhood as a social threat or a social problem.

Note

1 In this chapter, following UK academic convention, we use 'lone motherhood' as a generic term covering divorced, separated, widowed and never-married mothers, with 'single mothers' specifically referring to never-married mothers (which in itself includes both previously cohabiting and never-cohabiting mothers). In media reports, however, the terms 'single mother' or 'single parent' tend to be used generically (and are often preferred by lone mothers themselves – see Duncan and Edwards 1999).

References

Bradshaw, J., Kennedy, S., Kilkey, M., Hutton, S., Corden, A., Eardley, T., Holmes, H. and Neale, J. (1996) *The Employment of Lone Parents: a Comparison of Policies in 20 Countries*, London/York: Family Policies Study Centre/Joseph Rowntree Foundation.

Burghes, L. (1993) *One Parent Families: Policy Options for the 1990s*, London/York: Family Policy Studies Centre/Joseph Rowntree Foundation.

Burghes, L. and Brown, M. (1995) *Single Lone Mothers: Problems, Prospects and Policies*, London: Family Policy Studies Centre.

Dowler, E. and Calvert, C. (1995) *Nutrition and Diet in Lone Parent Families in London*, London: Family Policy Studies Centre.

Driver, S. and Martell, L. (1997) 'New Labour's Communitarianisms', *Critical Social Policy* 17(3): 27–46.

Duncan, S. (1995) 'Theorising European gender systems', *Journal of European Social Policy* 5(4): 284.

Duncan, S. and Edwards, R. (1999) *Lone Mothers and Paid Work: Gendered Moral Rationalities*, London: Macmillan.

Lewis, J. (1995) 'The problem of lone mother families in twentieth century Britain',

Welfare State Programme Discussion Paper 114, STICERD, London School of Economics.

Liddiard, M. and Hutson, S. (1998) 'Youth homelessness, the press and public attitudes', *Youth and Policy: The Journal of Critical Analysis* 59: 57–69.

Lister, R. (1998) 'From equality to social inclusion: New Labour and the welfare state', *Critical Social Policy* 18(2): 215–225.

Macnicol, J. (1987) 'In pursuit of the underclass', *Journal of Social Policy* 16(3): 293–318.

Morgan, P. (1995) *Farewell to the Family? Public Policy and the Family Breakdown in Britain and the USA*, London: Institute of Economic Affairs.

Morris, L. (1994) *Dangerous Classes: the Underclass and Social Citizenship*, London: Routledge.

Murray, C. (1990) *The Emerging British Underclass*, London: Institute of Economic Affairs.

Phoenix, A. (1996) 'Social constructions of lone motherhood: a case of competing discourses', in E. Bortolaia Silva (ed.) *Good Enough Mothering: Feminist Perspectives on Lone Motherhood*, London: Routledge.

Roseneil, S. and Mann, K. (1996) 'Unpalatable choices and inadequate families: lone mothers and the underclass debate', in E. Bortolaia Silva (ed.) *Good Enough Mothering: Feminist Perspectives on Lone Motherhood*, London: Routledge.

Sainsbury, D. (1994) *Gendering Welfare States*, London: Sage.

Sayer, A. (1992) *Method in Social Science: a Realist Approach*, (second edition), London: Routledge.

Segalman, R. and Marsland, D. (1989) *Cradle to Grave*, London: Macmillan.

Song, M. (1996) 'Changing conceptualisations of lone parenthood in Britain: lone parents or single mums?', *European Journal of Women's Studies* 3(4): 377–397.

Song, M. and Edwards, R. (1997) 'Comment: raising questions about perspectives on black lone motherhood', *Journal of Social Policy* 26(2): 233–244.

Stacey, J. (1996) *In the Name of the Family: Rethinking Family Values in the Postmodern Age*, Boston, Mass.: Beacon Press.

Stanley, L. and Wise, S. (1993) *Breaking Out Again: Feminist Ontology and Epistemology*, London: Routledge.

Taylor, D. (1998) 'Social identity and social policy: engagements with postmodern theory', *Journal of Social Policy* 27(3): 329–350.

Zulauf, M. (1997) 'Mother and baby hostels: a viable option for young single mothers?', *Research, Policy and Planning* 15(1): 13–18.

Chapter 16

They make us out to be monsters

Images of children and young people in care

Andy West

Children in care, and young people who have left care, say that the general public's perception of 'care'[1] is important if not crucial to their lives. When young care leavers across England conducted their own research on leaving care in 1995, they highlighted the importance of the public's attitude to children from care, and asked other care leavers questions about it. In the research, 70 per cent of respondents said that they never or rarely told anyone they had been in care (West 1995: 24). An open declaration of having a 'care' background has been referred to as 'coming out' by care leavers, an apparently deliberate reference to the phrase often used in an individual's public identification as gay or lesbian (see West 1998a). For young care leavers, the attitude of members of the public was found to be stigmatising at least, with individuals regarded as either a family-less foundling entitled to overly sympathetic attention or, more likely, a prostitute or criminal and therefore deserving of verbal abuse.

Children and young people currently in care speak of their bad experiences when others know of their care background – for example, that they live in a children's home (residential care) or even in a foster family.[2] They talk of being victimised and bullied by other children and by teachers, and of parents refusing to allow their children to play with them. Later in life, they may get refused jobs if they reveal their past as being in care (see West 1995: 14).

In talking about their experiences at school, children in care suggested that other children must get their ideas about care from their parents. But how do parents arrive at their opinions? And from where do teachers derive their views? This chapter will explore print media constructions of 'looked after' children in care and care itself, and the reactions of children and young people from care[3] to stories, and their views on media portrayals of them and their lives. It is necessary first to emphasise and briefly outline the importance of care and the complexities and subtleties of experience subsumed in that simple four-letter word.

Care

Between 60,000 and 70,000 children and young people are looked after by local authority social services and social work departments in Great Britain.

The figures for 1996 were 51,200 in England, 3,0225 in Wales, and for Scotland (1993 figures) 12,371 (Dunn and McCluskey 1997: 135–138). 'During the year ending 31 March 1996, 31,900 children started to be looked after while 31,600 ceased to be looked after . . . 61 per cent of children looked after are aged over ten' (Dunn and McCluskey: 135). These figures are important in indicating the numbers of children and young people who have experienced life in the care system, and those who are now adults must not be forgotten. Many more children were in care in the past: although numbers for Scotland fell slightly, the population of looked-after children in England dropped considerably 'from roughly 89,000 in 1982' (Coleman 1997: 10–12). But the figures by themselves do not tell the complex realities that make up 'care'.

Children and young people are looked after by local authorities for a number of formal reasons, which in England and Wales include:

> Those subject to an interim or full care order, those subject to police protection; those subject to an emergency protection or child protection order; those committed or remanded to local authority accommodation or made the subject of a residence requirement of a supervision order in criminal proceedings; those transferred to local authority accommodation under the provisions of the Police and Criminal Evidence Act 1984; those accommodated in community homes, having been sentenced under section 53 of the Children and Young Persons Act 1933.
>
> (Dunn and McCluskey 1997: 135).

This list indicates one of the problems important for the lives of children and young people in care and media representations of them. Being 'looked after' by the local authority does not distinguish between children who are the subject of criminal proceedings and children who are the subject of protection orders. Yet the majority of children looked after are under care orders or by voluntary agreements. In England in 1996 'the number of children accommodated compulsorily by local authorities was 620' (Dunn and McCluskey: 136) – that is, just over 1 per cent of children and young people who are looked after in that country.

Children may enter care for a variety of reasons, the most commonly cited being 'to give relief to the parents or families (29 per cent), . . . abuse or neglect (20 per cent), parents' health (14 per cent), and concern for the children's welfare (8 per cent)' (Dunn and McCluskey 1997: 137). These groupings made for the sake of brevity do, of course, mask the experiences of individual children and young people. One young woman, referring to her own early difficulties and tough time in care added, 'But mine wasn't bad compared to some. Some young people have had absolutely horrific lives'. As several writers have pointed out, while 'children and young people who are abused can, of course, come from a variety of different social backgrounds, . . . many will not be legally taken into care' and some children are taken into care because their parents cannot cope with their 'challenging behaviour', although in general 'young people who are taken into care are much more likely to come from socially and economically deprived backgrounds' (Coles 1995: 130–131) – they are the children of the poor, as a 1984 Social Services Committee Report put it (ibid.).

The experiences of children and young people when looked after by the local authority are also complex. The children may be placed with their parents or immediate family, an action encouraged and supported by the Children Act 1989 but questioned by some social work practitioners (Essex, Gumbleton and Luger 1997). They may be placed in residential care, an option less highly regarded in recent years, but importantly reinforced in the report by Sir William Utting at the end of 1997. Life experience in residential care may include many moves, perhaps over ten for a tenth of the population (see Who Cares? Trust 1998). Others may be placed with a foster family, a favoured option of the past decade. Many children and young people move in and out of care, have several placements, and a series of social workers. A number of local authority residential homes and services have been investigated in recent years, because of physical and sexual abuse of children in care, and allegations of abuse have also been made about some foster carers.

Approximately 8000 young people leave care each year to live independently. Most have left care before they are 18 years old and many leave care at the age of sixteen. They leave often with little or no support – and so it is perhaps not surprising that many go on to experience homelessness, rooflessness, and being without money (see Action on Aftercare 1996, West 1995 and 1998b). 'Between one quarter and one third of rough sleepers have been looked after by local authorities as children' (Hunter 1998: 8). In the early 1990s 'it was estimated that, on any given night, about 2000 people were sleeping on the streets of London' (ibid.: 8).

In short, the construction of care is complex, and the individual's experience of life being looked after by the local authority is varied and unique. Being or having been looked after affects thousands of children and young people currently in care and leaving care, although this is a small proportion of the total population of children and young people – in 1992 there were 11.8 million children under 16 in the UK (Dunn and McCluskey 1997: 21). But it also affects many thousand more adults who were in care in the past, especially because many more were taken into care in the past (see Coleman 1997). These adults will also read newspaper stories about children in care.

Newspaper representations of children and family

In order to comprehend fully the representation of children, young people and care, particularly in the tabloid press,[4] it is necessary to explore the general context of reporting on children and families. Children and young people feature a great deal in newspaper stories, but are frequently hidden under other guises. Young people, for example, appear daily on the sports pages, but as footballers, athletes, tennis players, and so on. Young women feature as models. Articles about education, from school standards to universities, are also about the lives of children and young people. Children appear centrally in the cast of stories about families and family life. Some newspapers produce their own supplement for children, such as the *Sunday Times* 'Funday' and the *Young Telegraph*, but these concessions to addressing children directly appear to be made only in the name of producing a newspaper for the entire family.

But in most newspaper stories concerning children where their age – their childhood or youth – is highlighted, the focus is on children out of place. That is, on children not behaving in accordance with the idealised and Western-centric conception of childhood, which strongly emphasises innocence (see, for example, Higonnet 1998; Holland 1992 on pictorial images of childhood and issues of divergence from the representation of innocence). This ideal is supported in the press, although it is largely constructed in the negative, through references to children involved in crime, teenage pregnancy, of the world turned-upside-down where teachers are scared of their pupils, and where children 'divorce' their parents. A few stories selected from the national press, mostly from a single month, illustrate some of these routinely rehearsed themes: 'Violent kids "a fashion"' (the *Mirror*, 18 April 1998), 'Youths jailed for shooting teenager' (*Daily Express*, 2 April 1998), 'Twins at 15 – but at least Emma is not planning any more' (*Daily Mail*, 25 April 1998), 'Children of 6 to get drug lessons' (*Daily Mail*, 25 April 1998), 'Ever younger drug abusers' (*Daily Mail*, 27 April 1998), 'Is the war on teenage drugs a sick joke' (*Daily Express*, 21 April 1998), 'Rule of the bullies – one in three pupils is victim of playground thugs' (*Daily Express*, 2 April 1998), 'In a class of his own, the boy who punched schoolmistress' (*Daily Mail*, 11 April 1998), 'Expelled from a school at age of 5 – tearaway barred after attacks on staff and other children' (*Daily Express*, 9 April 1998), 'Teachers call for parents to wallop young tearaway' (*The Times*, 18 April 1998), 'Five year olds' unwelcome lesson in living with divorce' (*Daily Mail*, 18 April 1998), 'Nagging for toys is child's play' ('nagging children get their own way' – *Daily Express*, 2 April 1998), 'Boy aged 13 is the youngest on sex pest list' (*Daily Mail*, 19 April 1998), 'Boy aged 3 faces quiz over death of a toddler' (*Daily Express*, 7 April 1998).

The ideal of childhood is also supported even through simple stories, such as the widely reported 'marmite kid', a child who apparently eats only marmite sandwiches (reported in most, if not all, tabloids on 9 April 1998). Although not a crime, it reinforces ideas about childhood now being different, through stories of children's unusual or unconventional behaviour. The media response to the killing of James Bulger emphasised the reliance on a particular construction of children and childhood (see Chapter 12). Subsequent ideas of childhood in crisis, played out in the media, have been documented (see

Scraton 1997). But this moral panic might also be seen as a surge of words, an increase in space and time devoted to the usual values of what is newsworthy, and the regular media theme that childhood is changing for the worse, and that children are out of control (Lumley 1998). These news values ensure that particular types of story about children and young people appear frequently, and occasionally achieve prominence as in the *Daily Express*' series in April 1998 on 'A generation betrayed – we live in a country where our children's freedom has been destroyed. Why do we accept it?' The article noted parents' fears of letting their children 'walk on the streets, play games in the park or stand too long at the school gate'. But these fears included fears of other children – bullies, and in the 'Opinion' piece, the newspaper contrasted the 'prison without locks and bars' of children with 'the youngsters having £5,000 a week spent on their care at Cookham juvenile prison in Kent [who] will not lack for things to amuse and entertain them – TVs, computer games, pool tables' (15 April 1998).

The key elements of the context for care involve conceptualisations of family and children's association with crime, resting on a nostalgic construction of childhood, and particularly the news value of children out of control. The *Daily Mail*, for example, under the headline 'Out of control, children who are spoilt by design' reported on 'The generation of "designer children" [who] get everything they want and have no sense of responsibility or discipline instilled into them' (9 April 1998). The notion that social life, and particularly family life, has deteriorated, with increased crime and poor schooling, resonates with Pearson's (1983) history of the fear of hooliganism and popular nostalgic ideas about life being better two decades ago, and two decades before that and so on. These notions are important in developing the framework within which stories about care are reported and a particular construction of children and young people from care is generated.

Family

The ideal of family is crucial to the media's preferred image of childhood and fundamental to children in care. Children from care themselves construct images of what they see as 'normal family life' and are very much aware that they are living outside the preferred biological family in residential care or in foster care (see West 1998a). The focus in the tabloid press is on a preference for two heterosexual (and preferably married) parents comprising a family, as an institution which is under threat of change by outside forces. The *Daily Mail* headline asked 'What have they got against the family?' above an article focusing on a series of stereotypical touchstones said to be destroying 'normality' and the family: the disparate list included homosexuality, broadcasters, the pill, the absence of 'loving discipline', drug taking and 'our rulers' (abuse of children within the family and domestic violence, although widespread, were not mentioned (20 April 1998). This idea of family is intimately associated with marriage: in a later edition the *Daily Mail* announced 'Married parents, a child's best start in life' (22 October 1997).

The family is central to care because, as Goldson notes, 'not all families . . . are considered as "suitable" in the raising and socialising of children and herein lies the determination of family versus state ownership and control of childhood' (Goldson 1997: 24). The family, however, is still pre-eminent, and important to the ideal of children, as Sgritta suggests: 'the argument that childhood constitutes a substantially passive phase of life and that children have no rights that are not mediated by the family, has a certain unadorned plausibility to common sense' (Sgritta 1994: 358). What of children living outside a family – how then are their rights mediated?

These readings of family life, however, are selective. As Davis and Bourhill point out, there is no moral panic concerning violence to children within the family. 'When children are killed within the family, the cases are often treated as routine' and 'Despite the frequency of such stories, a catalogue of abduction and mistreatment of children by adults, no moral panic is constructed. They are not accompanied by anguished media pronouncements warning of the collapse of society' (Davis and Bourhill 1997: 37). Given the moral panic of 1997–98 concerning paedophiles in the community, their statement was perhaps somewhat precocious (see Chapter 13). But what is pertinent is the lack of panic over mistreatment within the family. Indeed, many newspapers, through their support for 'smacking' and 'loving discipline', endorse a level of violence towards children.

Crime

Many stories with a focus on children and young people feature them as criminals or associated with crime and wrongdoing (see Chapter 11). Some of these stories challenge the ideal of innocence for all children (for example, *The Times*, 'Children can lie as soon as they talk' (13 September 1997) and 'Criminal tendencies evident in childhood' (16 January 1998)), while others challenge the ideal just for some children (for example, the *Sunday Times* 'Unruly under 10s target of new curbs' (23 January 1997)). Stories, often based on unnamed 'experts', raise and reinforce fears of children and young people. Under the headline 'The Crimebomb', for example, the *Daily Mail* declared that 'crimes will rise because of a sharp rise in the number of youths experts warned yesterday' (that is, for demographic reasons, an increase in births in over a short period) (8 April 1998). Many stories focus on individual children; the *Daily Mirror* headline 'The urban terrorist – 15ft [long] record of crook, 16' (27 February 1998), and 'Ratboy' and 'Spiderboy' of recent years, offer obvious examples. The *Daily Mail* in its report on 'Court puts a name to tearaway with 15ft crime record' noted that this boy, now 16 'in common with the two other tearaways who have terrorised Tyneside – Ratboy . . . and Spiderboy . . . [he] is the product of a broken home – his father left years ago' (27 February 1998).

Davis and Bourhill note that the 'media portrayal of children's involvement in crime . . . is central in creating and reinforcing public perceptions of childhood' (1997: 29): but the question 'which children?' is important, because another particular theme is the association of care and crime.

Constructing care

If the general context is that '*all* children are suspect' (Davis and Bourhill 1997: 48 emphasis in original), then it might be thought that, in this media construction, the case is proven against those children placed in care. The association is often direct, as the *Daily Express* front-page headline '54 crimes in fifty days – Police can't stop a city's young thugs' alleged that children had 'committed these crimes while held at a children's home in Nottingham' (Davis and Bourhill 1997: 49). The words of the Home Secretary, Kenneth Clarke, that 'courts should have the power to send really persistent nasty little juveniles away to somewhere where they will be *looked after* better' (quoted in Davis and Bourhill 1997: 50–51, emphasis added), helps reinforce the idea that children in care (most often associated with residential care, that is institutions) are bad, particularly with his words replicating the formal designation 'looked after' for children in care. The term 'in care' has connotations of being inside, that is in jail, and sounds like a truncation of incarceration, so it is not surprising that it was formally replaced – but it seems that associations, even if not deliberate, will continue to be made.

The association of care and crime means that stories about children in secure units, and about children's jails, will be conflated with care. This is difficult to escape since the formal reasons for being looked after include remand as well as abuse. But although the numbers are comparatively small, stories about crime and children's jails are more prominent, certainly than stories about everyday violence within the family. Where children associated with crime are from children's homes, this seems to be always reported. The *Daily Mail* story headlined 'Blip boy on the run – one-youth crimewave culprit is named after he escapes', was about a 'teenage burglar' who escaped from a young offenders' institute. But it included that he 'had previously gone on the run from institutions with limited security and when he was away at children's homes, having been sentenced by the courts, they would give him his train fare home so he could visit us at weekends. It was then he became mischievous and got into trouble' (26 November 1997). The undifferentiated association of crime ('a ruthless burglar'), secure units and children's homes, gives a particular meaning to care. Another article, 'Tearaways aged 12 warned: we'll lock you up before trial' was accompanied by a case study of 'a drug addict of 13' arrested 58 times, 'said to have carried out 114 burglaries', remanded into council care, who 'had absconded from children's homes many times before' (*Daily Mail*, 16 October 1997).

A key element in the construction of care is children being away from family. This places children in care outside conventional ideals of childhood spent within the family. Stories about family life, and problems when parents are not present, have implications for the way in which children in care are thought of, because they are regarded as without parents or certainly with absent parents. Under the heading 'Stay in for your sons', for example, the *Daily Mail* reported that parents should stay in when their children have a party, or the children will be tempted 'by drugs and casual sex' (3 April 1998).

For newspapers, being away from family not only means being in residential care. It is the biological family that is designated as important. The implication that foster children are also a problem is raised through stories which focus on, for example, 'Overdose tragedy of the teenager torn between her two families' where 'A teenager said to have been torn between foster parents and her natural family killed herself with an overdose of sleeping pills' (*Daily Mail*, 26 November 1997). The *Daily Mail* also reported 'the 11-year-old girl torn between the mother she loves and a new life of affluence' (the 'mother she loves and two Oxford academics who want to adopt her' and with whom she was placed in foster care) (26 October 1997).

Young women in and from care are often associated with sex and teenage pregnancy, in a way that ignores but contrasts with the abuse experienced by many children in care. Thus, 'Tragic baby's mother "may be only 13"', about an abandoned baby, reported that 'a schoolgirl could have secretly given birth' and police 'want to trace a teenager who went missing from a children's home' (*Daily Mail*, 20 October 1997). The headline story 'Care Girls in sex for sale scandal' (*Yorkshire Evening Post*, 17 August 1997) implied the association of care and sex work was not unusual by reporting that a manager 'denied the problem was widespread. One girl is believed to have been charged for persistent offending.'

Newspapers' construction of stories about care very much reflects the experiences of children and young people from care and the attitude towards them shown by members of the public. The views of some children in care and young people who have left care, on stories about care and the lives of their peers, are considered on pp. 262–265 after an outline of some different types of care story.

Care stories

There are several forms of newspaper story involving children and young people from care. The most obvious and striking are front-page headline articles such as those in the *Daily Express* or the *Yorkshire Evening Post* referred to above. The *Daily Mail* story headlined 'Police in 1000 calls to care home for children' told how 'Police have been called out 1,053 times in the last 20 months to deal with anarchy at a children's home . . . social workers have lost control and simply watch powerless as the tearaways run riot' (15 April 1998). This type of story is more often seen in local newspapers reporting on neighbours wanting to close a children's home or hostel, or campaigning against proposals to open such a home in their area. Here the *Daily Mail* went on to report that 'neighbours insist they have been "going through hell" for eight years. They say that the children, who are in care because they are orphans, have been abused, or because their parents cannot control them, never seem to go to school and regularly abscond'. The report continued by arguing against condemnations of a new children's prison by children's charities, by suggesting that such prisons were necessary for problem teenagers.

This direct link of children in care and children's prisons illustrates the kind of stories which focus on care and crime. Some of these have been raised above, but others include headlines and features on children's prisons. While the development of such prisons is welcomed in most of the press, the first built was largely denigrated as 'The Medway Hilton' with stories suggesting it was luxuriously appointed and highlighting an estimated cost of £5000 a week per child. The story in the *Express* was accompanied by a cartoon of a boy, cigarette in mouth, back-to-front baseball cap on head, smiling as he carried his case out of the terraced house towards the saluting chauffeur opening the door of the Rolls Royce: his mother proudly informing a passer-by that 'He's just off to do his 12 months at the Medway Secure Training Centre' (16 April 1998). The prison was also headlined the 'College of crime' by the *Mirror* which reported on children 'locked away in luxury' (14 April 1998).

There are smaller stories which include references, often apparently incidental, to children's homes or care, but generally associated with problems, such as the abandoned baby referred to above, or the links to crime. Some large feature stories, such as 'I found my missing daughter with a message on a bottle' (*Daily Mail*, 3 October 1997), also concern care. Here a double-page story about a missing person was about a young woman who went into care, living with foster parents and in a children's home, and then ran away and became a drug user and beggar. Other types of story include court cases, such as 'Judge lets two foster boys stay in the land they call home' (*Daily Mail*, 23 October 1997) and those noted earlier involving adoption and the coroner's report of the teenager who overdosed. These reports associating children from care with court reinforce the impression of children outside the family, children in care, being associated with trouble.

Most of the stories referred to here have been in the national press. Another source of media stories about children and care is the local press. As noted above, many of these focus on opposition to existing or proposed children's homes, such as '"You're not welcome", children's home sparks new row' (*Yorkshire Evening Post*, 1 July 1993), 'The sin bin – row over plans to re-open home for problem children' (*Yorkshire Evening Post*, 3 June 1997), '"We'll fire-bomb remand home" – angry residents issue warning to council' (*Yorkshire Evening Post*, 5 May 1993). Other stories are related, also concerning alleged criminal activities, 'Havoc of young crooks' (*Yorkshire Evening Post*, 3 April

1993, where neighbours call for home to be closed), 'Care girls "sex for sale" probe' (*Yorkshire Evening Post*, 16 December 1996 – a different story and date from that with a similar title noted above). Another local story reports on children 'out of place': '"Shame" of B&B children: foster care crisis leaves 15-year-olds in guest houses' (*Telegraph & Argus*, 19 September 1998). The wording of the headline associates shame with the children rather than the system of care.

The other main type of story deals with conditions in children's homes and reports of abuse. The release of the report by Sir William Utting in November 1997 was extensively covered in the broadsheet papers. Press reporting, however, served to emphasise the image of children in care as victims with a particular emphasis on paedophilia. The *Independent* reported the story highlighting the paper's six-year campaign against abuse in children's homes, and both the *Guardian* and *The Times* had the story of the report on the same page as news of a network of child prisons to be set up. Children and young people from care did not find this kind of story any different from others, in the image of care represented, and it is to their views we now turn.

The views of children and young people in care

The responses of children and young people from care, to media stories about care, focus on three main areas: the authenticity and integrity of these stories, their effect on readers and the public's attitude to children in care, and the impact on professional and policy responses to care. The strength of feeling about the media representation of care is indicated by the way children and young people discuss the press, relating stories to their own experiences, connecting newspaper images to their own lives. The fact and content of articles in the papers are very much part of their view and experience of reality. The reaction to press stories was similar to the description and discussion of other aspects of their lives, such as the doings of neighbours, events at school, and so on, which also turned upon their identity as a child in care, or a young person who had left care.

An early reaction in discussions was that newspapers were 'not telling the truth' about care. One young woman had seen an article on foster care in a local free newspaper, and said: 'did you see that story . . . a load of bull about foster care, half the kids in residential are from foster care anyway'. The article had apparently reported foster care a success, 'it's a lie, if that's the truth then we'd all be in foster care'. This perception that newspapers lied about care was a consistent theme, and one young woman's immediate response to raising the subject of the media, was that the press are 'very biased against us'. She felt that 'you could tell them one story and they'd print another. They make us out to be monsters, no hopers'.

One issue was that the newspapers failed to print positive stories about children in care. It was said that there 'are no role models' of people from care publicised and praised for young people to identify with. The care background of famous people, however, is often known to young people from care, although this fact may be disregarded by the general public. One front-page story about residential homes and the police was adjacent to the photograph of a well-known actor, with a short caption indicating a story inside: this was pointed out with the words, 'he's from care, but he said he had a good time. I don't believe it'. There was no mention of his care background in the story, and the irony of the juxtaposition of the two was enjoyed by young people.

Young people felt that the lives of children in care were not described, and the reality of care was ignored. The variety and complexity of life in care, and the heterogeneity of children living in care was pointed out. Alongside the lack of positive role models, it was suggested that there was a particular news agenda, that the press would not be interested in 'for example, my voluntary work'. The emotional experiences of being in care, 'like being away from your Mum and Dad – the trauma of knowing they may not want you' were ignored. This was said to be linked to a problem, reinforced by newspapers, that 'the public do not understand why they've come into care': that the 'public associate care with crime. A child could have been abused by six members of their family and come in, horrific lives . . .' Experiences in care offering contrasting views to the dominant story were also rarely reported. Reflecting on articles about police and residential homes, one young person commented 'why didn't they do an article on me, when I got my head split open when they [police] bashed it into a cell door'. There was, however, an awareness of the commercial motives behind press reporting of care and the way that press accounts both shape and reflect public views; 'the trouble is, changing the general story won't sell papers'.

But, the fact that newspapers did not 'tell the truth' was not simply an issue of newspapers misleading readers. Young people believed that both the public and the press preferred to have an inaccurate representation – 'they don't want to hear the truth – that taxpayers' money is going on care that isn't working'. This perspective is a fundamental part of children's and young people's analysis of the representation of care, and how it is connected to their own experiences.

Young people explained that the press presented a partial picture of children in care: 'newspapers aren't looking at the whole picture'. They said that stories focus 'on a few, they think we're all like that' and 'they make it sound like it's all of us'. The newspapers were 'not seeing all sides of the story. They make out that everyone in care is the same'. Children living in residential homes felt that 'they see us the same. They probably think we're in secure [units]. They try to pair us up'. The local press especially was said to make this connection between ordinary children's homes and special secure units: 'papers here do it all the time, link residential and secure. For example, when they were trying to re-open a kids' home'. The issue was that people 'get ideas from reports like that. They think everyone's the same [that all children in care are the same]'. The link meant that at very least 'they assume that children in care are a lot more misbehaved'. Children felt that what the press was doing was 'trying to pick out every child who has been bad and make it sound like us all'.

The outcome of all this was 'blame' which children and young people felt was heaped upon them. 'We get it from everywhere. From children down our street, from their parents, and from the papers.' The connection of blame, newspapers and neighbourhood, was a reflection of their life in the community, where newspaper versions of care were an extension of day-to-day life and contact with others. 'We get the blame for everything, because we're in a kids' home.' Another told of how 'every time something goes wrong on the estate, they come to us', and another that 'students at the back of us turn the music up loud. But we're the ones who get it.'

This stigmatisation extended deeply to other areas of their lives. Other children, from family homes, in particular were singled out: 'kids riding by and calling kids bastards'. This meant not merely the idea of illegitimacy, but here a particular insult of being without family. The stigmatisation also had an impact on life at school and was seen as having an effect on professionals, especially education and social work professionals. For example, 'some of the teachers act different to children in care than to other children'. One described how 'teacher picked me out of the whole class [in public] and asked me to write a story about being in care', an experience she felt was humiliating. Another explained how it was bullying and staff actions and attitude in children's homes that were the reasons why residents 'kicked off' and the police were often called out.

Young people clearly felt that this media construction of care, supporting, reinforcing or creating the public's perception, has a significant effect on their lives and on social policy. 'This is why young people [in care] get a hard time, because of the bad press.' They saw especial relevance to the scandals of violence and sexual abuse concerning some children's homes in recent years, in that this media and public representation of children in care made it easier for children's cries for help, and description of their experiences, not to be taken seriously. It was felt that children were ignored, partly because there was an idea that they 'deserved it'. While some children and young people from care accept they are 'not angels' – 'I've been in trouble with the police myself' – they denounce the characterisation of themselves which they see as appearing in the press.

This perceived caricature of themselves created problems; 'they think that young people [in care] don't deserve any help'. The reason why 'things go astray for children in care is, if a young person reports being hit in care, no one's interested. The public think it's OK because we're all little bastards anyway'. Newspapers are judged to present an unduly simple picture – 'what's wrong is wrong, right is right, there's no in-between'. They have 'different standards for different people', it was explained: 'if I hit you I get done for assault, because he's a "teenage thug" he deserves it'.

Children and young people felt there are, and have been, serious implications emerging from this representation of care. Children and young people in care and who have left care have been criticising the circumstances of life in care, and the process of leaving care, and describing their experiences, for many years. Their critique has been consistent and repetitive, but they feel that little or nothing has significantly changed. The representation of care is seen as being at the heart of this. 'You know the big scandals. Well no one takes any notice. [Young] people are disclosing [abuse] all the time. No one listens because it's acceptable.' That is, because of the association of care and crime, the children are not really believed, and are deemed to be of lesser worth. 'The public think, they don't mind [about what happens] because "they are the people who rob us" – they think so anyway'. 'The public see young people [in care] as shite – and it's wrong.'

Conclusion

The press reporting about care is part of a spectrum of stories about children and young people which ranges from illusory and nostalgic ideas of childhood to a notion, frequently surging to a full-blown moral panic, of children out of control. In this context, children and young people from care are particularly demonised, associated with courts and crime, portrayed as victims, burglars and prostitutes. During this process the nature of care is simplified and the characters of children in care homogenised.

For children living in care and young people who have left care, the press representation of care resonates with their experiences. The construction of 'blame' in the newspapers extends to their own lives, a stigmatisation frequently realised in the reaction to themselves and their homes by other children, adults in the neighbourhood, by their peers and teachers at school, by the unknown public met generally when out, and by some of the staff working with them. Children in care see parents as a source of such discrimination by other children, but see media stories as influencing adults in constructing and reinforcing their opinions.

Children in care see the media portrayals as an important part of a general representation of care that has denied and ignored the reality of their experiences of abuse, has not taken them seriously, and has failed many in the provision of care and of education. They also see a link between such representation and experiences of, for example, humiliation at school. Although children and young people from care are implicitly represented as different and separate from an approved ordinary family life, the popular construction of childhood depends very much on such a portrayal of children in care. As victims and as villains, children from care represent a negative of idealised children and childhood: through their representation in this way, the social norms emphasised in much of the press are articulated. But the consequences for the lives of thousands of children and young people are appalling.

Acknowledgements

I would like to acknowledge my debt to the many children and young people who have discussed their experiences and informed me about care issues. It is impossible to list them all, but I want to thank in particular Lindsay, Jim, Emma, Jay, Mark, Mandy, the Rights Thing Group in Hull and others who prefer not to be named.

Notes

1 'Care' is formally called 'being looked after' by the local authority. References are often made to 'looked after children', but such references are largely limited to professionals working in or associated with social services. In this chapter the term 'care' is predominantly used, as used by children and young people in and from care themselves, its use preferred in a spirit of sarcasm.
2 This chapter draws on conversations held with many children and young people, from different parts of England and Wales, over the past four years, in addition to group discussions and interviews held specifically on the subject of media portrayals of care.
3 The phrase 'from care' is used here to denote children and young people who are in care and those who have left care.
4 Within the tabloid press, the *Daily Mail* has taken on particular significance, with a circulation increasing since the early 1980s, and for the months of September and October in 1998 outselling the *Mirror* for the first time (*Guardian* 28 September 1998).

References

Action on Aftercare (1996) *Too Much Too Young*, London: Action on Aftercare Consortium.

Coles, B. (1995) *Youth and Social Policy: Youth Citizenship and Young Careers*, London: UCL Press Limited.

Coleman, J. (1997) *Key Data on Adolescence*, Brighton: Trust for the Study of Adolescence.

Davis, H. and Bourhill, M. (1997) 'Crisis: the demonisation of children and young people', in P. Scraton (ed.) *Childhood in Crisis*, London: University College London Press, 28–57.

Dunn, M. and McCluskey J. with Abrahams, C. *et al.* (1997) *NCH Action for Children Factfile '98*, London: NCH Action for Children.

Essex, S., Gumbleton, J., and Luger, C. (1997) 'Place of Safety', *Community Care*, 23–29 July, 23.

Goldson, B. (1997) '"Childhood": an introduction to historical and theoretical analyses', in P. Scraton (ed.) *'Childhood' in 'Crisis'?*, London: UCL Press Ltd, 1–27.

Higonnet, A. (1998) *Pictures of Innocence: the History and Crisis of Ideal Childhood*, London: Thames & Hudson Ltd.

Holland, P. (1992) *What is a Child? Popular Images of Childhood*, London: Virago.

Hunter, M. (1998) 'Are the answers in the tsars?', *Community Care*, 16–22 July, 8–9.

Lumley, K. (1998) 'Teeny thugs in Blair's sights: media portrayals of children in education and their policy implications', *Youth and Policy* 61: 1–11.

Pearson, G. (1983) *Hooligan: a history of respectable fears*, Basingstoke: Macmillan Education Ltd.

Qvortrup, J., Bardy, M., Sgritta, G. and Wintersberger, H. (eds) (1994) *Childhood Matters: Social Theory, Practice and Politics*, Aldershot: Avebury, Ashgate Publishing.

Scraton, P. (ed.) (1997) *'Childhood' in 'Crisis'?*, London: UCL Press Ltd.

Sgritta, G.B. (1994) 'The generational division of welfare: equity and conflict', in J. Qvortrup *et al.* (eds) *Childhood Matters: Social Theory, Practice and Politics*, Aldershot: Avebury, Ashgate Publishing, 335–363.

Utting, W. (1997) *People Like Us*, London: HMSO.

West, A. (1995) *You're On Your Own: Young People's Research on Leaving Care*, London: Save the Children.

West, A. (1998a) 'Family, identity and children's rights: notes on children and young people outside the family', in D.K. Behera (ed.) *Children and Childhood in our Contemporary Societies*, Delhi: Kamla-Raj Enterprises, 189–202.

West, A. (1998b) *Which Way Now? Young People's Experiences of Leaving Care*, London: Save the Children.

Who Cares? Trust (1998) *Remember My Messages*, London: Who Cares? Trust.

Index